Sexual Healing

BARBARA KEESLING, PH.D., has more than twenty years' experience as a sex therapist and surrogate partner. She has a doctorate in health psychology, teaches Human Sexuality at California State University, Fullerton, and maintains a private sexual therapy practice. Her experiences working skin-on-skin with hundreds of clients, together with her academic and teaching work, make her uniquely qualified in the fields of human sexuality and sexual pleasure.

Dr. Keesling is the author of many popular sexuality titles that have sold over a million copies worldwide. They include *Sexual Pleasure, Sexual Healing, Making Love Better than Ever, How to Make Love All Night (and Drive a Woman Wild),* and *The Good Girl's Guide to Bad Girl Sex.*

Dr. Keesling has appeared on numerous television and radio shows, including *Geraldo, Montel,* and "Howard Stern." Due to the high quality of the information in her books and her credentials as a human sexuality expert she is also frequently interviewed for *Playboy, Men's Health, Psychology Today, Redbook, Cosmopolitan, Glamour,* and *Marie Claire.*

Reviews for SEXUAL PLEASURE

"Finally, here is a look at the overwhelmingly positive effects of sexual expression in our lives, including increased self-esteem, feelings of personal fulfillment, and sexual ecstasy. Simplify your sex life and breathe some life back into that divinely sensual body." — WHOLE LIFE TIMES

"For anyone who wishes to increase [the] ability to experience sensual pleasure." — YOGA JOURNAL

"The real beauty of this book lies in the fact that it treats physical pleasure and intimacy as inseparable, mutually heightening ways to experience sexuality and to bond with your partner." — THE LAUNCH PAD

This book is dedicated to my clients.

Ordering

Trade bookstores in the U.S. and Canada please contact:

Publishers Group West
1700 Fourth Street, Berkeley CA 94710
Phone: (800) 788-3123   Fax: (800) 351-5073

Hunter House books are available at bulk discounts for textbook course adoptions; to qualifying community, health-care, and government organizations; and for special promotions and fund-raising. For details please contact:

Special Sales Department
Hunter House Inc., PO Box 2914, Alameda CA 94501-0914
Phone: (510) 865-5282   Fax: (510) 865-4295
E-mail: ordering@hunterhouse.com

Individuals can order our books from most bookstores, by calling
(800) 266-5592, or from our website at **www.hunterhouse.com**

Project Credits

Cover Design: Brian Dittmar Graphic Design
Book Production: Hunter House
Copy Editor: Kelley Blewster
Proofreader: John David Marion
Indexer: Nancy D. Peterson
Acquisitions Editor: Jeanne Brondino
Editor: Alexandra Mummery
Publicist: Jillian Steinberger
Customer Service Manager: Christina Sverdrup
Order Fulfillment: Washul Lakdhon
Administrator: Theresa Nelson
Computer Support: Peter Eichelberger
Publisher: Kiran S. Rana

Sexual Healing

The Completest Guide to
Overcoming Common Sexual Problems

third edition

Barbara Keesling, Ph.D.

Hunter House
PUBLISHERS

Hunter House Inc., Publishers
PO Box 2914
Alameda CA 94501-0914

Library of Congress Cataloging-in-Publication Data
Keesling, Barbara.
    Sexual healing : the completest guide to overcoming common sexual problems / Barbara Keesling.— 3rd ed.
        p. cm.
    Rev. ed. of: Sexual healing : how good loving is good for you—and your relationship.
    Summary: "A guide to every known sexual problem and all possible treatments, both new and experimental, with over 125 exercises to heal specific problems as well as maintain an intimate bond in relationships"—Provided by publisher.
    Includes bibliographical references and index.
    ISBN-13: 978-0-89793-465-7 (pbk.)
    ISBN-10: 0-89793-465-2 (pbk.)
    1. Sex (Psychology)—Health aspects. 2. Intimacy (Psychology)—Health aspects. 3. Sex instruction. I. Title.
    RA788.K38 2005
    613.9'6—dc22   2005013713

Printed and Bound by Sheridan Books, Inc.

Manufactured in the United States of America

9 8 7 6 5 4 3   Third Edition   08 09 10 11 12

Contents

Part II: Sexual Problems

Part IV: Healing Specific Sexual Problems

Part V: Advanced Sexual Healing

Important Note

The material in this book is intended to provide an overview of techniques for improving sexual health and functioning. Every effort has been made to provide accurate and dependable information. However, you should be aware that professionals in the field may have differing opinions, and change is always taking place. Any of the treatments described herein should be used under the guidance of a licensed therapist or health-care practitioner. The author, editors, and publisher cannot be held responsible for any outcomes that derive from use of any of these treatments in a program of self-care or under the care of a licensed professional. The treatments in this book should not be used in place of other medical therapies.

List of Exercises by Chapter

Introduction

Is your sex life a source of confusion or pain? Do you have sexual problems that prevent you from making love the way you imagine you could? Does sexuality cause you anxiety rather than pleasure? *Sexual Healing* is a self-help book that can address your concerns. It contains detailed, practical exercises for you alone or for you and a partner that can help heal you of your sexual problems.

The Evolution of Sexual Healing

My background and the topics addressed in this book have become intertwined over the past twenty-five years. In 1980, I was working for the U.S. Postal Service in southern California when I read a newspaper article about surrogate partners—men and women who work directly with people who are experiencing sexual problems. I decided to train as a surrogate partner and to begin college at the same time. I worked as a surrogate partner for twelve years, until 1992. During that time I also earned several college degrees, including a doctorate in health psychology, a field of psychology that studies the interaction between the mind and the body. In 1990, the first edition of *Sexual Healing* was published. It was based on my experiences as a surrogate partner and dealt with common sexual problems, such as erection problems, premature ejaculation, and problems with orgasm.

After 1992, I worked as a sex therapist rather than a surrogate partner. In 1996, the second edition of *Sexual Healing* was released. Although it had the same title as the original, its content was quite different. It focused very little on specific sexual problems and more on using lovemaking to heal people's bodies, minds, and relationships. It was based on some amazing, life-changing experiences I witnessed in my work as both a surrogate partner and a therapist. Around that time, I also began teaching at a university and writing many other books on sexual topics. Because of the demands of my writing and my university job, I quit my clinical practice as a sex therapist several years ago. When my publisher approached me about writing a third edition of *Sexual Healing*, I was ready.

This edition of *Sexual Healing* harkens back to the first edition in that it contains mostly material on treating specific sexual problems. Yet it also includes content on using sexuality to heal one's body, mind, and relationship. What I have done here is combine the content from the first two editions. I have also added a lot of new material, mostly in the areas of problems with desire, problems with anxiety, and sexual pain. I've updated the treatments for many of the sexual problems, based upon our continually growing knowledge in this area. This third edition of *Sexual Healing* represents twenty-five years of accumulated knowledge and experience in the field of sexuality.

Throughout the years, I have used the phrase *sexual healing* to mean many things. The following are some of the term's many connotations:

* Healing specific sexual problems

* Using sexuality to heal the body

* Using sexuality to heal the mind

* Using sexuality to heal a relationship

* Being healed of the effects of past sexual abuse

* Healing compulsive sexual behaviors, such as sexual addictions

This edition of *Sexual Healing* addresses the first four issues. It does not deal directly with the effects of sexual abuse or sexual addiction, although I believe that many of the techniques described here could be used as part of a treatment program for abuse and addiction.

Who Can Benefit from Sexual Healing?

Anyone who wants to make love and feel better can benefit from following a program of sexual healing. The primary audience for this book is people who suffer from specific sexual problems. The exercises have also proven very helpful for couples who have a strong intimate bond and would like to use that intimacy to bring strength to or heal other aspects of their relationship. Sexual healing is also helpful for people in relationships that no longer include lovemaking, and for people of any age with physical conditions that they believe prevent them from making love. There are even many exercises included in these pages for people who don't have partners.

I have written this book with heterosexual couples in mind because these are the people I've worked with the most. Unfortunately, the scheme used by most therapists to diagnose sexual problems is very biased toward the experiences of heterosexuals. However, with 3 to 4 percent of the male population and 1 to 2 percent of the female population exclusively homosexual, I believe it is important to acknowledge the fact that people who are attracted to the same sex can also experience sexual dysfunctions. Most of the sensate-focus exercises in *Sexual Healing* can be used by people of any sexual orientation.

Another population I don't specifically address in *Sexual Healing* is older adults. Studies show that many older people are sexually active or would like to be. The percentage of the population over age fifty is growing at an enormous rate. Sexual dysfunctions affect people of all ages. Erection problems are especially prevalent as men get older. Most of the exercises in *Sexual Healing* can be used by people of any age. Many of them are great for older people, especially the exercises for female arousal and male erection. Medical conditions such as arthritis that are common in older people may limit a person's ability to do some of the exercises, so as with any exercise program, consult your physician if you have concerns about your physical abilities.

Professionals, such as sex therapists and psychotherapists, may also benefit from reading this book and/or recommending it to their clients.

How This Book Is Organized

Sexual Healing is divided into five sections. Part I contains introductory material about common sexual problems, basic sexual anatomy and physiology, anxiety, and sexual positions. Part II includes chapters on each of the nine sexual problems that are commonly called *sexual dysfunctions*. Part III contains information about sensual touch, exercises you can do by yourself, and basic touching exercises you can do with a partner. Each chapter in Part IV deals with healing a specific sexual problem. Part V is devoted to using sexuality to heal your body, your mind, and your relationship.

Embarking on the Sexual Healing
Journey: How to Use This Book

If you would like to use *Sexual Healing* to heal yourself of a specific sexual problem or problems, first read through the entire book to get the big picture about sexual problems. Then go back and read in detail the chapters about your specific concerns. Next, begin the relaxation exercises in Chapter 16, the sexual fitness exercises in Chapter 17, and the self-touch exercises in Chapter 18. These are all exercises you can do by yourself, and many of them (particularly the relaxation exercises and pelvic muscle exercises) should be done every day, not only while you are going through the sexual healing program, but for the rest of your life as part of your commitment to sexual health.

Please don't be afraid of the word *exercise*. The activities in *Sexual Healing* are fun and don't require a high level of physical fitness. If you have a lot of anxiety about sex, the descriptions of some of the exercises may scare you. Try not to worry. If you have anxiety, I provide many strategies so you can break the exercises down into smaller steps. That's why it's important to read through the whole book before you start any exercises.

After you have started a program of self-touch, you can do the exercises in Chapters 19 through 22 with your partner. These are basic touching exercises that will also relax you. If you can't do a particular part of an exercise (for example, if your partner can't insert a finger into your vagina because you have muscle spasms), don't worry. The chapter devoted to that specific problem will explain what to do.

After you have done the basic partner touching exercises, you can move on to whichever chapters in Part IV apply to your problems or those of your partner. Once you have experienced healing of your particular sexual problems, you might want to try some of the exercises in Part V, "Advanced Sexual Healing." These are optional, and they don't have to be done in any particular order.

No Special Equipment Required

You don't need any expensive accessories to be able to go through the program outlined in this book. Most of the exercises take a half hour to an hour and a half. For most of them you will need a towel, some baby powder, and some form of sexual lubricant that you and your partner both like. A few exercises recommend the use of sex toys such as dildos. When that's the case, I'll tell you in the exercise's description. Sex toys range from simple and inexpensive to fancy and pricier. For our purposes, simple and inexpensive will work just fine. For a list of retailers who sell these sorts of accessories, see "Sources for Sex Toys," located at the back of the book.

The Healing Mindset

Although you don't need any expensive equipment to experience sexual healing, there is one thing you will need, and that is an attitude I call the "healing mindset." You need to go into each exercise in a positive frame of mind in which you say to yourself, "I know I will experience healing of my sexual problems," and, "I know I can be a sexual healer for my partner." I'll have more to say about the healing mindset in Chapter 14, "The Healing Touch."

A Word about Safe Sex

Any modern book on sexuality needs to deal with the issue of safe sex. Many of the exercises in *Sexual Healing* involve oral sex and intercourse, both practices in which bodily fluids may be exchanged. If you are in a committed, monogamous relationship, these exercises will be safe for you. If you are not in a committed, monogamous relationship and you would like to do these exercises, you should use condoms to protect yourself.

Congratulations! By reading the first few pages of this book, you've taken the very first step in your sexual healing journey. If you keep reading, you'll find that the whole spirit of the sexual healing program is to move forward one step at a time, and to make each step as small as it needs to be to give you the best chances of succeeding. My hope for you is that you will choose to tap into the awesome power of sexual healing to enhance your sex life, your health, your emotions, and your relationship—one step at a time.

Part I

THE BASICS OF SEXUAL HEALING

In this section you'll find introductory material on sexual problems, as well as a review of sexual anatomy and physiology, a description of the role of anxiety in sexual problems, and a review of sexual positions.

chapter 1

Sex Problems

Having a sexual problem can be scary. In this chapter I would like to begin to demystify the most common sex problems. I'll start by putting sex problems in perspective for you.

Types of Sexual Dysfunction

Currently, specialists recognize three types of sexual problems that can become so severe and cause such serious personal distress that they qualify as full-blown psychological or psychiatric problems. Before I list them, let me share with you how psychologists (mental-health professionals with Ph.D.s who study the mind) and psychiatrists (medical doctors who study the mind) diagnose mental problems in general. They don't use some kind of magic or voodoo (although they certainly use intuition). Instead, they use a book. It's called the *Diagnostic and Statistical Manual of Mental Disorders*. It has been revised several times over the past forty years or so. The current version, which was published in 2000, is called the *DSM IV–TR (TR* stands for *Text Revision)*. Psychologists and psychiatrists refer to the book simply as the "DSM."

The DSM contains information about all known mental problems, including mood disorders like depression; serious disturbances of thought, feeling, and behavior like schizophrenia; substance abuse disorders; and many others. For each mental problem, the DSM also contains information about causes, prevalence, and related conditions, if such information is available. The current DSM lists three types of sexual problems that could become severe enough to be classified as mental disorders: gender-identity disorders, paraphilias, and sexual dysfunctions.

A person is said to have a gender-identity disorder if his or her psychological sense of being male or female is different from his or her genital organs. You may have heard these individuals referred to as transsexuals. Paraphilias are persistent and recurrent uncontrollable urges to perform sexual behaviors (often with inanimate objects) that most people consider unusual, to say the least. Included here are things like exhibitionism (exposing your genitals to an unsuspecting person), voyeurism (spying on people when they are undressing or having sex), sex with animals, and sex with children under the age of puberty, as well as other compulsions.

The third type of sex problem included in the DSM is sexual dysfunction. Sexual dysfunction includes all problems that involve the failure of the genitals to work right. For example, most people believe that a man's penis should become erect so he can have sexual intercourse and that a woman's vagina should lubricate so she can enjoy intercourse. If these natural responses don't happen, it can be a problem. The current DSM identifies nine different sexual dysfunctions. I've listed them below with a short description of each. Chapters 5 through 13 describe each of these dysfunctions in more detail and discuss their possible causes.

The following are the nine types of sexual dysfunction:

* **Hypoactive sexual desire disorder (HSDD):** low sexual desire characterized by an absence of sexual interest or fantasy .

* **Sexual aversion disorder (SAD):** a fear of some aspect of sex characterized by an avoidance of sexual situations and activity

* **Female sexual arousal disorder (FSAD):** failure of a woman's genitals to lubricate or to engorge (swell) in a sexual situation; also, a woman's subjective lack of feelings of arousal

* **Male erectile disorder (MED):** inability of a man to achieve an erection ·

* **Premature ejaculation (PE):** a condition in which a man ejaculates before he wants to or after very little sexual stimulation ·

* **Male orgasm disorder (MOD):** a condition in which a man has difficulty reaching orgasm or ejaculating

* **Female orgasm disorder (FOD):** a condition in which a woman has difficulty reaching orgasm even after normal arousal, lubrication, and genital swelling

* **Vaginismus:** a contraction of the muscles surrounding the opening of the vagina, preventing penetration ·

* **Dyspareunia:** psychologically based pain experienced during sexual intercourse .

There is another problem that is dealt with quite frequently in sex therapy, although it's not considered a sexual dysfunction as such. It's called *protracted virginity*. It means that a person has reached a relatively late age without having had sexual intercourse or, in some cases, without having had any sexual experience with a partner. Most people in the United States have had sexual intercourse by the end of their teenage years, although there's no rule that says you have to. Having sexual intercourse for the first time in your forties or fifties can pose some challenges that I believe this book can help with.

The sexual dysfunctions are the focus of most of *Sexual Healing*. Also included are sections on using your sexuality to heal physical, emotional, and relationship problems. This book does not address the paraphilias or gender-identity disorders. The sexual dysfunctions (which I usually refer to throughout the book as "sex problems") are extremely common. Recent surveys show that up to 40 percent of Americans will experience one of these problems in a severe enough form to cause personal distress. It's also possible to have more than one of the dysfunctions.

When a sex therapist begins work with a new client, in addition to making a specific diagnosis of one of the above nine problems, the therapist also makes other distinctions about the problem. The following distinctions have implications for deciding on a proper course of treatment:

Is the problem lifelong or acquired? A lifelong problem is one that has existed ever since the person first started having partner sex. Lifelong problems are also called *primary problems*. A person with an acquired problem, by contrast, functioned well in the past but at some point developed the problem. Acquired problems are also called *secondary problems*. Obviously, acquired problems are much easier to treat. Generally, if a person functioned well in the past, he or she can learn to function well again.

Generalized or situational? A sex problem is generalized if it occurs in all situations. For example, a man with generalized erection problems can't have an erection during sleep, with masturbation, or with a partner. A situational sex problem is specific to certain contexts, activities, or partners. For example, some men can have erections with their mistresses but not with their wives (or vice versa). Situational sex problems are easier to treat than generalized problems. If a person can function in one situation, usually he or she can learn to transfer that ability to other situations.

Physical or psychological? Professionals who treat sexual dysfunction also make a distinction between problems that are totally psychological in nature and those that are caused by a combination of physical and psychological factors. Physical problems are also called *organic problems*. This distinction has huge implications for treatment, because it would be a waste of time to try a psychologically based intervention if the problem is largely physical. To continue with the erection example, many medical conditions exist that can cause erection problems (see Chapter 7). It wouldn't do any good to use psychological sex therapy with a man who has severely compromised blood flow to his penis.

Also included in the definition of each of the sexual dysfunctions is the idea that it must cause "marked interpersonal difficulty" in order to be considered a problem. This implies two things: that sexual dysfunctions are couple problems, and also that you don't have a sexual problem unless you think you have one. There are many people out there who don't function very well by most standards, but who aren't really bothered by that fact.

The Role of Anxiety

In Chapters 5 through 13, I'll discuss all the factors I know of that can cause specific sexual problems. Sex problems have what are called *distal* and *proximal causes*. Distal causes are things that occurred far in the past that can contribute to sex problems, such as a restrictive sexual upbringing. Factors in a person's present situation also contribute to the problem. These are the proximal causes. The biggest proximal cause of sex problems is anxiety.

Anxiety has both physical and mental symptoms. The main physical symptom of anxiety is rapid heart rate. The main psychological symptom is worry. All of the sex problems I deal with in this book are caused to some degree by anxiety. Sometimes the anxiety is overt and sometimes it is less obvious, but the key to healing any sex problem is learning to identify, deal with, and reduce anxiety. Symptoms depend in part on when during a sexual encounter the anxiety hits. If the anxiety hits before a sexual encounter starts, the resulting problem is generally low desire, sexual aversion, or vaginismus. If it hits toward the beginning of a sexual encounter, it usually causes female arousal problems or erection problems. If it hits once intercourse has started, it usually results in dyspareunia. If it hits right before orgasm, it causes male or female orgasm problems or premature ejaculation.

Because anxiety is such an important factor in causing sexual problems, reducing anxiety is crucial for sexual healing to occur. In Chapter 3, I'll go into much more detail about the different types of anxiety that can affect your sex life.

A Brief History of the Treatment of Sexual Problems

Many historical accounts of sexual problems exist—mostly accounts of erection problems in men, which used to be called *impotence.* Some of the earliest attempts at treating sexual problems involved the use of aphrodisiacs: foods or potions made from animal parts that were purported to increase sexual desire and ability. (In fact, to my knowledge, no true aphrodisiacs exist.) One of the earliest treatments suggested for erection problems was to have the impotent man sleep with an attractive young woman.

Sex manuals have been around for many centuries. The most famous of these is probably the Indian *Kama Sutra,* which contains illustrations of unusual sexual positions. The fields of sex therapy (treating sex problems scientifically) and sexology (sex research) developed in the late 1800s. In 1886, Richard Krafft-Ebing wrote *Psychopathia Sexualis,* a collection of case histories of people with unusual sexual desires, such as fetishes. Sigmund Freud was one of the first to recognize the importance of psychological factors in sexual problems. During Freud's era (very roughly from about 1880 through the 1930s), experts began to recognize that men could experience erection problems and premature ejaculation, and that women could experience low sexual desire, difficulty becoming aroused, and difficulty reaching orgasm. In Freudian theory these problems were believed to stem from childhood sexual abuse or from unconscious conflicts. The treatment of choice for these problems was psychoanalysis (the "talking cure"), with the goal of bringing up unconscious material that was causing the sex problems. I'm not aware of any good evidence showing that psychoanalysis is effective in treating sex problems.

Major breakthroughs in treating sexual problems were made in the middle of the twentieth century. The Kinsey reports on male sexuality (1948) and female sexuality (1953) revealed that many people were ignorant of some of the most basic aspects of sexuality. The Kinsey reports also gave us information about things like how long the average man lasted during intercourse. The Kinsey reports counteracted some of the popular marriage manuals of the 1920s, 1930s, and 1940s, many of which were full of laughably inaccurate information.

One of the first attempts to treat a specific sexual problem occurred in the 1950s. The stop-start technique for treating premature ejaculation was described in 1956 by James Semans in the *Southern Medical Journal*. The biggest breakthrough in treating sexual problems in the twentieth century was the work of sex researchers William Masters and Virginia Johnson. Their first major work was *Human Sexual Response* (1966), in which they described their research on the sexual response cycle (a very brief description of which is included in Chapter 2). Based on their findings, Masters and Johnson developed treatments for all of the sexual dysfunctions. In contrast to psychoanalysis, which at the time was really the only other treatment available for sexual problems, Masters and Johnson's treatment followed a "cognitive-behavioral" approach. This means that rather than focusing on childhood issues or repression, they focused on thoughts and behaviors that cause people's natural sexual responses to shut down before or during a sexual encounter. Masters and Johnson's treatment involved specific touching exercises and sexual techniques. An irony about treating sexual problems is that even though Masters and Johnson focused only on improving mechanical sexual functioning rather than on healing sexual issues, the techniques they promoted ended up helping thousands of people who had sexual problems.

In 1974 Helen Singer Kaplan published a book called *The New Sex Therapy*. Her treatment for sexual problems involved a combination of psychoanalysis and cognitive-behavioral strategies. In the 1980s Dr. Ruth Westheimer became famous as a media personality with a television show on sexuality. She worked as a sex therapist for many years and popularized many of the field's concepts. The American public's idea of what sex therapy is about probably comes largely from Dr. Ruth.

Most people have heard of Masters and Johnson. Their contributions to sex therapy really can't be overestimated. Most people have probably never heard of Jack Annon. In 1974 he published a book called *The Behavioral Treatment of Sexual Problems*. In it, he built on the work of Masters and Johnson and formulated his own treatment model, which he called the *PLISSIT model*. PLISSIT stands for *permission, limited information, specific suggestions,* and *intensive therapy*. The main idea of the PLISSIT model is that people with sexual problems may need help at several different levels. Some people are afraid to try new sexual activities and really only need a therapist to give them permission to do so. Others have a lack of knowledge about sexual matters and just need some information, often the same type of information one could get from taking a college course on sexuality. Still others will benefit from specific suggestions: detailed techniques for touching the genitals that can improve one's ability to become aroused. And, of course, there are some people whose sexual problems genuinely result from past sexual trauma or deep-seated personality issues. These individuals will benefit from intensive therapy. When I was studying to become a surrogate partner and later a sex therapist, I read the works of Masters and Johnson, Helen Singer Kaplan, and Jack Annon, among many others. The work that was most helpful to me over the years was Annon's.

What is the current state of sex therapy? Most psychologically based sex therapies still rely on treatment concepts that began with Masters and Johnson. Cognitive-behavioral sex therapy has had very good treatment success. However, in the last ten to twenty years, sex therapy has become increasingly medicalized. The introduction of Viagra and other medical treatments for sex problems has taken the focus off psychology.

Where This Book Fits In

Like Kinsey's work, *Sexual Healing* provides you with facts about sexuality. It builds on the work of Masters and Johnson because it is behavioral in approach by virtue of its reliance on exercises. In terms of Annon's PLISSIT model, *Sexual Healing* addresses sexual problems at the first three levels: permission, information, and specific suggestions. I give you permission to take action to heal your sex life. Some readers may need only limited information about sexuality, such as the role of anxiety in sexual problems; this book provides such information. The main thrust of *Sexual Healing*, however, is to offer help in the form of specific suggestions, the third level of Annon's model. The majority of the book's content consists of practical, easy-to-understand exercises that you can do alone or with a partner to heal your sex life.

Although this book may give you some insight into what has caused your sexual problems, if your problems are very serious and long-term there's no substitute for intensive therapy. If that's the case, I encourage you to find a professional to help you explore your sexual history in depth.

What Happens in Sex Therapy?

Sex therapy is a narrowly focused professional specialty that deals with the treatment of sexual dysfunctions. Typically, a couple would be referred to a sex therapist by a marriage counselor or physician. Sex therapy is meant to be short-term—usually a few weeks to about six months or so. It is behavioral. Clients are asked to do specific homework assignments that involve touching.

Most sex therapists treat couples, because sexual problems generally occur in the context of a relationship. When a couple first visits a sex therapist, the therapist takes a detailed sex history from each partner. This can be in the form of an interview or a written questionnaire. During the course of the sex history, the couple will list their present complaints, which could be any of the sexual dysfunctions. A person could have more than one sexual dysfunction, and both members of a couple can have problems.

Based on the couple's sex histories and current complaints, the sex therapist forms a treatment plan that usually includes bonding and touching exercises (called *sensate-focus exercises).* These start with sensual touching and relaxation exercises and gradually progress to exercises that include oral sex, high levels of arousal, and intercourse, if all of these are agreeable to both members of the couple. In most cases a couple meets with the therapist once a week. The therapist gives the couple a touching assignment to do at home. When the couple returns the following week, they discuss how the assignment went. The therapist then outlines a new homework assignment and also deals with any concerns the couple has. When a married couple comes in for sex therapy, the focus is on keeping the couple together. No reputable sex therapist or marriage counselor would try to split up a couple, except in cases of abuse. Certainly, no therapist would advise one member of a couple to have sex with a third person! Instead, sex therapists ask couples to do certain touching exercises together in the privacy of their own home or another private place, such as a hotel room.

All of the exercises in this book are based on sex therapy exercises. You'll find treatment programs here that therapists would use for all of the most common sexual problems. The book allows you to set up your own personal program of touching exercises so you can be your own sex therapist.

Much of my training in sex therapy was as a surrogate partner. Surrogate partners work with single clients who have sexual problems but don't have a partner available to work with. I'd like to explain to you what surrogate partners do so you will be confident that I have the experience you can draw upon to help you solve your own problems.

How Surrogate Partners Heal

When a single person comes to a sex therapist for a problem such as lack of desire or difficulty with orgasm, arousal, or erection, he or she is in a bind. He or she needs to do the same exercises a couple would do but has no partner to practice them with. To address single people's needs, some sex therapists work with trained, professional surrogate (substitute) partners, who act as the client's partner during therapy. Professional surrogates always work under the supervision of a licensed therapist.

For twelve years, from 1980 to 1992, I worked as a professional surrogate partner. I personally treated hundreds of sex therapy clients, mostly men suffering from erection problems or premature ejaculation, although I also worked with some women who experienced problems with arousal and orgasm. It was during those years that my colleagues and I developed and refined many of the exercises included in this book. I was inspired to become a surrogate partner so that I could help to heal others. It is a helping profession, akin to teaching or nursing. In fact, it has much more in common with professions like nursing and counseling than it does with prostitution or other sex-industry occupations, although surrogate partners are often considered "sex workers." I also became a surrogate partner because I believed that sex therapy worked, and that it changed lives. I believe that in certain relationships lovemaking can be a life-affirming and potentially life-changing experience.

The therapy practiced by surrogate partners is powerful and unique, but many misconceptions exist about what surrogate partners do. Many people consider surrogate partners essentially prostitutes who are paid to have sex with people they don't know. In fact, nothing could be further from the truth. Based on my years of experience as a surrogate partner, I strongly believe that the relationship between a client and a surrogate is a healing one. It is not the best of all healing scenarios, since neither person is the other's physical choice or emotional mate, and the relationship is somewhat artificial because it is time-limited. Nevertheless, a great deal of emotional, physical, sexual, and spiritual healing has taken place in client–surrogate relationships. I've even known people whose lives have been changed dramatically by one episode of lovemaking.

So what do surrogates and their clients actually do? In the first session, I would begin by sitting and talking with the client, kind of like a first therapy session or a first date. Then, usually during the first session, we would take turns doing a sensate-focus touching exercise called the face caress, which you will learn in Chapter 19. The client and I would meet with his therapist before and after our session, which usually lasted about an hour. By the second session, most clients were comfortable with nudity, so we would take off our clothes and do a back caress (Chapter 20). If the client were comfortable, the next session would include a front caress, and then a genital caress (Chapters 21 and 22). Depending on the client's problem, we would then progress to the more advanced sensate-focus exercises for specific problems that you will read about in Chapters 23 through 31.

As a surrogate partner, it was my job to create a relaxing atmosphere for my clients. As you can imagine, they were very nervous. I taught them all how to breathe, relax their muscles, and do pelvic muscle exercises (Chapters 16 and 17). Meanwhile, I had to be alert for any signs that they were anxious. If a client became too anxious, we would stop the exercise and back up to a more comfortable activity. I also had to figure out whether the client was responding normally or had some kind of physical problem. There were multiple things going on that I had to be aware of. In addition, I had to be ready, willing, and able to do an exercise when I came to work—but I also had to be myself and not fake a response.

Since surrogate work is a healing profession, practitioners are very subject to burnout. My work as a surrogate partner meant a lot to me, but it is the type of job most people cannot do forever. I eventually reached a point where I couldn't do it anymore. Most people think I stopped working as a surrogate because I got tired of impersonal sex. Actually, the opposite is true—it's too personal. You run the danger of caring too much about your clients and taking their problems home with you.

What You Can Learn from My Experience as a Surrogate Partner

Either as a person who needs sexual healing or as a beginning sexual healer, what can you learn from my experience as a surrogate? Some of the things you can learn are very concrete, and some are intangible. The first seems pretty basic, but it eludes a lot of people. That is, if you want to be healed or be a sexual healer for yourself and your partner, you must schedule a time to do exercises together, and you must both agree to honor that scheduled time. Second, if you agree to the scheduled time, you should be ready to fully engage in the exercises—mentally, physically, and emotionally. If you and your partner are not emotionally or physically prepared to do so, recognize this fact and don't pursue the exercise; if you have already begun, stop and backtrack. Third, for sexual healing to take place, you should have a comfortable room that is completely free of distractions. All of these points relate back to the healing mindset I mentioned in the Introduction.

The intangibles also relate to the healing mindset, starting with attitude. You can heal yourself and your partner if you stay in that mindset., which involves several things. As a surrogate partner, I always did my best to nonverbally convey the expectation that the client would be fine and everything would be all right. A big part of the attitude is also what you don't convey: You don't convey anxiety or performance pressure about desire, arousal, or erections. The best way to describe my professional healing experience is to say that for one hour at a time my client and I were absolutely absorbed in and involved with each other. As lovers, you and your partner will experience the added force of working to be sexual healers for and with each other.

The sexual activities you will learn in this book will promote confidence and self-esteem. You will feel better about yourself not only because you have learned to enjoy sexual expression, but also because you know your partner enjoys what you do and is able to become sexually aroused with you.

How can I make these claims? When I worked with clients, I often saw people who were extremely anxious and depressed, not only because of their sexual problems, but also because of their lack of a satisfying intimate relationship. One client in particular stands out in my mind. I'll call him Gary. The first time I met Gary he entered the room hunched over and could not look me in the eye. He stammered when he talked and looked as if he wanted to run away. He was one of the most anxious and withdrawn people I had ever met. It was extremely gratifying for me to see that after only a few sessions of therapy, Gary walked into the room with perfect posture, exuding self-confidence. He looked his therapist and me in the eye and talked animatedly. He had even bought new clothes!

I hope that interacting with your partner in a healing way and learning to communicate honestly about your sexual experiences will have some of the same effects on you. I believe this is possible, and that is why I wrote this book. Join me now on the journey of sexual healing.

chapter 2

Sex 101

L et's begin your sexual healing process with a review of sexual anatomy and physiology. This chapter is based on a lecture I give to my university class on human sexuality. You probably already know about the genital organs and their functions, but I've included this chapter as reference material, and I've focused on the significance of the genital organs for sexual healing. I've also included information about medical problems with the genitals that can complicate sexual problems.

Although in this chapter I've focused on the genitals, there is certainly much more to sexual functioning and enjoyment than just the genitals. People receive sexual pleasure from touch on other areas of the body, such as the breasts, the back of the neck, or the anus. Anal sex, especially, has become increasingly popular in recent years. Studies show that between 20 and 40 percent of heterosexual couples have experimented with some form of anal sex. I don't include in this book a section addressing anal sex practices because there are no specific sexual dysfunctions associated with anal sex. If your sexual repertoire includes anal sex, or if you would like for it to, many of the sensate-focus exercises included in this book can be adapted for anal sex practices. The anal area can be caressed just like any other body area.

At the end of the chapter I've included a section on Masters and Johnson's sexual response cycle: the physical changes that men and women go through when they receive sexual stimulation. As you've read, Masters and Johnson were quite influential in developing many of the techniques for solving sexual problems that I've built upon in this book.

Male Sexual Anatomy and Physiology

The penis is the male organ that is used for sexual intercourse and to convey both urine and semen outside the body (see Figure 1). If you look at a penis, you'll see that it has two structural divisions: the shaft and the head. The

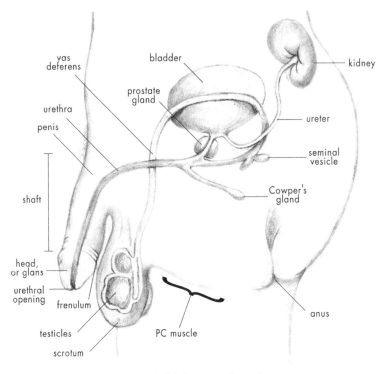

Figure 1. Male sexual anatomy

head of the penis is very sensitive because it contains many nerve endings. The shaft of the penis does not contain muscles or a bone. Instead, it contains three cylinders of erectile tissue—tissue containing many tiny blood vessels that fill when a man has an erection. The two cylinders on the sides of the penis are called the *corpora cavernosa* (Latin for "cavernous bodies") and the cylinder that runs along the bottom of the penis is called the *corpus spongiosum* (Latin for "spongy body"). Assuming a man has the normal ability to have an erection, these cylinders fill with blood when he receives either direct physical stimulation or mental stimulation. Male erectile disorder occurs when this response does not happen.

The penis itself does not contain muscles. However, a very important muscle group runs from the pubic bone, in the front of the body, to the tailbone (coccyx), in the rear. This muscle group is called the *pubococcygeus* or *pubococcygeal muscle group*—*PC muscle* for short. It supports the whole pelvic floor. In order for an erection to occur, this muscle has to relax to allow blood to flow into the penis. The PC muscle is very important for sexual healing in several ways. Many men experience erection problems because they have chronic tension in their PC muscle, which prevents blood flow into the penis.

The PC muscle is also the muscle that spasms when a man has an orgasm and ejaculates. Spasms in the part of the PC muscle called the *bulbocavernosus (BC) muscle* cause semen to be expelled from the penis. Sexual problems can occur when the BC muscle spasms out of control following minimal stimulation, resulting in premature ejaculation. The opposite problem, male orgasm disorder, can occur when a man consciously or unconsciously tightens his PC muscle as he nears orgasm, causing him to be unable to reach orgasm and ejaculation.

The testes are the male reproductive organs that are housed in a skin pouch called the *scrotum,* which hangs outside a man's body between his legs. The testes produce both sperm, for reproduction, and the male hormone testosterone, which is responsible for the male sex drive. Several problems can occur if a man does not produce enough testosterone or if for some reason he can't use the testosterone he does produce. For one, it can cause a loss of the sex drive, which, as you read in Chapter 1, is called *hypoactive sexual desire disorder* or *low sexual desire.* Testicular cancer, which is obviously a very serious medical condition, can cause swelling in a testicle, a lump in a testicle, or a sense of heaviness or dragging in a testicle. It can cause pain during sexual arousal or intercourse. In many cases of testicular cancer a testicle must be surgically removed, which need not affect sexual functioning if replacement hormones are administered.

Another male organ that's really important in terms of sexual functioning is the prostate gland. Although the prostate gland is not directly involved in reproduction, it can have an effect on whether or not a man has sexual problems. The prostate is a walnut-sized gland located near the bladder. The urethra, the tube that travels through the penis and carries semen and urine outside the body, passes through the prostate. The prostate gland contributes some of the liquid content of semen. Sexual problems can occur if the prostate becomes enlarged, which tends to happen in older men. An enlarged prostate can cause difficult or painful urination or ejaculation, as well as erection problems.

Because it is made up of glandular tissue, the prostate is highly susceptible to cancer. Many cases of prostate cancer are readily curable, but, unfortunately, many of the treatments for it can have a serious effect on a man's sex life. For example, if a man has his prostate gland surgically removed due to cancer, some of the nerves that trigger erection may be damaged, causing him to be unable to have an erection. Furthermore, a man whose prostate gland has been removed will probably be unable to ejaculate (although he will probably still be able to have an orgasm). Even the other treatments for prostate cancer, such as chemotherapy and radiation, can affect a man's ability to have an erection and ejaculate. The good news is that many medical solutions are available to help men who have erection difficulties due to prostate problems. You'll read about these in Chapter 24.

Two other potential problems with the male genitals can cause sexual problems: phimosis and Peyronie's disease. When boys are born, a flap of skin called the *foreskin* covers the head of the penis. In many cultures the foreskin is surgically removed in an operation called *circumcision.* In uncircumcised boys and men, sometimes the foreskin is too tight and can't be retracted behind the head of the penis for urination; this condition is called *phimosis.* When a boy with phimosis reaches puberty and his penis enlarges in size, erections can be painful; he may need to undergo circumcision to allow for pain-free erections.

In Peyronie's disease the erectile tissue develops sections of calcified plaque, which cause the penis to bend in one direction. (Hardly any man's penis is perfectly straight. Most normal penises curve to one side or the other.) If there is only one small plaque, it can be removed to straighten the penis. More than one plaque can cause quite a bit of pain and can limit a man's ability to have an erection. Peyronie's disease can result from injury to the penis, or it can occur for no apparent reason in older men.

Female Sexual Anatomy and Physiology

The term *vulva* refers to the female external genitals (see Figure 2). The vulva includes the clitoris, the inner and outer vaginal lips, and the vaginal opening. A girl's clitoris grows from the same embryonic tissue as a boy's penis. Like the penis, the clitoris has a head, shaft, and hood. It contains two rather than three cylinders of erectile tissue. When a woman receives stimulation, blood flows to the clitoris and to the inner and outer vaginal lips, causing them to swell. A failure of this normal arousal response is called *female sexual arousal disorder.*

When female babies are born, a membrane called the *hymen* partially covers the vaginal opening. Injuries can tear the hymen, but sometimes it remains intact until the first time a woman has sexual intercourse. A medical

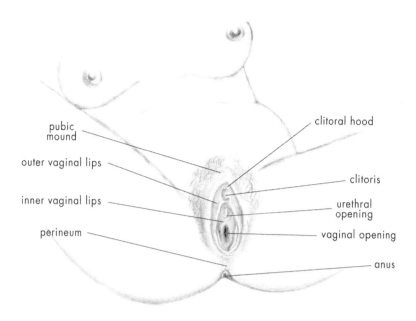

pubic mound

outer vaginal lips

inner vaginal lips

perineum

clitoral hood

clitoris

urethral opening

vaginal opening

anus

Figure 2. Female external sexual anatomy

condition called *imperforate hymen* can cause either vaginismus or sexual pain; the condition occurs when the hymen is too fibrous and doesn't tear during intercourse. Sometimes it has to be surgically removed.

Like men, women have a pubococcygeus muscle that supports the pelvic organs. The PC muscle is very critical to female sexuality. It is the muscle that spasms when a woman has an orgasm. Having a weak or out-of-shape PC muscle can cause a woman to experience difficulty reaching orgasm. At the opposite end of the spectrum, anxiety that causes an uncontrollable spasm of the PC muscle and prevents penetration results in the condition known as vaginismus.

The inner female genitals include the vagina, the cervix, the uterus, the fallopian tubes, and the ovaries (see Figure 3 on the next page). The vagina is the tubular sex organ that is used both for sexual intercourse and as the birth canal. It therefore must be very muscular. The vaginal canal has muscular ridges called *rugae* that run along its walls. If you looked inside a vagina, you would see that the walls have a striped or corrugated appearance. When a woman receives stimulation, blood flow to the vaginal walls causes them to lubricate. If this does not happen, a woman has arousal problems.

Several areas inside the vagina are sensitive enough that stimulating them can often lead to orgasm. The anterior fornix, or A-spot, located on the upper front wall of the vagina, is one such spot. It is believed to be

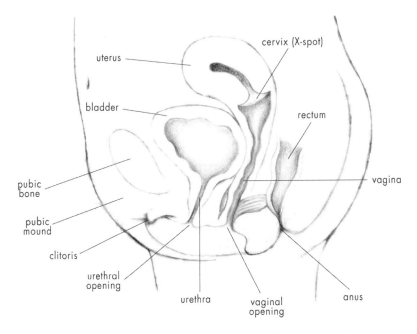

Figure 3. Female internal sexual anatomy

responsible for most of a woman's vaginal lubrication. The Gräfenberg spot, or G-spot, is located on the front wall of the vagina behind the pubic bone. Stimulation of the G-spot causes some women to release a great deal of fluid. This is called *female ejaculation.* Some women enjoy stimulation of the cervix, which is the opening to the uterus. Positioned near the cervix is the end of the vagina, called the *cul de sac.* When a woman becomes intensely aroused, the muscles that support her uterus tighten and cause the uterus to lift up, exposing the cul de sac. Many women report that penetration into the cul de sac is intensely pleasurable.

Speaking of orgasm, there are many areas on a woman's body that can trigger one. In fact, some women can have orgasms without even being touched. In the genital area, the sites that most commonly trigger orgasm are the clitoris, the PC muscle, the G-spot, the cervix, and the cul de sac. Some theorists think in terms of two types of female orgasm: clitoral and vaginal. A clitoral orgasm is one that results from stimulation of the external genitals, and a vaginal orgasm is one that results from stimulation of the internal genitals. Sometimes a clitoral orgasm is called a *vulval orgasm* and a vaginal orgasm is called a *uterine orgasm.* There's also such a thing as a *blended orgasm,* which occurs when a woman has an orgasm while receiving stimulation both inside the vagina and on the clitoris.

The ovaries are the female reproductive organs. In addition, they produce hormones, including the hormone testosterone, which is essential for sexual desire, even in women. The adrenal glands, which lie atop the kidneys, also produce some testosterone. If a woman has glandular problems that cause her body to produce insufficient amounts of testosterone, her sex drive will suffer.

The fallopian tubes convey eggs into the uterus, and if an egg is fertilized, the uterus carries the developing embryo. The fallopian tubes and the uterus don't really have any direct bearing on sexual dysfunctions, although surgery to remove the uterus and/or ovaries can result in unintended nerve damage or problems with blood flow. Both of these could affect a woman's ability to become aroused.

There are many health problems involving the genitals that can affect a woman's sex life, especially in terms of pain during intercourse. I cover many of these issues in Chapter 13, on sexual pain.

Intersex Conditions

About one in two thousand children are born in the United States each year with genitalia that are ambiguous enough to create problems accurately identifying the child as male or female. Medical conditions that cause ambiguous genitalia are called *intersex conditions.* There are many types of intersex conditions—in fact, too many to list here. Intersex conditions can result from problems with chromosomes, prenatal hormones, or internal or external organs.

An example of an intersex condition that affects some men is Klinefelter's syndrome, in which a boy is born with an extra X (female) chromosome. If the condition is recognized before puberty, it can be treated with hormones. But if a man has this problem in adulthood, it can cause an abnormally small penis and lack of sex drive.

An intersex condition that can affect women is called *congenital adrenal hyperplasia (CAH).* In CAH, a female embryo is exposed to male hormones before birth. When the baby girl is born, her clitoris is so enlarged that it could be mistaken for a penis.

In terms of sexual healing, some intersex conditions affect sexual functioning and some do not. You can see that Klinefelter's syndrome would affect sexual functioning, but CAH would not (although it would almost certainly affect body image). Although this book is not directed specifically toward people with intersex conditions, I believe it can be of use to many such individuals.

The Sexual Response Cycle

In the 1960s, sexologists William Masters and Virginia Johnson conducted research that involved volunteer subjects visiting their laboratory and agreeing to have recording devices attached to their bodies. The devices recorded things like respiration rate, blood pressure, and even genital blood flow. Some people came into the laboratory alone, and some came in as couples. The single people were instructed to masturbate and the couples to have sexual intercourse. As the volunteers became sexually stimulated, often all the way to orgasm, Masters and Johnson monitored the changes in their bodies. The result of these studies was the first clinically defined model of the sexual response cycle, which is the series of physiological changes that occur in the human body as it becomes aroused and reaches orgasm.

The sexual response cycle has four stages: excitement, plateau, orgasm, and resolution (see Figure 4). I'll briefly summarize the physiological changes that happen in men and women as they go through each stage.

In the excitement phase, men get a partial or full erection, and their scrotum and testes swell and move closer to the body. Women also experience blood flow to the genitals, including the clitoris, inner and outer lips, and vagina. Blood flow to the vagina causes vaginal lubrication. In both sexes, blood pressure, respiration, and heart rate start to rise. Both men and women may experience nipple erection and the "sex flush": redness on the chest, face, and neck.

The plateau phase occurs when a person reaches a high level of arousal and stays there for a while. On a scale of 1 to 10, with 10 being orgasm, the plateau phase would correspond to about a level 8. Men experience a very strong erection during the plateau phase. Due to blood flow to the penis, the head of the penis may turn a dark color. The scrotum and testes continue to move close to the body. The Cowper's glands, which are located at the base of the penis, may secrete a couple of drops of clear fluid that appear at the tip of the penis.

In the plateau phase, women may experience engorgement of the areolas of their breasts. The inner third of the vagina may tighten and grip the penis. The muscles that support the uterus contract and cause the uterus to lift up. This opens the back area of the vagina, the cul de sac. The

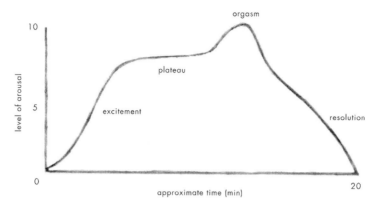

Figure 4. Masters and Johnson's human sexual response cycle

Bartholin's glands, located under the skin of the inner vaginal lips, may secrete a couple of drops of lubrication. A woman may experience "sex skin," which occurs when the inner lips of the vagina turn a very dark color due to blood flow.

In both sexes, blood pressure, respiration, and heart rate continue to rise and then plateau at a high level. Both men and women may continue to experience the sex flush, as well as muscle spasms in the hands, feet, or face.

As stimulation continues, a person may enter the orgasm phase. Orgasm occurs when blood flow and muscle tension reach a peak in the genitals. It is a reflex that dissipates the blood flow and muscle tension. Masters and Johnson judged that a woman had had an orgasm if her PC muscle spasmed rhythmically and her heart rate reached a peak. They judged that a man had had an orgasm if his PC muscle spasmed rhythmically, his heart rate reached a peak, and he ejaculated. In fact, however, in a man, orgasm and ejaculation are not exactly the same thing. Ejaculation is the localized genital response in which semen leaves the penis. Orgasm is a full-body or systemic response that includes changes in blood flow, muscle tension, and the brain. The distinction between ejaculation and orgasm is important for treating male orgasm disorder, as I'll explain in Chapter 10.

When you have an orgasm, muscles in your body contract, especially in the genital area, although many people also experience muscle spasms in their legs, arms, and face. For most people, the mental experience of orgasm runs anywhere from a pleasant feeling to intense pleasure or an almost altered state of consciousness. When you reach high levels of arousal and then have an orgasm, your brain secretes endorphins, which are chemicals that kill pain and cause pleasure. After orgasm, most people experience a sense of closeness or intimacy with their partner.

During the resolution phase, the body returns to its normal, unaroused state. The man loses his erection, and blood leaves the female genitals. Many men experience a refractory period, during which they are unresponsive to sexual stimulation for some time after ejaculation and orgasm.

The sexual response cycle has its problems and critics. It has been augmented over the years. For example, in the 1970s Helen Singer Kaplan added a desire phase to the beginning of the cycle. She theorized that some kind of motivational factor must be present in order for stimulation and excitement to take place.

The significance of all this for sexual healing is that Masters and Johnson's sexual response cycle has been highly influential in how we view and treat sexual problems. The sexual dysfunctions I briefly described in Chapter 1 are usually grouped according to the sexual response cycle. For example, sexual aversion disorder and low sexual desire are problems with the desire phase; male erectile disorder and female sexual arousal disorder are problems with the excitement phase; and premature ejaculation, male orgasm disorder, and female orgasm disorder are problems with the orgasm phase. (The sexual pain disorders are not grouped according to the sexual response cycle. They fall at different phases for different people.)

Earlier in this chapter, I described sexual problems in terms of what anatomical structures or physiological functions they involve. Another way of looking at sexual problems is to use Masters and Johnson's sexual response cycle as a guide. I described Masters and Johnson's plateau phase as about a level 8 on a 1-to-10 scale. The program in *Sexual Healing* uses two different 1-to-10 scales: a physical arousal scale, which measures either a man's erection or a woman's lubrication/swelling response, and a subjective psychological or emotional arousal scale, which measures perceived closeness to orgasm. This system is a good one for healing many of the problems you'll read about in this book.

For now, let's take a closer look at anxiety. As I pointed out in Chapter 1, anxiety is a contributing factor in all of the sexual problems addressed in this book. The next chapter introduces some simple and effective strategies for reducing anxiety during sexual activity.

chapter 3

Dealing with Anxiety

Many of the sexual dysfunctions are affected by anxiety. Before you read in detail about the different sexual problems and before you try any exercises, I would like to give you some ideas for how to deal with any performance pressure or anxiety you might feel.

In our society, we tend to view sexuality—and much else—as a performance. We wonder constantly if we could "do it better." We also tend to think of a sexual problem as something "missing." In fact, if you experience problems with your sexuality, you probably need to *subtract* stress or anxiety rather than *add* props such as X-rated videotapes, exotic clothing, or other erotica to your sexual encounters.

How to reduce and eventually eliminate sexual anxiety is one of the most important things you can learn from this book. The sensate-focus exercises (which, if you remember from Chapter 1, are touching and bonding exercises you do with your partner) are designed to teach you, step-by-step, how to identify and deal with anxiety during the course of a sexual encounter. If you have been experiencing sexual anxiety for a long time, even the earliest and most basic sensate-focus exercises may make you anxious. Do not blame yourself for this. Even fairly mild levels of anxiety take time and practice to overcome completely as you work to undo the results of years of fearful reactions to sexual encounters.

Remember, though, that the exercises will not help you if you remain anxious while you do them. You will do yourself more harm than good if you attempt to disguise your anxiety just to get through an exercise. It is extremely important that you stop any exercise that makes you anxious; if you continue, you will only reinforce your fear.

The Physiology of Anxiety

What is anxiety? It is a mind-body phenomenon that occurs because of the way our nervous system is set up. (I'm sorry that the explanation is about to get a bit technical, but I hope it will help to demystify anxiety for you.) The body's nervous system allows all of the parts of the body to communicate with each other. At its most basic level, the nervous system includes the brain and spinal cord. This is called the *central nervous system*. In addition to the central nervous system, we have the peripheral nervous system, which includes all the nerves that go from the spinal cord to the rest of the limbs and organs.

The peripheral nervous system has two parts: the skeletal nervous system and the autonomic nervous system. Sometimes the skeletal nervous system is called the *voluntary nervous system* and the autonomic nervous system is called the *involuntary nervous system*. The skeletal nervous system provides nerves to limbs like your arms and legs. We call it the voluntary nervous system because your ability to activate these nerves and move your limbs is under your control.

The autonomic nervous system provides nerves to your internal organs, such as your heart, diaphragm, intestines, stomach, and genitals. We generally do not have much control, if any, over the responses of these organs. Their activities are largely reflexive. The presence of food in the stomach, for example, triggers a series of reflexes that cause digestion. We can't make it stop or cause it to happen any faster. The same thing is true of the genitals. A touch on the penis can trigger a reflexive erection, or a touch to the opening of the vagina can trigger reflexive vaginal lubrication.

The autonomic nervous system has two divisions—the sympathetic nervous system (the SNS) and the parasympathetic nervous system (the PNS). The function of the SNS is to expend energy rapidly. It is responsible for initiating the stress response (also known as the fight-or-flight mechanism). The SNS functions when you are faced with a major threat to your safety. When your SNS is activated (which happens within a split second), your eyes dilate, your heart pounds, and blood rushes away from the center of your body toward your limbs so you can fight or run away. The action of the PNS is the opposite. Its function is to conserve energy for use at a later time. The PNS is active when you are asleep, digesting, or just resting. Many sexual phenomena are functions of the PNS. For example, the early stages of erection and arousal occur when the PNS is active. The activity of the PNS is also called the *relaxation response*.

It is probably becoming clear to you by now what causes anxiety. Anxiety occurs when something happens that really doesn't threaten your life, but still your body overreacts to it with full sympathetic-nervous-system activity. Physical signs of anxiety include cold hands and feet, tensed muscles (especially in the thighs and abdomen), rapid and shallow breathing, rapid heart rate, and a feeling of nausea or nervous stomach.

Because of the way the autonomic nervous system is organized, you cannot be relaxed and anxious at the same time. You gain control of your anxiety by consciously promoting relaxation. One way to reduce anxiety is through repetitive, slow, nonthreatening touching. Another way is through deep, slow, rhythmic breathing. If you are gradually taught to respond in a relaxed way to a previously anxiety-producing stimulus, relaxation will carry over to other anxiety-producing situations in your life.

How Sensate-Focus Exercises Help to Reduce Anxiety

The sexual healing program offers a series of sensual exercises that gradually become more sexual. The first few exercises are nonsexual and nonthreatening. You are simply training your body to relax. By the time the exercises become more sexual, you will be able to respond to a sexual situation with relaxation rather than anxiety. The process I recommend has much in common with that described by Herbert Benson in his book *The Relaxation Response*. According to Benson, four things are necessary for the relaxation response to occur: a mental device, quiet, a comfortable position, and a receptive or passive attitude. In the exercises that appear throughout this book, focusing on the sensations of touch provides the device that keeps your mind occupied. You will take a passive role during part of each exercise, and you should do the exercises in a quiet room and a comfortable position. As a bonus, learning how to decrease your anxiety by sustaining the relaxation response helps more than just your sexual functioning. It will also benefit your physical and mental health in general.

If you have a sexual problem, you have learned to associate sexual activity with the bodily changes produced by anxiety. In the program outlined in this book, you will learn three basic steps to dealing with the anxiety you may feel before or during a sensate-focus exercise. First, concentrate on the touch in order to occupy your mind. Second, breathe properly. When you become anxious, you hold your breath or you breathe too shallowly. To counteract this tendency, take deep, slow breaths that you can feel all the way down into your stomach (belly breaths). Third, consciously relax the muscles in your thighs, stomach, and buttocks. Even momentary tightening of those muscles can cause anxiety and interfere with your natural sexual arousal response.

Some people can experience very severe forms of anxiety, called *panic attacks, panic reactions,* or *phobic reactions.* (A phobia is a learned fear that is experienced to an incapacitating degree, such as a fear of heights, fear of snakes, or fear of being in enclosed spaces.) You may have a phobic reaction to the whole idea of sexual contact, or just to some element of the sexual encounter. Signs of this kind of severe anxiety reaction include profuse sweating, paleness, an extremely rapid heart rate, breathing difficulties, a feeling of tightness in the chest, and nausea, vomiting, or diarrhea. These sensations are usually accompanied by a feeling of unreality, extreme dread, or even the feeling that one is about to die of fright.

Psychologists have made great strides in the treatment of phobias, and even this very severe type of anxiety is usually completely treatable. I have successfully used the sex therapy program for anxiety outlined in Chapter 29 to treat many people with very severe sexual fears. However, if your sexual anxiety is quite severe, you might want to seek the assistance of a qualified therapist rather than attempt to deal with the anxiety yourself. You may need some antianxiety medication before you can begin healing your sexual problems.

If you do decide to heal your own problems, when you become anxious during any touching exercise, you will learn to tell your partner that you feel uncomfortable, and you will back up to an earlier exercise with which you felt comfortable. Only after you feel relaxed with one exercise should you add in elements of a new exercise.

You will also want to know how to respond if your partner becomes anxious during an exercise. If you are touching your partner as part of any exercise, you should be able to notice if your partner is anxious or tense. Obvious signs of anxiety include rapid and shallow breathing, a jumpy or quivering stomach, and muscle tension in the thighs and abdomen. If during any exercise you notice these signs in your partner, slow your touch down. Continue to touch your partner as slowly as you can. If the signs of your partner's anxiety don't go away, encourage your partner to take deep breaths. If necessary, stop the exercise and back up to a previous exercise with which you both felt comfortable.

When you are touching your partner, he or she may tighten up the leg muscles, especially during touching of the genital area. This muscle tightening is a learned habit that causes sexual problems and makes them worse.

For example, in men who have problems with erections, tightening the leg muscles steals blood away from the penis. In men with premature ejaculation, tightening the leg muscles can trigger ejaculation. In men and women who have difficulty reaching orgasm, tightening the leg muscles can prevent orgasm. If you notice your partner tightening his or her legs, give the legs a very light tap or pinch to remind your partner to relax those muscles. If you notice yourself tightening up, consciously relax your legs. Three to five instances of your partner reminding you to relax during an exercise will usually take care of this habit.

Performance Anxiety

A particular form of anxiety is unique to sexual situations. It's called *performance anxiety*. It stems from our fear of being watched or evaluated. Men, particularly, tend to think of a sexual encounter as a "performance." A man might say, "I was with a woman, but I was unable to perform," meaning, of course, that he didn't have an erection. Thinking of sex as work or as some kind of performance put on for the benefit of your partner is an attitude that can only detract from your enjoyment of a sexual encounter.

In most areas of life we are trained to achieve. Those who work hard and succeed on the job or in school are valued in our society. They are the go-getters and the self-made successes. And from childhood on, we are encouraged to compete, an attitude that often helps us achieve work or school goals (although possibly at the expense of our mental health). Sexual activity, however, is an area in which this performance orientation has only negative effects. For example, men who have been successful in work often encounter difficulties with erections as they age. Success in business often means thinking many steps ahead of what you are doing in the present. In sexuality, thinking ahead leads to feelings of anxiety and pressure to perform, which can result in erection failure and other sexual problems.

There are many features of the sensate-focus exercises that can help you learn to take the pressure off yourself and decrease your anxiety. For example, the use of "active" and "passive" roles in the sensate-focus exercises is designed to make it difficult if not impossible for you to maintain a performance orientation toward sex. There is no point in working to please your partner if you know that he or she has been instructed not to provide you with any verbal feedback. The person in the active role has no real choice but to act for his or her own enjoyment.

As you do the exercises in this book, watch yourself for signs of performance orientation. If you catch yourself thinking, "I tried so hard, but the exercise just didn't come out right," recognize that you are looking at the activity as a performance situation. Stop trying. Experience yourself rather than judge yourself. Your sexual responses will happen normally if you relax, allow yourself plenty of time, and avoid putting pressure on yourself.

Which brings me to my next point: Don't hurry through the exercises. You have been conditioned by our culture to believe that moving quickly wins you the most rewards. But if you rush through this program, you will not learn what you need to learn from each exercise, and you will have to repeat each exercise more times. Paradoxically, the more slowly you proceed with these exercises and the less you plan or think ahead, the sooner you will find that your problem is a thing of the past. You will benefit more if you start the program with the thought, "I will have fun and enjoy myself," rather than, "I will get better (or better at it) as soon as possible."

Learning to relax during sexual activity and ceasing to view sex as a performance will also benefit other areas of your life. Clients have often reported to me that sensate-focus techniques helped them relax and concentrate in other areas, such as studying, listening to music, or cooking. Other clients have said they were actually more productive at their jobs because they learned to concentrate on the task at hand and no longer made themselves anxious by thinking ten steps ahead. There's no room for multitasking during a sexual encounter.

Spectatoring

The term *spectatoring* was coined by Masters and Johnson. Spectatoring is one of the leading causes of performance anxiety. It means you're thinking when you should be feeling or experiencing. An example would be a man who is receiving a caress. As his partner's touch moves toward his penis he thinks, "I wonder if it will get hard. I bet it won't get very hard. Uh-oh, it's going down now." Spectatoring does not mean literally watching your sexual performance with your eyes, but rather being unable to put a stop to obsessive thoughts about your response. Women, especially those who have difficulty reaching orgasm, can also be prone to this type of thinking. Maybe a woman is receiving a genital caress. As her partner moves closer to her clitoris, she thinks, "I wonder if I'm starting to lubricate. It feels a little wet down there. I wonder if I'll have an orgasm this time." As the stimulation becomes more intense, her thoughts switch to "I'm getting kind of close. I wonder if I'll have one this time. Wait, now it's slipping away. Darn, I was so close!"

Spectatoring tends to be a concern in men with erection problems and in women who have problems with orgasm. It rarely occurs with premature ejaculation, since the ejaculation is often over before the man has time to think about it.

Our society overemphasizes a visual-logical-verbal processing of sensory information, a pattern that can cause a person to be prone to spectatoring. The sensate-focus exercises you will learn in this book will return you to the tactile-emotional way of receiving and expressing information about your world that you used naturally when you were a child. The exercises will also help you become acquainted with your partner on a body level as well as on a mental level. The cure for spectatoring, therefore, is additional practice with sensate-focus techniques—in fact, overpractice. If your mind is totally focused on the touch, you will be unable to comment internally on your "performance." Practicing sensate focus will help you learn the difference between focusing on your response and worrying about it. If spectatoring is a severe problem in any given exercise, back up to a less threatening exercise in which it was easy for you to pay complete attention to the point of contact between your skin and your partner's skin.

Pressuring Your Partner

Throughout this book I will suggest many ways to stop putting pressure on yourself to perform sexually. However, your sense of being pressured to perform may not be all in your mind. For example, if your partner ever says things to you like "Did you come yet?" "Are you close?" "Why aren't you hard yet?" "Can't you last longer?" or even, "I want you to come now," you are justified in feeling that you are being pressured.

If you are in the habit of saying things like this to your partner, please stop. If your partner says things like this to you, ask him or her to please stop. You may not have realized that these simple questions can create tremendous psychological pressure. Chapter 15 contains guidelines for giving verbal feedback to your partner—constructive, positive, and pressure-free ways for each of you to communicate your feelings about your sexual activities.

Although direct and overt performance pressure is fairly easy to recognize, pressure conveyed through nonverbal cues may be more subtle. Picture a sexual experience in which everything seems to be going fine, in the sense that both partners are functioning well and doing activities that they enjoy. Yet for some reason both feel uneasy. They may start to search for something to which they can attribute their negative or confused feelings: "I must be in a bad mood," or, "I guess I'm just not feeling sexual right now." What is more likely is that they have become caught up in a widening spiral of interpersonal performance expectations, each picking up on the fact that the other is thinking or worrying rather than enjoying the experience.

Let's say a man is giving an oral genital caress to a woman. If he is enjoying himself and concentrating on exactly what he is doing (in other words, if he is focused on the sensations), then his partner is also free to enjoy herself and to focus on her own pleasure. However, if the man thinks, "I wonder if she's enjoying this" or "I wonder how much longer I'm going to have to do this until she has an orgasm," the woman will pick up on his attitudes and will realize that her partner is no longer concentrating on the touch but is instead having performance-related thoughts.

Your partner cannot read your mind, but he or she can tell if you are concentrating on what you are doing and if you are enjoying it. You may not know exactly what is going on, but you realize that something isn't right because you feel uncomfortable. In that sense, anxiety can be a good thing because it alerts us to the fact that we need to refocus. In fact, we are picking up our partner's nonverbal cues, which are often more honest than the activities that are taking place. We may attribute our feeling of discomfort to a thought like, "Something is wrong with me or my sexual response," when instead we need to recognize that there has been a subtle shift in the quality of the sexual encounter. What will happen in the situation I have just described is that the woman will think to herself, "Uh-oh, he's expecting me to have an orgasm pretty soon. I better fake it." At this point, the sexual interaction becomes based on expectations, worries, and performance pressure, rather than on sensate focus and mutual enjoyment.

In another example, a woman might be caressing the genitals of a partner who has difficulty having an erection. Instead of enjoying what she is doing and concentrating on how her hand feels on her partner's genitals, the woman may think—briefly—"I wonder when he's going to get hard." Her partner will instantly pick up on the fact that something is not right. The quality of her attention has changed. He may then think, "Uh-oh, she's getting tired, she's getting bored, why am I not getting hard?" Needless to say, if this situation isn't remedied his problem will only become worse, because the performance anxiety will begin earlier and earlier in each subsequent sexual encounter.

Another source of sexual pressure is the idea that you are somehow responsible for your partner's enjoyment. You need to take responsibility for your own arousal and enjoyment and learn to please yourself while accommodating your partner's needs so that both of you can become aroused together.

How do you avoid these pitfalls of unwittingly putting pressure on your partner or of succumbing to sexual pressure your partner puts on you? First, become aware of the problem. If you feel pressure, any pressure, it means the pressure is real. At this point it doesn't matter what caused it—you just need to get rid of it. If your first reaction is to think, "There is something wrong with me," redefine the situation as, "I am feeling pressured due to something that is going on in this situation." Then you can see the solution: to make sure you truly enjoy what you do by doing only what you enjoy. By practicing the sensate-focus techniques, you will learn what kinds of sexual behaviors you enjoy. Staying focused on what you are doing will increase your enjoyment, and your enjoyment in turn will leave your partner free to enjoy himself or herself. If an activity or situation is so uncomfortable or anxiety provoking that you can't focus on it, stop and do something else with which you are comfortable.

❧

You may be surprised to learn that the sexual positions you and your partner choose can have an effect on your sexual healing process. That is the topic of the next chapter.

chapter 4

Sexual Positions

There are many positions in which couples can have sexual intercourse. None of them are inherently good or bad, or right or wrong. However, some of them are more healing than others. In general, the face-to-face intercourse positions have more potential to help your sexual healing process because they are more intimate. In addition, some positions are better than others for dealing with specific sexual problems. In all of the treatment chapters (Chapters 23 through 31), whenever I recommend an exercise that includes intercourse, I'll give you suggestions about which position I believe to be the best for that exercise.

The following are the main types of sexual positions. For each group of positions, I'll tell you how to do the positions, the pros and cons from a physical standpoint, and the pros and cons from an emotional standpoint.

Male-Superior Positions

This is the group of positions many of us are most familiar with. Being the most traditional, they are the sexual positions that are typically depicted in Hollywood movies. In the basic missionary position, the woman lies flat on her back and her partner lies on top of her. There are several variations. The man can support himself on his elbows and knees or even on the palms of his hands and his toes, if he's agile enough. Another version of this position is called the *coital alignment technique,* or *CAT.* In this variation, the man pulls himself up and forward toward the woman's shoulders, causing his pubic bone to rub against her clitoris, and his penis to go in and out of her vagina more vertically than horizontally.

Another variation of the male-superior position is called the *butterfly position.* The woman lies on her back, but she tilts her pelvis so that her vagina is pointing almost straight up. This position can be varied a good deal depending on the positioning of her legs. She can bend her knees and spread her legs, raise them into the air, or wrap them around her partner's waist. In this position, the man kneels in front of the woman.

For a man, any version of a male-superior position is usually very arousing. These positions contribute to a feeling of bonding and intimacy because the couple can easily make eye contact, talk, and kiss. We tend to idealize the male-superior position in this culture because it reflects our conception of traditional male and female roles—that the man is the sexual initiator and the woman is the receiver. Many people find it a turn-on when the man is the more dominant partner.

The straight missionary position is one of the least effective positions for clitoral stimulation, whereas the CAT version is used specifically for clitoral stimulation. Some men find it difficult to delay ejaculation in the male-superior positions, and say that supporting their weight in these positions can be tiring. The straight missionary position doesn't give very much depth of penetration; therefore, in this position it's difficult for a woman to receive stimulation of her G-spot and the other erogenous zones deep in her vagina.

As I'll explain later in some of the chapters on healing specific sexual problems, certain positions are recommended for certain problems. The straight missionary position is good for couples who need help with intimacy or desire issues. The coital alignment technique is good for women with female sexual arousal disorder because it provides a lot of stimulation to the clitoris. The butterfly version of the male-superior position is excellent for female arousal and orgasm problems because it allows stimulation of both a woman's internal and external orgasm triggers.

Since the male-superior positions usually are very arousing for men, I initially advise a man with premature ejaculation to stay away from them while he is learning ejaculation control. That said, within this group some positions are better than others for helping a man learn ejaculation control. For example, it's much easier for a man to maintain ejaculation control in the butterfly position than in the straight missionary position. The male-superior positions are also good for men with male orgasm disorder (difficulty ejaculating). In the butterfly position, the man has a very exciting view of his partner's breasts and of his penis going in and out of her vagina. Men with erection problems generally also do well in the butterfly position. In this position, if you feel your erection go down, it's easy to take your penis out of your partner's vagina and stimulate yourself.

Female-Superior Positions

These are the woman-on-top positions. In the most commonly used version of the position, the man lies on his back while his partner kneels on top facing him. Her legs can be placed in several different ways. She can lie on top of her partner in such a way that they have total body contact. Or she can squat over her partner's body with her knees on either side of him. In this way she can raise her body so she is almost sitting up.

The female-superior positions are great for female arousal and orgasm because they give a woman so much control. She is in charge of the speed of intercourse as well as the depth and angle of penetration. In this position it's easy to maintain eye contact and intimacy. There can be full body contact. It's easy for either partner to caress the other's body. Either the man or the woman can stimulate the woman's clitoris to help her get aroused and have an orgasm. Or she can use a vibrator on her clitoris in this position. From an emotional standpoint, the female-superior position has often been considered a "bad girl" position, and for that reason a lot of people find it especially arousing.

From a negative standpoint, some men are uncomfortable with their partner appearing dominant or aggressive, and some women are equally uncomfortable appearing or feeling dominant. Some women don't like the way they look and feel in this position because they believe their bodies jiggle and sag when they're sitting upright and moving rapidly.

The female-superior position is highly recommended for women who have desire, arousal, and orgasm problems. I wouldn't generally recommend it for men with male orgasm disorder, because most men need to be more active in order to ejaculate. When men have erection problems, sometimes it's difficult to maintain an erection when their partner is on top of them.

Side-to-Side Positions

In the side-to-side positions, both partners lie facing each other, and one person puts a leg over the other's hip. There are several variations. In one of them, called the *scissors position,* the man lies on his side, while his partner lies on her back perpendicular to him. The couple interweaves their legs so their genitals meet.

The side-to-side positions are very relaxing because they don't require either person to support his or her body weight. Many people find that these are great positions first thing in the morning, when neither partner is in the mood for major sexual acrobatics. Many people like the eye contact and sense of intimacy these positions provide. With a couple of small bodily adjustments, these positions allow for the possibility of the man sucking and kissing the woman's breasts. The side-to-side positions tend to be the least genitally stimulating for both sexes because they are so relaxing. They don't allow much depth of penetration, so they are not generally stimulating to the woman's internal orgasm triggers like the G-spot, cul de sac, and cervix.

Because they are not physically strenuous, the side-to-side positions are often recommended for older people or for people who have physical limitations like arthritis. These positions are very good for men who have erection problems, because the penis doesn't have to be super-hard to penetrate the woman's vagina. In fact, a man can penetrate in these positions without even having an erection at all. These positions are also very good for men with premature ejaculation, because they allow a man to spend time inside his partner's vagina without moving, just getting used to the warmth and containment. Because these positions are relaxing rather than stimulating, I don't recommend them for men who have difficulty reaching orgasm.

Although the side-to-side positions tend not to be stimulating for the deeper areas inside a woman's vagina, I definitely recommend them for women who have difficulty with arousal and orgasm, because either the woman or the man can reach down and manually stimulate the woman's clitoris. These positions are also good for both vaginismus and sexual pain, because it's easy to lie in these positions with the man's penis held against the woman's vagina, without actual penetration.

Rear-Entry Positions

In the basic rear-entry position, the woman kneels on the bed on all fours, while the man kneels behind her. The variation I recommend is one in which the woman kneels at the edge of the bed and the man stands on the floor behind her. She puts her folded arms on the bed so she can rest her head on them. This is more comfortable than kneeling on all fours because due to the change in the angle of penetration, the mattress rather than the woman's back absorbs the energy of the thrusting. In another version of this position the woman lies flat on her stomach and the man lies on top of her.

These positions may feel primitive and animalistic, and for this reason they can be an exciting turn-on for many people. They sometimes turn people off for the same reason. Some people say that the rear-entry positions feel too impersonal. It's more difficult to kiss and make eye contact in these positions, although for that to happen all the woman has to do is turn her head. Then her partner leans over so she can see his face.

The rear-entry positions are the best for fast stroking and depth of penetration. They're also great if the woman likes to have her cervix stimulated, and they offer some of the best ways for the penis to make contact with the woman's G-spot. While in one of these positions, if a woman chooses she can shift her arms and hands so that she can easily stimulate her clitoris.

The rear-entry position is a rather advanced position that I don't recommend for the early stages of most sexual healing programs. It's good for women who have difficulty with arousal, because of the possibility of intense stimulation to the G-spot and the cervix. However, I don't recommend this position for men with erection problems, because the angle of penetration is a little tricky and can cause some "entrance anxiety." I do recommend it for men who have difficulty reaching orgasm, because in the early stages of learning to ejaculate more easily during intercourse, sometimes it works well for a man to use a more impersonal position. Getting to the point where they can enjoy intercourse in this position can be a real breakthrough for women who have successfully dealt with vaginismus or sexual pain, because it's the position in which the woman has the least amount of control over penetration.

⚬

In addition to the four major categories of positions, you can combine positions from different categories. For example, you could combine the rear-entry and side-to-side positions, so that the man lies on his side behind the woman, who is also on her side. That way you get the stimulation of the rear-entry position but neither person has to support his or her own weight. Or you could do a combination of the rear-entry and female-superior positions in which the man lies on his back and the woman straddles him facing away from him. Combining positions gives you the advantages of both.

Theoretically, the number of position variations is infinite. Every time you move an arm, a leg, or even a finger, technically it's a different position. But when it comes to using sexual intercourse to heal your problems or doing it just for sheer enjoyment, there's more to it than just positions. Your healing capacity and potential enjoyment depend on comfort and predictability as well as novelty. For your sexual healing process, comfort and predictability are probably more important than novelty. Once you are more confident in your sexual abilities and in your ability to enjoy intercourse, then it's time to branch out into some of the more exotic positions.

Part II

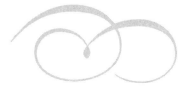

SEXUAL
PROBLEMS

In this section you'll find detailed descriptions of each of the nine sexual dysfunctions, along with information about what causes them.

chapter 5

Low Sexual Desire

In the DSM, low sexual desire is called *hypoactive sexual desire disorder,* or *HSDD.* A former name for this condition was inhibited sexual desire. Low sexual desire can affect both men and women, although it is more common in women. The DSM defines low sexual desire as "persistently or recurrently deficient (or absent) sexual fantasies and desire for sexual activity." This diagnosis has to be made by a clinician based on factors that affect sexual functioning, including age and the context of the person's life.

In cases of lifelong low sexual desire, a person has never felt sexual desire for someone else. This is extremely rare. Most people experience the desire to have sex with another person at some time in their lives, even if they never act upon it. In acquired low sexual desire, the person at one time had what would be considered a normal level of sexual desire, but no longer experiences desire. In generalized low sexual desire, a man or woman does not experience desire in any situation—that is, he or she doesn't have the desire either to have sex with a partner or to masturbate. In situational low sexual desire, a person may experience sexual desire with one partner but not with another.

What's Normal?

This is a really tough question to answer. I'm going to start with the simplest possible explanation and say that I think it's normal to feel sexual desire for another person at some time in one's life. I believe this experience is common to the vast majority of people throughout the world.

Yet low sexual desire is extremely common, especially among women. In fact, in the 1980s, inhibited sexual desire (as it was called then) was thought to be of epidemic proportions. But a diagnosis of low sexual desire is fraught with complications. When Helen Singer Kaplan modified Masters and Johnson's sexual response cycle and added a desire phase into the model, unfortunately she was unable to adequately define sexual desire, and nobody has really been able to do so since. It's clear that sexual desire has at least two components, and probably more. The physiological component, which I call sex drive rather than desire, is a result of testosterone, a hormone produced by both men and women. If you don't have testosterone, you don't have a sex drive. The presence of testosterone is a necessary condition for sexual desire, but by itself it isn't enough to create sexual desire. There's another aspect of sexual desire, especially for women, that is highly psychological.

The most common form of low sexual desire is acquired. In other words, a person felt desire in the past but no longer feels it. This is often transitory—the result of stress or overwork. There is nothing wrong with you sexually if you feel no desire when you are tired and overworked! If you have ever felt sexual desire (as you understand it) in the past, you can feel it again—if you take the time to create the conditions to allow yourself to do so. Following the program I describe in Chapter 28 will almost certainly restore your feelings of sexual desire, just because committing yourself to a program will force you to set aside time for yourself.

In a less common but more severe case of low sexual desire, a person may say that he or she is just not interested in sex. It is actually very rare for a person to have never felt any sexual desire whatsoever. The person who says he or she is not interested in sex is more likely to mean that he or she is not interested in doing a particular activity with a particular person at a particular time (for example, intercourse, with you, right now). You do not need to feel any sexual desire to do any of the exercises described in this book. You only need a willingness to spend time touching. "I guess I'm just not interested in sex" may have been a good enough excuse for avoiding sexual activity with your partner in the past, but it is no reason to avoid the exercises outlined in this book. Doing the exercises will increase your level of desire.

An expressed lack of sexual desire may in fact more accurately be described as a desire discrepancy: One partner desires sexual activity more often than the other. When it comes to sexual frequency (how often a person wants to engage in sexual activity), the range of what is considered normal is broad. One partner might like sexual activity many times a day, while the other may feel sexual desire only a few times a year. Both are quite normal. But it can become a problem if long-term partners have highly discrepant desire patterns. If your partner feels little sexual desire and is not interested in treatment, you will have to decide whether you want to stay with a person who does not even want to attempt to feel greater sexual interest in you. Often, people who feel they have no desire simply suffer from lack of knowledge or a lack of experience. They have never engaged in activities that were really stimulating and memorable. This program includes a range of such activities that you can try.

Finally, there is the rare case in which an absolute lack of sexual desire is caused not by fatigue, repression, or inexperience, but by physiological problems such as a lack of the necessary hormones or brain damage. Of all the clients with whom I have worked, I have seen only two for whom this was the case.

Changes in Thinking about Sexual Desire

As I've mentioned, in the 1970s noted sex therapist and researcher Helen Singer Kaplan added the concept of sexual desire to Masters and Johnson's model of the human sexual response cycle. The diagnosis of low sexual desire or inhibited sexual desire became very popular in the 1980s. It was thought to be quite widespread and was known as the "yuppie disease." The idea was that people didn't want sex because they were all working so hard. Back then the theories about the causes of and remedies for low sexual desire were pretty unsophisticated. The main insight was that overwork and stress could cause low sexual desire. The recommendation was that a couple take a weekend off, go to a hotel, turn off the phone, and have sex all weekend. Another insight was that sometimes what looked like low sexual desire was really desire discrepancy: a case in which one partner wanted sex significantly more often than the other partner did (or significantly less often than the other partner did, if you want to look at it that way). Treatment (or, as clinicians sometimes call it, "intervention") for couples most often included examination of the power struggles involved in scheduling sessions of sexual intercourse, and introduction of communication techniques for compromise in agreeing how often to have sex.

In the 1990s, the thinking about low sexual desire became much more sophisticated. The role of testosterone was recognized. A baseline level of testosterone is necessary for sexual desire, especially in women. It began to be recognized that many of the hormonal events that women undergo (such as long-term use of oral contraceptives) can cause low testosterone. During this period I used the following conceptualization of low sexual desire to help my clients: I thought of causes for low sexual desire as falling into three categories, ranging from the not-so-serious to the very serious. I based these categories on psychological causes for low sexual desire. I believe that the first thing anyone experiencing low sexual desire should do is to have his or her testosterone level checked. If your testosterone level is low (or nonexistent), no amount of psychological intervention is going to help.

In the *not-so-serious* category, I listed things like overwork, boredom, stress, lack of stimulating activities, poor time management, and lack of sexual knowledge or education. I call these not-so-serious because they are fairly straightforward and the solutions are easy to understand (even if they're sometimes difficult to implement). These are the cases where the advice to take a vacation, get away from the kids, rent a hotel room, and turn off the phone makes sense. Often people who experience low sexual desire due to one of the above causes really just need to set aside some time to reconnect with each other. Stress caused by overwork can be very serious. In addition to reducing your sex drive, it can affect your physical health in the form of psychosomatic illnesses. Often, once you have gotten yourself into workaholic mode, it can be difficult to change. But it can be done. Other solutions for problems in this category include reading books about sexuality (such as this one) or taking classes. Behavioral contracts or agreements about time management can also be helpful. Sometimes couples are so strung out and overworked that they actually need to make agreements about when to see each other. It also helps to give up expectations about sex happening spontaneously.

More serious causes of low sexual desire include clinical levels of anxiety or depression, or relationship problems. One of the most common symptoms of depression is low sexual desire or lack of interest in sex, and anxiety is the most common cause of low sexual desire. Sometimes a person needs a little help in the form of the temporary use of antianxiety or antidepressant medication. Similarly, if you are having major problems in your relationship, your level of sexual desire is going to be affected. If you are angry at your partner because of dishonesty, abuse, adultery, or any number of other serious problems, it is usually really difficult to feel desire for that person. In cases like this, marriage counseling, family therapy, or some other form of relationship counseling is the treatment of choice rather than sex therapy. The low sexual desire in this case is a direct result of other problems in the relationship rather than a sexual problem as such.

Finally, *much more serious* causes of low sexual desire include reactions to past events such as sexual trauma. I have seen many cases in which a woman suffered rape or incest in her early life and as a result was unable to experience sexual desire as an adult. Often the past abuse was repressed, and the woman wasn't even really aware of what sexual desire felt like. This experience isn't unique to women, but it is more common in women. Since these sorts of causes of low sexual desire are lifelong and are pretty much built into someone's personality, I believe the only solution is intensive individual therapy. Sadly, many people with these issues have experienced the problems for so long that they really don't want to seek treatment.

This scheme for viewing low sexual desire served me well in the 1990s. It helped me decide which couples would benefit from psychological treatment and which should be referred to relationship therapists or medical doctors. In the past few years, however, a lot of information has come to light about other causes for low sexual desire, especially in women. I'll list these in terms of causes of low sexual desire that are common to women, causes of low sexual desire that are common to men, and causes of low sexual desire that are common to both men and women. These lists come from different sources, including everything from scientific studies to anecdotal reports. There is obviously some overlap between male and female issues, but I've sorted them according to the things people most commonly report.

Causes of Low Sexual Desire in Women

Women experience a number of hormonal events throughout their lives that can cause low sexual desire. Most of them are temporary. They include childbirth, breastfeeding, the use of oral contraceptives, and menopause. All of these can cause low testosterone. Body-image issues can also cause low sexual desire. The most common of these is feeling fat. Related to this is lack of exercise, which can cause low levels of dopamine, a brain chemical that is highly related to being able to experience feelings of pleasure. Some women experience low sexual desire when they feel that their partner focuses sexually on a certain part of their body that they're uncomfortable with.

Women are very susceptible to being influenced by their partner's personality or mental state. Women have reported feeling low sexual desire because their partner is controlling and tells them what to do. Other issues include experiencing their partner as jealous or possessive, being patronized or talked down to, feeling that their partner doesn't love them, feeling that their partner lacks commitment to the relationship, or feeling that their partner is moody and withdrawn and doesn't want to communicate. Other issues reported by women include their male partner's habit of telling unfunny sexual jokes, his being prejudiced (especially homophobic), or his making promises he doesn't keep (such as promises of financial commitment).

Some women admit that they consciously sabotage a situation that could turn sexual. They purposely wait until their partner is too tired to have sex, or they wear something unappealing to bed. Other women report that having a television on in the bedroom turns them off to sex.

Of course, a woman's sexual history has a huge effect on her desire for sex. Having a bad first experience of sex can set the stage for a lifetime of low sexual desire. A history of any form of sexual coercion (including molestation, incest, or rape) can shut down a woman's sexuality. Women also have more fears and anxieties about sex in general than men have. Sex has the potential to be more dangerous for a woman than for a man. Women worry about being sexually abused and they worry about getting pregnant. It's easier for a woman to catch a sexually transmitted disease from an infected man than vice versa.

Lack of understanding of the male sex drive can also be a problem. Sometimes women are turned off because their partner wants sex so much more than they do. Other women are turned off because their partners learned to have sex from watching porno movies. They resent that their partner's idea of sex is focused only on the genitals instead of on full-body sensual contact. Other women are freaked out if they find out their partner has paraphilic interests—that is, an interest in what most people would consider unusual sexual activity. Maybe they discover a hidden collection of erotic materials that they find disgusting.

Causes of Low Sexual Desire in Men

For men, some of the biggest causes of low sexual desire include low testosterone, stress, anxiety, and depression. Work setbacks, such as job loss, also disproportionately affect men. The existence of other sexual problems, like premature ejaculation and erection problems, can also cause low sexual desire in men.

In the past, an unacknowledged homosexual orientation was often a cause of low heterosexual desire in men. This is less common than it used to be, now that same-sex behavior is no longer illegal and a homosexual orientation is no longer considered a mental disorder.

Causes of Low Sexual Desire in Both Men and Women

The following are some other causes people have cited for low sexual desire in both men and women. I've listed them in order from what I consider least serious to most serious.

* Boredom

* Lack of knowledge about sex

* Overwork

* Laziness

* Difficulty finding a partner

* Fear of sexually transmitted diseases

* Lack of opportunity to have sex

* Relationship problems

* Crowding in the house

* The presence of young children in the house

* Taking drugs like Prozac (the SSRIs, or selective serotonin reuptake inhibitors)

* Fear of intimacy or commitment

* Lack of interest or involvement in any area of life

* Feelings of intimacy and attachment as the primary focus of the relationship, to the exclusion of sexual feelings

* Traditional religion that produces guilt about sex by teaching that sex is wrong

* Unhappiness

* Conflict, power struggles, and criticism in the relationship

* Poor health

* Avoidance of sex due to phobias

✳ Addiction issues

✳ Lack of trust between partners, especially due to unfaithfulness

✳ Being asexual

✳ Grieving or serious personal loss

It's quite a list, isn't it? And it goes on. Isn't it amazing how many things that don't seem like they would have anything to do with sex can have such a profound effect on your sex life? With everything that can go wrong, it's remarkable that anyone wants to have sex at all. The good news is that because so many disparate things can affect your sex life, there are an infinite number of possible solutions to your desire problems, many of which I'll discuss in Chapter 28. Low sexual desire presents a huge number of opportunities for sexual healing on many different levels.

Differences Between Men's and Women's Sexual Desire

To add even more confusion to the issue, in general, men and women tend to differ somewhat in the many components of sexual desire. Some of these differences may seem like clichés, but most have been supported by research. I include these potential areas of difference here so you can see if any of them strike a chord with you, and thus can help you pinpoint specific areas of sexual desire with which you might have a problem.

The biggest difference is that men's sexual desire appears to be controlled by nature and women's by culture. A woman's sexual desire is more influenced by context, situation, and environment than a man's is. A man's main motivation for having sex is horniness or sexual release; a woman's main motivation for having sex is feeling that she is in love or feeling that she is emotionally connected to her partner. For women, romantic love and sexual desire appear to be the same for all intents and purposes. Sex for women is more about intimacy, or the emotional part of an encounter. It's a cliché, but both my work with clients and surveys I've taken in my classroom support this. (Remember that we're talking in generalities here; these statements may not be true for all women or for all men all the time.)

For women, sexual desire is more likely to have a particular object (a person). When a woman thinks about whether she desires sex, she thinks about whether she desires sex with a particular person. In the 1970s, with the advent of the women's liberation movement, many women made the mistake of trying to define their level of sexual desire using male criteria: testosterone, a feeling of horniness, or itching in the genitals. In fact, however, women may need to be in love first in order to feel sexual desire. A woman's sense of sexual desire may be a desire to seduce or be penetrated rather than a desire to have intercourse as such. This is the distinction between what's called *proceptive sexual desire* and *receptive sexual desire.* Proceptive desire is the urge to seek out and initiate sexual activity. It is probably more common in men and seems to be caused by testosterone. Receptive sexual desire is the capacity to become aroused upon encountering certain sexual stimuli. What happens is that a woman becomes aroused, and that causes her to have more desire, rather than vice versa. This pattern is probably more common among women because it's associated with estrogen.

Men often aren't aware of or won't admit to what could be causing them to go through a bout of low sexual desire. Women are the opposite—they'll obsess about what could be causing low desire to the point that they might ignore an attractive potential partner.

A large component of sexual desire seems to be the ability to fantasize. Men and women differ somewhat in their fantasy lives—why they fantasize and what they fantasize about. While the most common fantasy for both men and women is having sexual intercourse with someone they are in love with, women are more likely to fantasize about sexual encounters with past and present partners. Men are more likely to fantasize about genital contact with partners they don't know.

Surveys show that women seem to understand sexual desire better than men do. Women seem to have a better grasp that there's something psychological involved. In surveys, many men admit that they don't have a clue about whether their partner desires them sexually or why. Women have more potential turn-offs than men and are more susceptible to them. Because women's sexual desire is heavily influenced by culture, women have more ways in which their level of sexual desire could potentially be manipulated. Women define desire in terms of the pursuit of interpersonal goals. Men are more likely to define desire in terms of purely sexual goals, like pleasure. Women's sexual desire is heavily influenced by whether they feel their intellectual and spiritual needs are being fulfilled. And although women's sexual desire is more determined by cultural factors, they undergo more lifetime hormonal events (like childbearing and menopause) that have the potential to affect their sexual desire.

Measuring Sexual Desire

One of the difficulties in figuring out whether someone has a problem with low sexual desire is that we really don't have a good way to measure sexual desire. Synonyms that have been used for sexual desire include *sexual interest, lust, romantic love, passion, libido,* and *attraction.* Sometimes sexual desire has been defined as sexual satisfaction or sexual arousal, even though these appear to be conceptual opposites of sexual desire. Plus, to me, there's a lot of potential ground between "sexual interest" and "lust."

Sexual desire has been measured by the calculation of vaginal or penile blood flow using special instruments. These are actually measures of arousal, not desire, but the assumption was that if you could get aroused, you must have desired sex, which is not necessarily true.

I'm aware of two questionnaires that measure sexual desire. However, they confuse sex drive (the physiological component) and sexual desire. They also confuse the frequency of sexual desire and sexual behavior. For example, common measures of sexual desire include the questions "How frequently do you want to have sexual intercourse?" and "How often do you think about sex or think about wanting sex?" My point here is that it's no wonder if you are confused about whether you have an abnormally low level of sexual desire—even the experts have problems with the issue.

Asexuality

Related to the problem of low sexual desire is a concept called *asexuality.* A person is defined as asexual if he or she has never had sexual desire for anyone of either sex. I don't think this is a great definition. There are many people with a strong sex drive who don't want to have sex with other people; they only want to have sex with themselves or with inanimate objects.

The concept of asexuality has not been studied in depth. Here's what we do know: It may affect 1 to 2 percent of the population. It's related to gender—more women than men report being asexual. Other factors that appear to be related to asexuality are poor health, short stature, going through puberty at a later age, religiosity, and lower socioeconomic status.

Some people who seek out sex therapists for the treatment of low sexual desire may actually be asexual. The main difference that I can see between someone who has low sexual desire and someone who is asexual is that the typical person who sees a sex therapist for low sexual desire has felt desire in the past and knows what it feels like, so they know what they're missing. The typical person who is asexual senses that they are not like other people, but they really don't know what the fuss is all about. They generally are accepting of their status.

The Relationship of Low Sexual Desire to Other Sexual Problems

A final concern is that many people who seek sex therapy for low desire actually have other problems. A woman who has difficulty becoming aroused or having an orgasm may develop low sexual desire as a defense mechanism. So could a man who has premature ejaculation or erection problems. Women with vaginismus and sexual pain also often exhibit little or no desire for sex. We call this "low sexual desire secondary to other sexual dysfunctions." That's why, as a sex therapist, it's important to recognize that people can have more than one sexual dysfunction. If I see a client who claims that he or she has low sexual desire, I can't really take the client's self-diagnosis at face value. It could very well be that some other dysfunction occurred first that has caused the client not to want sex. The following are two patient stories illustrating this fact:

Ron

Ron, in his early sixties, stated that his main problem was low sexual desire. When I took his sex history, it was clear he'd had significant erection problems for many years. (This was well before Viagra was introduced and before erectile dysfunction was regularly discussed in the public forum.) I asked him, "If you knew that you could have a rock-hard erection whenever you wanted, and you knew that you could have sex with any woman you wanted, do you think you would want to have sex?" He looked at me like I had lost my mind and said, "Well, yes! Of course!"

Ron's problem was clearly not low sexual desire. He clearly was still extremely interested in sex. In sex therapy we usually find that other sexual problems are masquerading as low sexual desire. That's why it's important to treat the first (primary) problem rather than low sexual desire, because often the low desire is not the more significant problem.

Mary Ann

Like Ron, Mary Ann came to see me with a complaint of low sexual desire. She was in her late thirties. (I saw quite a few clients with this complaint in the 1980s, when the issue received a lot of press and many people were going to sex therapists with a self-diagnosis.) She complained that she used to feel sexual desire for her husband but didn't feel it anymore. Her sex history seemed to indicate that she didn't have any other sexual dysfunctions. However, her relationship with her husband was a mess. He had cheated on her, refused to work, and verbally abused her. And yet she was convinced there was something wrong with her because she didn't want to have sex with him! (I would have said there was something wrong with her if she did want to have sex with him!) I asked her who her favorite male celebrity was. She said she really had a thing for Harrison Ford. (This was in the Indiana Jones era.) I asked her, "If Harrison Ford asked you out on a date, would you want to have sex with him?" Again, she looked at me like I had lost my mind and said, "Of course! I'd cut off my right arm to have sex with him!"

Mary Ann clearly did not have low sexual desire. Her observation illustrates the fact that people often feel they have low sexual desire when what they really have is a problem with the object of that desire rather than with the level of desire itself. I referred her to a marriage counselor because I didn't really think low desire was her main problem. Her relationship with her husband was clearly a more pressing concern.

სა

If you picked up a copy of *Sexual Healing* because of issues with low sexual desire, by now I probably have you really confused. What I'm trying to convey is that if you would like to benefit from the healing of your problem with desire, you will first have to figure out if that's actually the main issue. Here are some questions to ask yourself to determine whether low sexual desire is your root problem:

❋ Is your testosterone level low or nonexistent? This is the first thing you should have checked if you are experiencing a lack of desire.

* Are you on medications such as antidepressants, antianxiety agents, or birth control pills? Any of these could cause low desire.

* Do you have other sexual problems such as difficulties with arousal or erections? Your desire problems could be a result of other accompanying sexual problems.

* Would you desire sex if you were with a different partner? If the answer is yes, you may have relationship issues that are interfering with your desire.

* Finally, do you think you would desire sex if you knew you could function well whenever you wanted to? If so, low desire probably isn't your most pressing sexual problem.

The program described in Chapter 28 for healing desire problems will work very well for you if desire is the main problem, if you basically have a good relationship, and if you are motivated to increase your desire. If you have examined yourself and realize that your desire issues are actually secondary to another sexual problem, then you should try healing the primary problem first. Also, recognize that your problem could be medical: the result of low testosterone, other hormone problems, or prescription drugs.

chapter 6

Sexual Aversion Disorder

According to the DSM, sexual aversion disorder (SAD) is "persistent or recurrent extreme aversion to, and avoidance of, all (or almost all) genital sexual contact with a sexual partner." The DSM also says that sexual aversion disorder may range from "moderate anxiety and lack of pleasure to extreme psychological distress."

In lifelong sexual aversion disorder, the person has experienced anxiety ever since he or she began to attempt partner sex. In acquired sexual aversion disorder, the person functioned without anxiety in sexual situations at some point, but cannot do so now. In generalized sexual aversion disorder, a person exhibits anxiety during a variety of different sexual situations, or during all sexual situations. In situational sexual aversion disorder, the person exhibits anxiety during a particular sexual behavior, or while having sexual contact with a particular person.

With sexual aversion disorder, as well as with many of the other sexual dysfunctions addressed in this book, we have some problems with the definition. As you read in Chapter 3, *all* of the sexual dysfunctions are caused by anxiety. A person will exhibit different symptoms depending on when in the sexual encounter the anxiety hits. With sexual aversion disorder, the anxiety symptoms are usually the entire problem. SAD is not a sexual dysfunction as such—the genitals are probably functioning fine in terms of erection, arousal, and orgasm. The problem is that the person experiences such intense anxiety in a sexual encounter or at the thought of a sexual encounter that he or she can't function physically at all.

There's also a definition problem with the words *anxiety, aversion,* and *avoidance,* all of which have been used interchangeably to describe this condition. In fact, these words don't mean the same thing. In Chapter 3 I presented a definition of anxiety. It's a mind-body phenomenon in which a person experiences physical symptoms, like rapid heart rate, and mental symptoms, like worry. It involves arousal of the sympathetic nervous system when there's really no physical threat. I think the concept of fear is very close to the concept of anxiety. The difference is that although both fear and anxiety produce the same physical symptoms, fear occurs in the presence of a genuine threat.

Aversion is a feeling of repugnance or disgust toward something. It's an attitude, a negative evaluation of an object or behavior. Avoidance is the behavioral manifestation of aversion. If you have a negative evaluation of something, you usually do your best to stay away from it.

Here's our problem from the standpoint of trying to understand sexual dysfunctions: Some people have an aversion to sex. They think it's disgusting in some way, but they don't experience anxiety symptoms when confronted with it, and they may not even try to avoid it. They may just sort of grin and bear it, or allow their partner to have sex with them. There are other people who like the idea of sex—they don't find it repugnant at all— yet when confronted with a sexual situation, they experience intense anxiety symptoms. Some people avoid sex for reasons that have nothing to do with anxiety, such as religious reasons. They avoid sex so they won't be tempted, because having sexual contact with another person goes against their belief system in some way. Still other people have all three symptoms. They are disgusted by sex, they have anxiety symptoms when confronted with a sexual situation, and they try to avoid sexual situations.

To add to the confusion, there's a personality trait called *erotophobia,* which is fear of sex. An erotophobe finds everything about sex fearful—not just potential sexual contact with a partner, but hearing about sex, reading about sex, viewing sexually explicit materials, or anything else having to do with sex. Erotophobia usually includes the whole gamut—fear, anxiety, aversion, and avoidance. Being a personality trait rather than a sexual dysfunction as such, erotophobia is very resistant to change. (The opposite of erotophobia is *erotophilia.* This personality trait describes someone who loves everything about sex.)

What's Normal?

As I did with sexual desire, I'm going to be very broad in deciding what "normal" means. I think it's normal for a person to have a sexual relationship that doesn't involve any overt anxiety symptoms. I believe this is the case for most people.

However, let me add another term to our vocabulary of *aversion, anxiety,* and *avoidance.* That term is *anticipation.* It's normal to feel a little bit nervous about having a sexual encounter with someone who excites you, someone with whom you've never had sex, or someone with whom you're in love. Most of us have experienced that "butterflies in the stomach" sensation. It's perfectly normal to feel that sensation when you're in love or when you're anticipating your first sexual encounter with a new lover. It doesn't mean you have an anxiety problem. When you're in love, it's also normal to feel negative sensations, such as anxiety, at the thought of possibly losing your partner. Again, this doesn't mean you have sexual aversion disorder.

So what constitutes the problem known as sexual aversion disorder? Having worked for many years with people with sexual dysfunctions, I believe that sexual aversion disorder should be referred to as sexual anxiety disorder or sexual phobia. I think the problem is best described by using the terminology of anxiety symptoms. One of the reasons I believe this is because, from a treatment standpoint, working with overt anxiety symptoms is better than trying to deal with aversion or avoidance. But for the purposes of this book, I'll call this condition sexual aversion disorder because the DSM does. As you read, keep in mind that I'm describing anxiety.

Types of Anxiety

There are many different types of anxiety, any of which could be associated with sexual aversion disorder. These forms of anxiety are not unique to sexual concerns; people can develop any of them in response to any stimulus they learn to be afraid of. Here's a list of the most common forms of anxiety. In my experience, these are the forms that are most often associated with sexual problems.

* Generalized anxiety disorder (GAD)

* Posttraumatic stress disorder (PTSD)

* Panic attack

* Specific phobia

* Social phobia or social anxiety

* Obsessive-compulsive disorder (OCD) or obsessive-compulsive personality disorder

In generalized anxiety disorder, a person experiences a low to moderate anxiety level most of the time. Sometimes this is called *free-floating anxiety* because it's so pervasive that it seems to be able to attach itself to just about any stimulus. People with generalized anxiety disorder are afraid of a lot of different things and are pretty much anxious all the time. Sex is a very common source of anxiety for these people. Symptoms are mainly rapid heart rate and worry.

Posttraumatic stress disorder is caused by being the victim of an unusually serious source of stress, the type that most people don't experience in their lifetime. Examples would be wars, plane crashes, violent crimes, sexual trauma, or natural disasters. Symptoms of posttraumatic stress disorder include insomnia, hypervigilance, and flashbacks to the original trauma. You can see that these would all interfere with the ability to be intimate with another person, which could certainly have an effect on one's sex life. Rather than causing sexual aversion disorder, posttraumatic stress disorder is likely to cause difficulty with arousal and orgasm.

Panic attack or panic disorder is a very severe, debilitating form of anxiety. A person with panic disorder experiences rapid heart rate, sweating, dizziness, a feeling of choking, chest pain, shortness of breath, chills or hot flashes, feelings of unreality, and fears of losing control, going crazy, or dying. Panic attacks can be so severe that they can cause nausea, vomiting, or diarrhea. I have seen many clients who had panic attacks in sexual situations. Panic attacks also involve what's called *anticipatory anxiety*. This means the person learns to fear having the panic attack itself, rather than just fearing the stimulus (in this case, a sexual encounter).

A phobia is a specific, irrational fear. The following is a list of some common sexual phobias. I got this list from *Sexual Aversion, Sexual Phobias, and Panic Disorder,* by Helen Singer Kaplan. I have seen all of these phobias in clients.

* Fear of the genitalia of the opposite sex

* Fear of the patient's own genitals

* Fear of being penetrated

* Fear of penetrating

* Fear of heterosexual activity

* Fear of homosexual activity

* Fear of sexual fantasies

* Fear of sexual secretions and odors

* Fear of sexual failure

* Fear of sexual arousal

* Fear of orgasm

* Fear of breast touching

* Fear of kissing

* Fear of partner rejection or belittlement

* Fear of undressing or being seen nude

* Fear of seeing the partner undressed

* Fear of oral sex (giving or receiving)

* Fear of anal sex (penetrating or being penetrated)

* Fear of pleasure

* Fear of commitment

* Fear of intimacy and closeness

* Fear of falling in love or being loved

* Fear of being sexually coerced or forced to have sex

* Fear of contracting a sexually transmitted disease

* Fear of becoming pregnant

Social phobia is a specific phobia that involves fear of interacting with other people in some way. Obviously, sexual aversion disorder involves a component of social phobia for most individuals. People generally are more afraid of aspects of sex with another person than they are of sex with themselves. The main features of social phobia are a fear of being observed by other people and being humiliated, or a fear of one's performance being judged. Other forms of social phobia, besides sexual fears, include a fear of public speaking and stage fright.

Obsessive-compulsive disorder is characterized by obsessions (uncontrollable disturbing thoughts) and compulsions (uncontrollable disturbing behaviors, such as counting, cleaning, or repeating words). The obsessions cause anxiety and the compulsions relieve it. I have seen obsessive-compulsive disorder most often associated with fears of touching or fears of body odors or secretions. Obsessive-compulsive personality disorder (OCPD) is somewhat different. The anxiety symptoms are not as overt, and the person is more preoccupied with perfectionism or organization. This could manifest itself in problems such as only being able to have sex a certain way, and it also interferes with intimacy in interpersonal relationships.

I know this is a lot of information to throw at you. For our purposes, I'll simplify it as much as I can and say that from my standpoint the most important issue with sexual aversion disorder is the level of the anxiety symptoms. In my experience, most cases of sexual aversion disorder involve either mild to moderate levels of anxiety (as in GAD) or severe levels of anxiety (as in panic attacks). This distinction is important because it helps a clinician decide whether or not a person needs medication and, if so, what kind. A person with sexually derived panic disorder often can't even experience psychological treatment without some type of antianxiety medication.

Also important is whether you are having active anxiety symptoms because of sexual activity or have avoided sex for a long time. People with fears tend to avoid the situations that cause the fears. An analogy would be fear of flying. If you never fly because you are afraid to, you can't actually say that you experience fear in a flying situation, can you? The same thing is true of sex. Before attempting to heal yourself of sexual aversion disorder, you need to recognize whether you have avoided sex for so long that you don't really know what sensations to expect in terms of anxiety. Believe it or not, it's actually easier to treat someone with overt anxiety (including panic attacks) than it is to treat someone who has avoided sex for a long period of time. It just takes longer to treat the person who has avoided sex.

The sexual healing program described for sexual aversion disorder in Chapter 29 can be adapted for different levels of anxiety. The level of anxiety is more important in determining the specific treatment course than the specific phobia is. You can use the treatment program in Chapter 29 for any sexual phobia.

Causes of Sexual Aversion Disorder

Simply saying that anxiety causes sexual aversion disorder doesn't tell us a lot, does it? Anxiety is the most obvious proximal cause, but what caused the anxiety in the first place? A number of factors could be relevant. One is that anxiety disorders tend to be hereditary. They run in families. This is especially the case for generalized anxiety disorder and panic disorder. There seems to be some genetic predisposition for panic disorder. People with panic disorder appear to have an abnormally elevated startle response and a tendency to pay excessive attention to body states such as rapid heart rate. They are oversensitive to bodily cues that many of the rest of us ignore.

Physical or biological factors can also trigger anxiety, which can manifest itself in sexual situations. The use of stimulants, even relatively mild ones like caffeine and nicotine, can cause anxiety. Hyperthyroidism (an overactive thyroid gland) can cause it. Any cardiovascular problem that causes irregular heart rate can trigger anxiety. So can heavy alcohol use, due to withdrawal symptoms.

Family background and upbringing can often predispose a person to sexual aversion disorder. People who grow up in families that don't show affection often develop phobias about touching. A strict religious background in which sex is forbidden or not mentioned at all can also predispose a person to sexual aversion disorder. Sexual trauma is a huge cause of fear of sex. Childhood sexual abuse can cause lifelong sexual aversion disorder, and rape or sexual assault as an adolescent or adult can cause acquired sexual aversion disorder.

Of course, it's also possible that some factor in a person's current interpersonal relationship could contribute to sexual aversion disorder. Fear of intimacy or fear of commitment can trigger it. If someone's sexual partner becomes particularly unattractive in some way, this could cause aversion to that particular partner. We would call this situational sexual aversion disorder since it only applies to the one partner. It might actually be better treated as a low sexual desire issue or as a relationship issue.

In Chapter 1, I briefly discussed the difference between a psychoanalytic approach to treating sexual dysfunctions and a behavioral approach. Obviously, this book describes a behavioral approach to healing sexual problems. However, just for your information, you should know that in the psychoanalytic approach, anxiety is a very important concept. Psychoanalysts believe that people can learn to become afraid of almost any stimulus, especially sexual stimuli, because sexuality is an area that is threatening to many of us due to a restrictive upbringing. Other psychologists believe that sexual anxiety actually begins in childhood with separation anxiety: the fear of separating from our primary caregiver.

Alan

In my practice as a surrogate partner, I treated many clients with different levels of sexual anxiety. One of the most severe cases I saw was Alan, age fifty-two. He had several very strong phobias about sexual activity. I counted ten separate phobias, including fear of nudity and fear of being touched. He also had many nonsexual phobias, including a fear of going barefoot. His anxiety was on the level of panic disorder. He often became nauseous at the thought of sexual intercourse and suffered incapacitating stomach cramps. I took him through the program described in this book, starting with intensive daily relaxation exercises. It took several months, but he was finally able to have sexual intercourse without overt anxiety symptoms.

chapter 7

Erection Problems

P roblems with erections are currently called *male erectile disorder (MED)*, or *erectile dysfunction (ED)*. Some therapists and writers still use the older term for the problem, which is *impotence.* According to the DSM, erectile dysfunction is "persistent or recurrent inability to attain, or to maintain until completion of the sexual activity, an adequate erection."

What's Normal?

Erection is the filling of the small blood vessels in the penis that occurs in the excitement stage of the sexual response cycle. There are two types of erection, based on the cause or source of the erection: *reflexogenic erection* and *psychogenic erection.* A reflex is a very basic automatic bodily response that you don't have to learn. When a man's penis is touched, it triggers an impulse in a sensory nerve in the penis. The impulse travels into the spinal cord through an interneuron, and back to the penis through a motor neuron, causing an erection. For an erection to be triggered, the smooth muscle at the base of the penis (PC muscle group) has to be relaxed. A reflex erection occurs very quickly because the erection reflex arc is located very low in the spinal cord. A reflex erection doesn't require input from the brain. Teenage boys are likely to have unwanted reflex erections with very minimal stimulation, such as the touch of clothing on their penis.

Psychogenic erections involve mental input. A man has a fantasy or some type of sexual thought, and the nerve impulses travel from the brain down the spinal cord, gather at a nerve center in the mid-back area, then travel down to the pelvic (sacral) section of the spinal cord, and trigger the smooth-muscle relaxation and the activity of the motor neurons that cause erection.

The reality for most men is that their erections are not strictly reflexogenic or psychogenic; they're usually a combination of both. For example, a man might have some time on his hands and lie in bed and start to stroke himself or masturbate. This will usually trigger a reflex erection. But he'll usually start to fantasize also, which will give his erection a psychogenic boost. It works the other way around, too. A man might have an unbidden sexual thought, and if he's alone he'll probably reach for his penis, triggering the erection reflex arc.

Another factor in erections involves the sleep cycle. It's normal for healthy men with no disease processes to have several erections during the course of a night's sleep. To understand this, you need to know something about sleep. Sleep is not an all-or-none phenomenon. It progresses in a series of stages characterized by different types of electrical activity in the brain. In stage 1 sleep, you experience drowsiness but are easily awakened. In stages 2 and 3 you go deeper into sleep. Stage 4 is extremely deep sleep. After stage 4, you cycle back through stages 3 and 2 and into *rapid eye movement (REM) sleep,* in which your body is asleep but your brain shows characteristics of alert wakefulness. REM sleep is also called *dream sleep.* The significance of this for erections is that during dream sleep most healthy men have some degree of erection, whether or not their dream has sexual content.

Each full sleep cycle lasts about ninety minutes, meaning that if a man sleeps for seven hours a night, he will probably have four to five nighttime erections. These nighttime erections are called *nocturnal penile tumescence,* or *NPT.* I'm going into all this detail because NPT is very important for diagnosing erection problems. If you wake up in the morning in the middle of an REM segment of your sleep cycle, you may wake up with an erection. Some men call this a "piss hard-on," based on the misunderstanding that they have an erection because they have to urinate. This isn't really true; they have an erection that is a remnant of NPT from being awakened during an REM stage. Scientists don't really know why men have erections during REM sleep. It just seems to be the body's way of checking out the plumbing. (Women have them too; the clitoris engorges with blood, and the vaginal tissues swell and lubricate.) The absence of NPT can indicate a physical cause for erection problems. The REM sleep/erection phenomenon generally begins around puberty, but children as young as infancy appear to have reflex erections.

Levels of Erection

Like sleep, erections are not an all-or-none phenomenon. There are varying degrees of erections. It's helpful to think of the erection process as having several stages—initiation, filling, rigidity, and maintenance. Initiation is the phase that occurs in the brain. It usually involves a sexual thought as well as the awareness that it's okay to have an erection. This is the same as a psychogenic erection. Filling involves the first stages of blood flow into the penis. The penis thickens and becomes fuller and warmer. Rigidity occurs when enough blood has entered the penis to give it a "spring back" quality. Rigidity occurs because there are five valves in the blood vessels at the base of the penis that close and press up against the body, holding blood in the penis. This also accounts for maintenance, which is the ability of the penis to stay at a certain level of hardness.

Throughout this book, I'll describe erections using a simple 1-to-10 scale. A level 1 is no erection. Levels 2, 3, and 4 reflect filling. Levels 5 through 10 reflect increasing degrees of rigidity, with a level 10 being an extremely hard erection that is almost painful.

One of the problems with the DSM definition of erectile dysfunction is that it talks about a man's failure to have an "adequate" erection, but it does not define what an adequate erection is. This is because it does not describe erections in terms of different levels. In my experience, anything that is about a level 5 or above is adequate for intercourse, depending on the person. Some men are better at having intercourse with a relatively flaccid penis than others are. In my view, a man has erection problems if he cannot have or maintain some degree of rigidity. Having said that, there are other ways in which we can describe different degrees of erection problems.

Forms of Erection Problems

A man with lifelong total erectile dysfunction has never had an erection in his life. I've never heard of a case like this. It probably exists in conjunction with serious congenital malformation of the genitals. In acquired erectile dysfunction, a man functioned fine at some point but can no longer get erections. In generalized erectile dysfunction, a man cannot have an erection in any situation. He goes not have NPT or morning erections, and he can't get an erection with masturbation or any kind of activity with a partner, including manual or oral stimulation or intercourse. In situational erectile dysfunction, a man can have an erection in one context or with a particular person, but can't have one in every situation.

Of all of the above conditions, acquired situational erection problems are the most common, as well as the easiest to treat. The most common scenario is a man who has normal NPT and can have an erection with masturbation but has difficulty getting an erection with a partner. Another common problem exists in a man who can get an erection from oral sex but loses the erection at the point of penetration. You can see that both of these situations appear to be psychological. The presence of NPT means that the plumbing is working, which indicates that some psychological factor in the sexual situation is shutting the man down.

In another pattern of erectile dysfunction, a man can get a full erection rather quickly but then immediately loses it. In the absence of NPT, this is usually caused by a problem with leaky valves at the base of the penis. Other men can get a partial erection but not a full one, either during sleep or with a partner. This is usually a sign that the erection problem has physical (also called *organic)* causes. For a list of possible physical causes of erection problems, read on.

Physical Causes of Erection Problems

The most common physical cause of erection problems is cardiovascular disease. Anything that interferes with blood flow can have a negative effect on a man's erections. In fact, doctors now use erection difficulties as a warning sign of cardiovascular disease. Diabetes can also cause erection problems by destroying the nerves that trigger erection. Disorders of the nervous system, like multiple sclerosis, can interfere with erection.

Drugs are a huge cause of erection problems. Alcohol potentiates estrogen (a female hormone) in men, placing chronic alcoholics at high risk for erection problems. Nicotine and caffeine are stimulants that constrict the small blood vessels in the skin, especially in the lips, fingertips, and genitals. Any medications that lower blood pressure can affect erections, as can medications for ulcers. Even over-the-counter medications like antihistamines can temporarily interfere with a man's sexual arousal. Some men take illegal stimulants like cocaine and amphetamine because initially these drugs appear to make their erection response stronger, which is true. However, the long-term use of any illegal stimulants that I am aware of eventually destroys erectile tissue and degrades a man's erection response over time.

Prostate problems can interfere with erections. Benign enlargement of the prostate can cause erection problems, and surgery to remove a cancerous prostate can cause permanent erection problems. Acute infections of the prostate and other genital organs can cause erection problems.

Hormone problems can affect erections. The main male hormone is *testosterone*. Problems with testosterone usually affect sexual desire rather than erection. High levels of another hormone called *prolactin* can affect a man's erections, but this condition is rather rare.

If you are experiencing erection problems, it is important to figure out if your problems are physical, psychological, or some combination of both. In general, if you get nighttime or morning erections that are relatively hard but you have trouble getting or maintaining erections with a partner, your problems are probably psychological and will most likely respond well to the strategies outlined in this book. If you don't have nighttime or morning erections, your problem may be physical and you will need to see a urologist who specializes in erection problems to find out what's going on.

What will happen if you go to a urologist? The urologist may be able to diagnose a physical problem based on your description or your responses to a questionnaire. There are also several tests that can be performed to find out if you have problems with blood circulation to your penis. The simplest test is the penile/brachial index. The physician takes your blood pressure in your arm and in your penis and compares the two to see whether the blood pressure in your penis is abnormally low. Another test is also simple but not very pleasant. The physician sticks a small needle into the penis at various locations. This tests for nerve damage, which could be a sign of multiple sclerosis. The urologist will also likely want to perform a digital rectal examination of your prostate to find out whether it is enlarged. He or she will probably also order a prostate-specific antigen (PSA) test to screen for prostate cancer.

If your doctor suspects that you may have cardiovascular disease, he or she may order an angiogram or other diagnostic procedure to screen for it. Specific tests exist to determine blood flow to the penis. One of them is dynamic cavernosography. A dye is injected into the bloodstream and ultrasound is used to see whether the dye fills the erectile tissue in the penis. When a man with no physical problems has an erection, valves at the base of the penis close and press up against the body, holding blood in the penis. Dynamic cavernosography can help the urologist determine if you have a leaky valve. The most common behavioral sign of this complication would be getting an erection but losing it right away.

Some doctors inject special drugs into the penis to test for erection problems. These drugs are fast-acting localized vasodilators like papaverine and phentolamine. They expand blood vessels and draw blood into the penis. If you are injected with a drug like papaverine and don't get an erection, it could mean that there is damage to your erectile tissue.

Urologists who are very thorough will do many of these tests twice—once with no sexual stimulation, and once while the patient watches sexually explicit materials. During this type of test patients are provided with special glasses that display X-rated visual materials.

Finally, with some men it's difficult to tell whether or not their erection problems are physical, because they don't know whether they have nighttime erections. If that's the case, the urologist can rent you a device called the *Rigiscan,* which measures nocturnal penile tumescence (NPT). The device consists of a flexible loop that you put around your penis before you go to sleep. It's connected to a computer, and as you sleep, if blood flows into your penis, the loop stretches and the computer records the activity and prints out a record of it. You get a graphic record that shows the degree of erection and how long it lasted. Patients are usually directed to use this machine several nights in a row to make sure the readings are accurate. A potential problem is that the gauge can fall off the penis in the middle of the night and fail to provide a reading.

Medical solutions for erection problems are described in Chapter 24. In addition to pursuing a medical solution, you may want to try the exercises described in this book even though they are psychologically based. They can't hurt you, and they'll definitely create the optimal situation for pursuing medical solutions.

Psychological Causes of Erection Problems

The most common psychological cause of erection problems is anxiety. Remember that anxiety has both physical symptoms (rapid heart rate) and psychological symptoms (worry). The reason anxiety shuts down your erections has to do with the organization of the nervous system, which you read about in Chapter 3. To briefly recap, the sympathetic nervous system helps you disperse energy really quickly when you perceive a threat to your life. In contrast, the parasympathetic nervous system produces your relaxation response. Erection is a function of the parasympathetic nervous system. If your sympathetic nervous system is activated (in other words, you are anxious), it floods your bloodstream with adrenalin and inhibits erection. If you have a tendency to be concerned about erections, you need to learn how to relax and activate your parasympathetic nervous system. The exercises in Chapter 16 will show you how.

There's a specific type of mental anxiety that interferes with erections. It's called performance anxiety. I talked about it in Chapter 3. What you need to know for now is that men with erection problems think differently in sexual situations than men who do not have erection problems. Men with erection difficulties usually have a problem with what Masters and Johnson called *spectatoring:* They mentally watch themselves to see whether or not they are getting an erection.

Another major psychological cause of erection problems is depression. Depression is an overwhelming feeling of sadness, along with a loss of interest in activities that used to give pleasure, like eating and sex. In fact, erection problems are a common symptom of depression. Depression is usually temporary. If you are severely depressed, you may need medication to help you through it. If you are only mildly depressed but it's affecting your erections, the peaking process described in Chapter 24, on dealing with erection problems, can help. Peaking is an arousal technique that helps the secretion of endorphins in the brain. Endorphins are feel-good chemicals that can often benefit mild depression. One of the problems with depression is that it can diminish a man's nighttime erections. This could lead him to believe that he has physical erection problems when he really doesn't. When men who have been depressed start to feel better, their nighttime erections return.

Besides anxiety and depression, there are other psychological causes for erection problems. Sexual trauma or abuse in the past can cause them. So can being unsure of your sexual orientation. Problems in your current relationship or your current sexual situation can also be a factor. Some men don't receive enough stimulation from their partner and don't ask for it. As you get older, you generally need more direct physical stimulation of your penis in order to get an erection. Men often expect their bodies to function like machines. They expect to have an erection even when they're hungry, tired, stressed out, or afraid.

Expectations also shut a lot of men down. Especially harmful is a form of interpersonal expectation called the *self-fulfilling prophecy*. In this situation, a man worries about having an erection, and the anxiety in turn interferes with his ability to have an erection. This means that even one episode of erection failure can unfortunately set the stage for some major problems.

Remember, men's erectile ability varies tremendously. What feels like an adequate erection for one man may be a source of anxiety for another. You don't necessarily have a problem if you don't have reflex erections. There are many men (even young men) who always need direct physical stimulation in order to have an erection. It's probably unrealistic to expect that you will have an erection merely from viewing something that is sexually explicit, whether it is pornography or your partner's naked body. It's probably also unrealistic to expect that your erection will maintain the same level of rigidity throughout the course of a sexual encounter. It's normal for a man's erection to vacillate between several levels depending on the amount of stimulation he is receiving.

Here are a couple of case histories from my surrogate practice. The first illustrates psychologically based erection problems, and the second illustrates erection problems with a physical cause.

Larry

Larry's story illustrates a typical progression from perceived erection failure to anxiety to actual erection failure. At first, Larry, age forty-two, noticed that sometimes he would lose his erection after several minutes of intercourse with his girlfriend. He would start worrying about this as soon as intercourse started. Then he started worrying about it even before intercourse started, when his girlfriend did oral sex with him. Eventually he found he had a difficult time getting an erection at all. Soon he began to avoid any type of sexual activity or touching because of the anxiety it caused him. After about a year he entered therapy. He followed the program I will describe later in this book and regained the ability to have intercourse with his girlfriend. Their sex life now is better than ever. In therapy, Larry learned how to reduce the anxiety he felt in sexual encounters and how to cope with changes in his sexual response as he aged. He learned to relax his body and allow his natural sexual response to happen instead of increasing his anxiety by working at getting an erection.

Tom

Tom, age sixty-two, was a retired firefighter. He first noticed erection problems when he masturbated. He went to a urologist and was diagnosed with prostate cancer. He had his prostate gland surgically removed, after which he was unable to have an erection or ejaculate, although he could still reach orgasm with stimulation. Tom was lucky because several medical options were available for his situation. He tried some of them and found that the best option for him seemed to be a hormone suppository called MUSE. The suppository is inserted into the urethral opening before the man wishes to engage in sexual activity. You'll read about MUSE and other medical options in Chapter 24.

The cases of Tom and Larry illustrate something very important about erection problems: They aren't necessarily caused by deep, dark secrets in your sexual past. In Larry's case, he developed thought patterns that stood in the way of his getting erections. In Tom's case, his erection problems were due to a serious medical condition.

chapter 8

Female Sexual Arousal Disorder

According to the DSM, female sexual arousal disorder (FSAD) is "the persistent or recurrent inability to attain, or to maintain until completion of the sexual activity, an adequate lubrication-swelling response of sexual excitement." The older name for this problem was frigidity, a term that is rarely if ever used today because of its negative and sexist connotations.

Before the current DSM definition, there were two main criteria for diagnosing female sexual arousal disorder. One was failure to have the lubrication-swelling response, and the other was failure to feel a subjective sense of arousal or excitement. I believe this second criterion was a very important part of the definition of FSAD and I was sorry to see it taken out of the diagnostic manual. Here's why. In men, the physical erection response and the psychological or subjective sense of feeling sexually aroused pretty much go together. For women, typically that's not the case. Many different lines of research have shown that it's possible for a woman to lubricate but not feel sexually aroused, and also that it's possible for a woman to feel very sexually aroused but to experience very few lubrication- and swelling-related changes in the vaginal area. In fact, a woman can desire sexual intercourse very much, even beg for it, while knowing that she is not lubricating and that her vaginal opening is not expanding.

Another issue is that the DSM definition of women's arousal problems says that a woman fails to have an "adequate" swelling and lubrication response, but it doesn't define "adequate." Does adequate mean any lubrication at all, or does it mean enough lubrication to last a woman through an act of intercourse of average length? In order for a woman to become psychologically sexually aroused, it's not necessary for her to produce any lubrication at all. There are plenty of women who don't lubricate naturally; they use an externally applied lubricant and become aroused enough to have orgasms.

In my clinical experience the most common form of FSAD was in women who reported that their clitoris engorged and their vagina lubricated, but they just didn't feel turned on. It's clear that sexual arousal is a much more psychological process for women than it is for men, and the current DSM definition fails to recognize this.

What's Normal?

When a woman becomes sexually aroused, blood flows to her genitals, triggering a number of phenomena. Her clitoris, which contains erectile tissue just like the penis does, engorges with blood. Her inner and outer vaginal lips swell up and turn a darker shade of pink or red. Her vaginal opening expands. Most important, blood flowing into the middle layer of vaginal tissue forces fluid out through the vaginal walls. This is the source of most female lubrication. Although engorgement of a woman's genitalia can be thought of as an "erection" of sorts, it's very different from a man's erection. A woman's erection doesn't just involve the clitoris. The whole area of her body called the *vaginal sponge,* or *paraurethral sponge,* swells up. The vaginal sponge encompasses the entire area surrounding the urethra. It includes the clitoris on the outside, the G-spot on the inside, and all the tissue in between. Normal, healthy women with no disease processes experience the lubrication-swelling response during REM sleep the same way men experience nighttime erections. And as with men, this response in women has nothing to do with dream content.

It's normal for a woman to experience some degree of reflexive vaginal swelling if her genitals are touched, in a process that is similar to a reflexogenic erection in men. However, unfortunately there is about a thirty-year time lag between our understanding of male genital anatomy and physiology and our understanding of female genital anatomy and physiology. This means we still don't fully understand the contributions of spinal cord reflexes and the brain to female arousal. We do know that women have a reflex arc that goes from the genitals to the sacral area of the spinal cord and back out to the genitals. Stimulation of the female genitals triggers this reflex and causes the clitoris and other genital tissues to swell and the vaginal walls to lubricate.

There is also no doubt that women can produce genital arousal from the brain. I have read research confirming that many women can experience genital swelling and lubrication without having their genitals touched—for example, while reading a sexy story or hearing their lover whisper something sexy in their ear. This psychological aspect of female arousal is so important that I think it's a mistake for the DSM to ignore it.

There's a wide range of what's "normal" in terms of how women experience sexual arousal, both physically and psychologically. During sexual activity, some women experience very little overt genital sexual arousal but high levels of psychological arousal, and that's normal for them. There are also huge differences in the amounts of lubrication women produce. Some women produce a lot and some women hardly lubricate at all, and, again, that's normal for them.

Patterns of Female Sexual Arousal Disorder

In lifelong arousal problems, a woman has never experienced genital swelling or lubrication. In acquired arousal problems, a woman has experienced what she considered normal swelling and lubrication in the past but no longer does so. In generalized arousal problems, a woman fails to experience swelling or lubrication in any situation—not during sleep, masturbation, or any activities with a partner. In situational arousal problems, a woman may experience swelling and lubrication with masturbation but not with a partner; or with kissing, genital fondling, or oral sex but not with intercourse; or with one partner but not with another.

As I mentioned above, the most common complaint I've encountered regarding female arousal problems is that a woman swells and lubricates but doesn't feel psychologically aroused. Another common complaint is for a woman to experience swelling and lubrication with oral sex but not with intercourse. Most women who become psychologically aroused but don't lubricate very much usually don't consider this a problem. Many choices of artificial lubricant are available that can remedy a lack of vaginal lubrication. I'll discuss these in Chapter 26.

Physical Causes of Arousal Problems

Physical origins of female arousal problems are similar to the causes of men's erection problems, with some additional ones unique to women. Cardio-vascular problems can cause difficulty becoming aroused, because any problems with blood flow have the potential to affect the genitals. Diabetes and multiple sclerosis are huge causes of arousal problems in women. Another cause that is often overlooked is complication from pelvic surgery, such as hysterectomy or ovarian cyst removal. And cancer treatment that includes radiation of the pelvis can dry out the vaginal tissues.

Drugs, such as high blood pressure medications and ulcer medications, can cause difficulty with arousal. Over-the-counter weight loss supplements that contain stimulants can cause problems with lubrication, as can anti-histamines. Nicotine and caffeine can restrict blood flow to the genitals, and illegal drugs such as barbiturates can cause problems with arousal.

Women undergo many more hormonal events throughout their lives than men do, including puberty, monthly menstruation cycles, potential multiple pregnancies and childbirths, breastfeeding, and menopause. It's not unusual for women to report different abilities to become sexually aroused during the different stages of pregnancy. It's also unrealistic to expect the same degree of lubrication and swelling throughout the lifespan. After menopause, the lack of estrogen can cause a woman's vaginal tissues to dry out, which can cause problems with lubrication, resulting in painful inter-course.

Psychological Causes of Women's Arousal Problems

Anxiety and depression can cause women to have problems becoming aroused, as can past sexual abuse or trauma. A woman's lack of trust in her partner is another factor that can inhibit her arousal response. Perhaps some aspect of a woman's partner is a psychological or physical turn-off. In addi-tion, women often embrace a double standard for men's and women's sexual behavior. They may believe that "nice girls don't do that"—that is, don't lubricate or otherwise become turned on. Such a belief can cause mixed feel-ings about becoming excited and create a self-fulfilling prophecy in which a woman may fail to become aroused because she believes she can't or won't or shouldn't. Many possible factors in a woman's current sexual situation may cause her to have difficulty becoming aroused or may cause her arousal response to shut down when it reaches a certain level. She may be receiving sexual stimulation and find herself focusing on some kind of antiarousal cue, such as a basket of unwashed laundry, instead of on the pleasurable sensations.

The typical way in which men and women have sex may present arousal difficulties. The woman may not receive enough foreplay, such as kissing, genital fondling, or oral sex, before intercourse starts. The genital fondling she does receive may be done in a manner that's typical of an X-rated movie rather than in a sensuous manner. Her partner may fail to pay enough attention to her A-spot, which as we saw in Chapter 2 is the vaginal area that's responsible for most of a woman's lubrication. He may fail to stimulate the clitoris enough, or he may stroke it too hard or too fast. Failing to use external lubrication if it's needed or using condoms without lubrication can also cause arousal problems.

By far the biggest cause of women's arousal problems is the lack of a history of self-touch. Many women begin to have sexual intercourse with male partners before they have learned to touch themselves or before they have experience with what pleases and arouses them from a genital standpoint. Any program to heal female arousal problems (such as the one described in Chapter 26) begins with self-touch.

Diagnosing women's arousal problems is similar to diagnosing men's erection problems. If you go to either a urologist or a gynecologist who specializes in women's sexual problems, you'll undergo a series of tests designed to measure genital blood flow, lubrication, and swelling. Sometimes these tests involve stimulating yourself while watching and/or reading sexually explicit materials. Some urologists, such as Jennifer Berman, M.D., author of *For Women Only,* use very sophisticated devices to measure genital blood flow and sensation. She uses probes to measure vaginal lubrication, a balloon device to measure the ability of the vagina to relax, heat and cold sensation measures of both the internal and external female genitals, and ultrasound to measure vaginal blood flow when a woman is sexually aroused. She also takes a comprehensive sex history to determine if a woman's arousal problems might be psychological. This is clearly a very thorough approach to women's arousal problems.

Sherri

Here's a case history of a woman with arousal problems. Sherri, forty-two, was in serious trouble when she sought sex therapy. She was married, but she and her husband had not had sex for two years. She had been able to become aroused (and even reach orgasm) in the past, but her current problems dated from an extramarital affair she'd had three years previously. Her lover, who from her description clearly had sadis-

tic tendencies, injured her vagina by inserting objects into it without lubrication. She needed surgery to correct the injuries.

It was obvious that Sherri's problem with sexual arousal stemmed from several sources. In addition to the sexual trauma she had experienced, she was bored with her husband, who was rather mechanical about sexual activity and tended to prefer positions that were not very stimulating for Sherri. After her affair she went through a stage of apathy toward sexual activity, and when she and her husband tried to have sex, she found she couldn't get aroused at all—she didn't lubricate or feel any sense of excitement.

Fortunately, the sexual healing program worked for Sherri. She was afraid that she might have suffered some kind of permanent injury to her vagina, but that turned out not to be the case. Her psychological issues were shutting down her arousal, and when she worked through them she once again experienced the ability to become aroused.

chapter 9

Premature Ejaculation

Premature ejaculation is defined in the DSM as "persistent or recurrent ejaculation with minimal sexual stimulation before, on, or shortly after penetration and before the person wishes it." This condition used to be called *rapid ejaculation*. A clinician working with a client who complains of this problem has to take into account factors that affect arousal, such as age, novelty of the sexual partner or situation, and recent frequency of sexual activity.

Like so many sexual problems, premature ejaculation can be a matter of degree. Some men ejaculate with no physical or sexual stimulation at all. Others ejaculate when a woman rubs against them. (This is probably a reflex ejaculation that occurs without the pleasurable feeling of orgasm.) Some men ejaculate upon being touched by a hand or mouth, and some ejaculate immediately upon penetration. It is very common to ejaculate a few seconds after penetration. Some men experience premature ejaculation the first time they are with a new partner. Others ejaculate quickly during a first episode of intercourse, but last much longer if they have intercourse again during the same sexual encounter. Premature ejaculation may occur with any type of stimulation, or it may be specific to the vagina during intercourse.

Lifelong premature ejaculation means that a man has ejaculated quickly ever since he first attempted sexual intercourse. In acquired premature ejaculation, a man lasted what would be considered a normal amount of time during intercourse in the past, but ejaculates quickly now. In generalized premature ejaculation, a man ejaculates quickly in every situation. In reality, this means he ejaculates quickly with every partner. Men don't really complain about premature ejaculation when they masturbate because most men ejaculate more quickly with masturbation than they do with any partner activity. Generalized premature ejaculation also includes the understanding that a man ejaculates quickly with every type of partner activity, including manual stimulation, oral stimulation, and intercourse. In situational premature ejaculation, a man ejaculates quickly with one partner but not with others, or ejaculates quickly in some situations but not in others. Men with situational premature ejaculation tend to ejaculate more quickly when they are with partners they care more about or with whom they are more intimate. In this situation they experience more of a sense of psychological pressure and therefore more anxiety.

Confusion used to exist about the definition of premature ejaculation. Some authors tried to define it based on how long a man lasted during sexual intercourse before ejaculating. The problem was, nobody knew how short a time was too short. Back when the famous sex researcher Alfred Kinsey was conducting his research, the average man reported that he lasted about two to three minutes during intercourse before ejaculation. But what really constitutes a premature ejaculation? One minute? Thirty seconds? Attempts were made to define premature ejaculation by the number of thrusts a man was able to complete during intercourse before he ejaculated. This was problematic also, because not all thrusts are created equal. Some men tend to thrust with very short, fast strokes, and some men tend to thrust with longer strokes. Generally, a pattern of thrusting with short, fast strokes contributes to premature ejaculation.

Masters and Johnson believed that all sexual dysfunctions were couple problems. Therefore, they tried to define premature ejaculation partially according to the woman's response. I believe they said a man ejaculated too quickly if he didn't last long enough for his female partner to have an orgasm half the number of times they had sexual intercourse. This is a very misleading definition, as a woman's orgasmic response during intercourse is not dependent on how long intercourse lasts. It's dependent on a number of other, more important factors, such as how aroused she was before intercourse started.

Currently, premature ejaculation is not defined by the amount of time a man lasts, the number of strokes he has, or whether or not his partner has an orgasm. It's defined by the man's personal sense of ejaculating too quickly, ejaculating before he wants to, or lacking control of his ejaculation.

What's Normal?

The issue of what is normal in terms of ejaculatory control is a little trickier than trying to define how fast is too fast. Technically, male ejaculation and orgasm are reflexes, meaning they are involuntary reactions, and therefore nobody has control of his ejaculation. If you reach a certain critical level of genital stimulation, the ejaculation is going to happen no matter what, and it's beyond your control. So many men have problems lasting as long as they want to that, in a sense, premature ejaculation is the norm.

Most men gain a rudimentary sense of ejaculation awareness in adolescence or young adulthood based on their experience with masturbation. They learn to back off the stimulation slightly to last longer and to speed it up to ejaculate more quickly. This trial-and-error learning process usually carries over when they start having intercourse with women. However, for some men this learning process doesn't happen. You could make an analogy to swimming or riding a bicycle. Most people learn to swim when they're kids. Some people don't learn it, because maybe they didn't have the opportunity to be around water. You can still learn to swim as an adult. You may never be as good a swimmer as someone who learned when they were young, but you can still swim. The same thing applies to riding a bicycle. Most people learn to ride a bicycle when they're kids, but for some reason, maybe because their family couldn't afford bicycles, some kids don't learn this skill. You can still learn to ride a bicycle when you're an adult; you just may be a less confident bicycle rider than you would have been if you had learned when you were a kid.

It's basically the same story with ejaculation control. Many men (maybe even most) learn some rudimentary degree of ejaculation control and awareness when they're teenagers. Many men don't. You can still learn it when you're an adult. You may ultimately be less confident than someone who learned it early, but even then there are things you can learn to do to cope with the anxiety generated by a lack of confidence. I feel uncomfortable giving someone a stigmatizing label ("You're a premature ejaculator") when the problem is simply that they didn't learn something growing up that many other people did learn.

The pervasiveness of premature ejaculation is illustrated by the following. Remember that in Kinsey's day, the 1940s, men reported an average time spent in sexual intercourse of two to three minutes. In surveys taken in the 1990s, men reported average times of six to seven minutes, meaning that the average time spent during sexual intercourse doubled or tripled in about fifty years. However, if you ask most men how long they would *like* to last during intercourse, the desired average is about twenty minutes.

In the course of my research for this book, I used the Internet to look up articles published in the last few years on all of the sexual dysfunctions.

There are at least ten times more articles on premature ejaculation than there are on any of the other sexual dysfunctions. This clearly shows the extent of this problem, as well as the fact that many men are still very concerned about it. The good news is that the program for premature ejaculation described in this book (Chapter 23) has been shown to be very successful. Premature ejaculation has the second-highest treatment success rate of any of the sexual dysfunctions (lifelong vaginismus has the highest). I believe that the goal of lasting twenty minutes or more during sexual intercourse is attainable for most men. That has certainly been my experience in treating this problem.

Causes of Premature Ejaculation

The major cause of premature ejaculation is anxiety. It is almost never caused by a physical problem. The only medical conditions I know of that can cause premature ejaculation are alcohol withdrawal and opiate withdrawal. A man with premature ejaculation may not feel as if he is anxious—on the other hand, he may panic at the thought of any sexual encounter. Either way, his body has learned a response in which tensed muscles, irregular breathing patterns, and distracting thoughts are triggering his ejaculation. By learning to recognize both his level of anxiety and his level of arousal, he can learn to last as long as he would like.

If you have been experiencing a problem with rapid ejaculation, you may feel as if everything on your body is connected to your genitals. A kiss or touch anywhere on your body triggers a genital response and the accompanying panic. You may try to ignore your genitals and think of something else. You may find yourself masturbating to ejaculation several times a day in order to "wear down" your arousal level before you attempt sexual intercourse. (This usually doesn't work; all it does is get you used to ejaculating more frequently, which actually makes the problem worse.) You may worry constantly that you are not satisfying your partner and that she is going to leave you, and you may try to make up for your premature ejaculation in other ways in the relationship. When you are close to ejaculation, you may think "Oh no!" rather than feel pleasant anticipation.

Very severe premature ejaculation involves ejaculating with any kind of stimulation prior to penetration. Other cases are less severe. If you simply ejaculate sooner than you want to when you are inside your partner's vagina, your problem may be only that you are not having sexual intercourse often enough. Consider your body and how often you spontaneously have an erection and feel like ejaculating. If you have those feelings daily, but have intercourse only once a week, you may find that with more frequent intercourse you will not ejaculate as quickly. You might try having intercourse as many times as you would like to for a few days to find out what the optimum frequency of sexual intercourse is for you. (Of course this implies that you must have a willing partner.)

Robert

One of my former clients, Robert, age thirty-eight, was married for a number of years to a woman who constantly belittled him, but for whom he cared a great deal. After every sexual encounter she told him he had failed to satisfy her. He began to ejaculate sooner and sooner during intercourse, and eventually he began to ejaculate before penetration. His wife had a number of extramarital affairs and told him all of the details, including how well her lovers had satisfied her and how long they had lasted. Eventually she refused to have intercourse with Robert at all.

Robert tried to make up for his perceived inadequacies in other ways, such as buying his wife gifts. I say "perceived" inadequacies, because when Robert entered therapy after starting divorce proceedings, he found that after going through the program described in this book with a cooperative partner, he had no problems at all lasting as long as he wanted. Robert's story illustrates how a partner can contribute to sexual problems. His was a case of acquired situational premature ejaculation. Chances are that Robert never would have developed premature ejaculation if his partner had not exploited his self-doubt. In any event, he went on to a satisfying second marriage.

Albert

Here's a case of lifelong generalized premature ejaculation. Albert, forty-four, had one of the most severe cases of premature ejaculation I had ever seen. He ejaculated at a mere touch anywhere on his body, and had done so since he first attempted to have sexual intercourse more than twenty years before. Through the program of exercises I describe in this book, Albert learned to maintain intercourse for up to half an hour. Altogether he spent almost a year in therapy, but for a case of such severity and duration his progress was truly remarkable.

chapter 10

Male Orgasm Disorder

Male orgasm disorder is currently defined in the DSM-IV as the "persistent or recurrent delay in, or absence of, orgasm following a normal sexual excitement phase during sexual activity that the clinician, taking into account the person's age, judges to be adequate in focus, intensity, and duration." Older terms for this problem include *retarded ejaculation, ejaculatory incompetence, inhibited male orgasm,* and *inhibited ejaculation.*

Right away we see that there is a problem of changing definitions of male orgasm disorder. The DSM-IV basically defines it as having a problem reaching orgasm. Previous descriptions defined it as having a problem with ejaculation. Which is it? We know from Chapter 2 that orgasm and ejaculation are not exactly the same thing, although they occur together most of the time. Orgasm is a full-body response that includes rapid heart rate, increased blood pressure, rapid breathing, muscle contractions all over the body, and psychological sensations ranging from relief or release to intense pleasure. Ejaculation is a localized genital response in which the PC muscle spasms and semen is released from the penis.

This confusion about diagnosis makes it really important to figure out exactly what is going on with a man who suspects he has this disorder. In many cases a man with male orgasm disorder cannot have either an ejaculation or an orgasm. In some cases, a man can have an orgasm but not an ejaculation. Getting proper treatment depends on knowing exactly what the nature of the problem is.

Although male orgasm disorder is much more rare than premature ejaculation or erection problems, I have treated enough cases of it to have an opinion about what constitutes it. I see it as a problem with ejaculation rather than orgasm. I think it should still be called inhibited ejaculation.

Patterns of
Male Orgasm Disorder

In lifelong male orgasm disorder, a man has never been able to ejaculate at all with any type of stimulation. I've never heard of a case like this. During adolescence, more likely than not a boy will have an ejaculation (a nocturnal emission, or wet dream) as a result of the erections that occur during REM sleep. In acquired male orgasm disorder, a man has been able to ejaculate in the past, but has difficulty doing so now. In generalized male orgasm disorder, a man cannot ejaculate under any circumstances—not during sleep, with masturbation, during genital fondling, oral sex, or intercourse. Again, this is extremely rare. In situational male orgasm disorder, a man can ejaculate with some forms of stimulation but not with others, or with some partners but not with others. In the most common form of situational problems with ejaculation, a man can ejaculate with masturbation but not with any partner activities, or he can ejaculate with all sexual activities except intercourse. Men who have this problem can sometimes reach orgasm without ejaculation. This usually becomes an issue if the man's partner is trying to become pregnant, and many men put off solving the problem until a pregnancy is desired.

Followers of some Eastern religious traditions believe that ejaculating is physically bad for a man because it depletes his chi or vital essence, so they try to avoid ejaculating during sexual activity. Instead, they train themselves to experience intense sexual pleasure (including orgasm) without ejaculation, and they don't consider the absence of ejaculation a problem.

Supposedly, male orgasm disorder is more prevalent among homosexual men than among heterosexual men, although I haven't read any theories about why this might be the case, and I have no personal experience working with this population.

What's Normal?

Some men who subscribe to Eastern religious traditions believe that it's normal to ejaculate very infrequently, or that it's normal to regularly have orgasms without ejaculating. These men constitute a minority. I would have to say from everything I've read that it's normal for a heterosexual man to be able to ejaculate during sexual intercourse with a woman within about twenty minutes. This seems to be the most common pattern of ejaculatory behavior.

Physical Causes of Ejaculation Difficulties

Alcohol consumption can cause a man to have difficulty ejaculating. So can the use of illegal stimulants like amphetamines and cocaine. In fact, men often take these substances on purpose to delay ejaculation. Some antidepressants (particularly those that are in the classes called *monoamine oxidase inhibitors, or MAOIs)* can cause a man to have difficulty ejaculating. The antianxiety agents known as the selective serotonin reuptake inhibitors (or SSRIs) can also cause a man to have difficulty ejaculating. These include commonly prescribed drugs, such as Prozac, Paxil, and Zoloft, as well as other, newer drugs in the same class. In fact, the SSRIs are notorious for causing difficulty with ejaculation. Physicians should never prescribe them for a man who already has tendencies toward delayed ejaculation, but this is done all the time.

Prostate problems such as benign enlargement of the gland can cause difficulty with ejaculation or painful ejaculation. Often, men who've had their prostate glands removed due to cancer can have orgasms but can no longer ejaculate. Nervous-system disorders such as multiple sclerosis can also slow down the ejaculatory reflex.

Psychological and Behavioral Causes of Male Orgasm Disorder

Based on my observation, the biggest behavioral cause of male orgasm disorder is a man's masturbation habits. A man who becomes accustomed to masturbating frequently and for a long period of time using a very hard, fast stroke runs the risk of experiencing delayed or absent orgasm during sexual intercourse. He has accustomed himself to a high degree of stimulation that his partner's vagina cannot duplicate.

Another behavioral factor is the regular use of the withdrawal method of birth control (which isn't a reliable method, by the way). This practice involves the man's pulling out of his partner's vagina when he senses that he is about to ejaculate, and then masturbating until he ejaculates outside of the vagina. This habit can cause a man to develop the inability to ejaculate during intercourse. I treated a man named Robert for male orgasm disorder. Ever since he'd begun having sexual intercourse, in high school, he had used the withdrawal method. By the time I saw him in his mid-forties, he could not ejaculate with intercourse at all and was starting to develop erection problems on top of his ejaculation problems. Through the use of the exercises outlined in this book, he learned to ejaculate with intercourse.

A sexual trauma can cause an inability to ejaculate. Another sex therapist once told me of a case involving a man in his early twenties who was making love with his girlfriend at her parents' house when the parents were out of town. The two were going at it on the couch when the parents came home unexpectedly and threw the door open just as he reached his climax. He jumped off the couch naked and ejaculated right in front of the parents. He was so mortified by the experience that he suffered a temporary inability to climax at all. Fortunately, sex therapy exercises helped him relax and regain his ability to ejaculate.

Another cause of difficulty with ejaculation, especially during intercourse, is developing a mentality of working at ejaculating rather than enjoying the sensations of intercourse. The man starts anticipating his ejaculation and orgasm before he is really close. In other words, he doesn't wait until arousal level 9 to start thinking about ejaculating. He's gotten into the habit of thinking about it at around level 6. As part of this pattern, he starts to thrust harder and faster and either consciously or unconsciously tightens his PC muscle, which in turn delays the ejaculation he seeks even more.

Other writers often cite the so-called delivery-boy mentality as a cause of problems with ejaculation. This term refers to a man who is more concerned with his partner's pleasure than his own pleasure, especially during intercourse. He sees it as his job to deliver orgasms to his partner as part of a compulsive need to please her. Holding off ejaculating on purpose as part of this mindset can create problems with ejaculation.

Other writers cite "automatic erections" as a contributor to orgasm problems. Some men experience very hard erections very quickly, even when they aren't psychologically aroused. They have intercourse but they can't ejaculate because they're not even close to orgasm on the arousal scale. In my experience, this hasn't been a very common contributor to problems with ejaculation.

In the psychoanalytic view, which is no longer very popular, premature ejaculation is thought to be caused by a fear of women, and inhibited ejaculation is thought to be caused by anger at women. In this view, a man has an unconscious motivation to punish his female partner by withholding ejaculation. From a conscious standpoint, this doesn't make a lot of sense, because if he withholds ejaculation, he's punishing himself, not his partner. However, as I describe in more detail below, a man's anger at his partner or at women in general can often be deeply unconscious.

Sometimes a man becomes afraid to ejaculate because a partner in the past has berated him for ejaculating too quickly. One of the most common causes of inhibited ejaculation is a fear of premature ejaculation, even when a man doesn't have this problem. This can cause a man to overrely on strategies to delay his ejaculation, which in turn can cause him to be unable to ejaculate at all.

Men often try to learn about women's sexual desires by watching pornographic movies. Doing so can lead to inhibited ejaculation because pornographic movies generally show scenes of intercourse that go on for abnormally long times (if you think of the average time frame of intercourse as being about six to eight minutes, as the most recent surveys show). Men who watch a lot of pornography can become convinced that women prefer intercourse to continue for twenty minutes or more, when in fact this is not necessarily the case. (When was the last time you saw a pornographic movie that showed a man ejaculating within a minute of penetration? It doesn't happen, although from a statistical standpoint this is much more true to life than an intercourse scene that lasts twenty minutes or more.)

A problem with inhibited ejaculation is defined not so much by the lack of ability to ejaculate as it is by the man's feelings about ejaculation. As I mentioned earlier, psychologically based inhibited ejaculation usually involves the feeling of "working at" ejaculating rather than enjoying the sensations of intercourse. Frequently, the cause of frustration for the man is the fact that he is working at it, rather than the inability to ejaculate itself. He may sense that his level of physical arousal has remained high during intercourse, but that his emotional arousal has remained at or backed off to a low level.

Treatment Outlook

Male orgasm disorder is one of the more difficult sexual dysfunctions to treat in therapy. That's because many men with this problem just live with it and don't seek treatment, so we hardly ever see the "easy" cases that could be resolved in a few sessions. The men who have such a severe problem with ejaculation that they seek treatment often have waited twenty or more years to do so, and by then the problem is pretty well entrenched. In my view, a lifelong inability to ejaculate during sexual intercourse is very difficult to treat, especially if a man is in his forties or fifties. On the other hand, acquired problems with ejaculation are highly treatable. The ability to ejaculate with masturbation but not with sexual intercourse is also highly treatable, as is the inability to ejaculate because of unusual masturbation habits. My general rule of thumb is that if a man was able to ejaculate successfully with sexual intercourse at any time in the past, he can most likely learn to do so again.

Most men with an inhibited ejaculation problem are able to ejaculate with masturbation if they want to, but are unable to ejaculate in their partner's vagina during intercourse. Or maybe a man has the ability to ejaculate during intercourse with one woman but not with another. Like other sexual problems, inhibited ejaculation usually builds up gradually. As a man experiences the inability to ejaculate more and more often, and as he withdraws to masturbate outside the vagina, the problem worsens. He needs to reverse the process and move closer and closer to ejaculating in a vagina rather than further and further away from doing so.

A short-term case of inhibited ejaculation, in which the problem has occurred for less than a year, can usually be treated quickly with sex therapy techniques and will respond extremely well to the exercises described in Chapter 25. A long-standing case of inhibited ejaculation, as I have said, can be one of the most difficult sexual problems to deal with. I have seen it take a long time (sometimes years) for a man to learn to ejaculate in his partner's vagina. It is particularly difficult to heal a problem that has been going on for a long time (twenty years or more) and that is fueled by anger toward women in general or toward a specific female partner. A man may not experience this anger on a conscious level. When I worked with men who had this type of problem, I often saw that the anger had become such a part of their personality that they were unaware of it; most of them denied that they were angry with their partners and insisted that they liked women and liked sexual activity. If you are unable to ejaculate because of repressed anger, you may still be able to learn to ejaculate through the exercises described in this book, because they are quite powerful. The healthiest way to deal with long-standing anger, however, is to work on the underlying issues with a competent therapist.

In my practice, I have noted two specific types of inhibited ejaculation. Some men experience difficulty ejaculating due to their having worked to control their ejaculations, generally over a period of years. In other words, they tried to avoid premature ejaculation and overdid it. Dealing with this type of problem is a relatively straightforward matter, for which the treatment options described in Chapter 25 work very well. In other cases, a man has developed a problem with ejaculation as a result of anger against women or against a specific woman. This anger, which may be of long duration, destroys the intimacy in their relationship. While the man may maintain an erection for long periods of time, his feelings are so dulled that his penis has literally "numbed out."

If you are experiencing inhibited ejaculation, you may have some of the following experiences. You may accept that you have a problem but rationalize it by saying, "Well, most women like a guy who can last a long time." You may even be proud of yourself for lasting longer than you perceive that other men last. You may have intercourse steadily for over an hour and yet still have to leave the room and masturbate in order to ejaculate. You may feel that you have lost the sensation in your penis or that it is no longer a part of you. You may or may not be aware that you are angry, or you may be unaware of the source of the anger you feel.

If you are experiencing the first type of inhibited ejaculation I described (holding back), it should be a fairly easy and enjoyable process for you to relearn how to ejaculate during intercourse, though it may take a few weeks. If you are experiencing the type of inhibited ejaculation related to anger, you may need to consult a qualified therapist to help you deal with the psychological aspects of the problem.

For example, you will have to confront the fact that, while some women do enjoy prolonged intercourse, few women like intercourse without intimacy, and that may be what they have been experiencing with you. You will have to confront the fact that instead of thinking what a great lover you are, the women you have been with may have been thinking, "Isn't he ever going to come?" If you are willing to confront and deal with these issues, you have an excellent chance of learning to experience intimacy, learning to feel your body again, and learning to ejaculate during intercourse, though you may require the help of a qualified therapist. You will have to decide whether learning to ejaculate during intercourse is worth truly sharing yourself with your partner in such intimate behaviors as kissing, talking, and passively accepting stimulation.

I'm not trying to discourage you, but I want you to have realistic expectations. As I've said, in my experience this type of inhibited ejaculation is the most difficult sexual problem to deal with. In fact, many clients quit therapy rather than face up to their problems. For some men, remaining unable to ejaculate with a partner is preferable to experiencing vulnerability and intimacy. But if you are motivated to deal with your problem and are willing to do the sensate-focus exercises, your chances of learning to ejaculate with a partner are good and the outlook is positive.

Don

I have treated many men with inhibited ejaculation. One of them was Don, thirty-eight. Don's inhibited ejaculation was of the first type that I described, the result of consciously holding back ejaculations for a number of years to avoid impregnating his wife. In therapy, Don learned sexual activities that promote intimacy, such as kissing and sharing feelings. He learned to relax his body when he felt close to ejaculation, and he began to feel sensations in his penis again.

Steve

Steve, age sixty, had a more severe problem with inhibited ejaculation, worsened by other factors in his relationship with his wife. He had never forgiven her for an extramarital relationship she'd had in the early years of their marriage, and his inability to ejaculate with her dated from that time. By the time he sought sex therapy, more than twenty years later, his wife had refused to have sexual relations with him for five years, and she had developed a number of psychosomatic illnesses. Steve developed problems with his erections in addition to his difficulty with ejaculation. However, he could masturbate to ejaculation in front of a partner, and there was an excellent chance that he could have learned to ejaculate again during intercourse. But he decided to quit therapy, saying that sex with his wife was just not worth being intimate with her in other ways.

chapter 11

Female Orgasm Disorder

Female orgasm disorder is currently defined in the DSM-IV as "persistent delay in, or absence of, orgasm following a normal sexual excitement phase." Another name for this condition is *inhibited female orgasm*. Older terms include *inorgasmia* and *anorgasmia*. The problem has also been called *preorgasmia*, reflecting a belief that all women are capable of having an orgasm, even if they haven't yet had one.

Although it is common for women to be unable to reach orgasm, you must keep in mind that women have wide variability in the type and intensity of stimulation that triggers orgasm for them. The clinician has to judge that the woman's orgasmic capacity is less than would be expected for her age, sexual experience, and the kind of stimulation she receives.

What's Normal?

This is a difficult question to answer, because, in theory, all women with intact genitals and no injuries to the nervous system or other physical problems should be able to have orgasms. In addition, women on average have a more diffuse orgasm ability than men—that is, they have the potential to experience orgasm from the stimulation of sites on the body other than the genitals. This means that many more women than men are able to have orgasms through psychological stimulation alone, or through touch to parts of the body that we don't normally think of as erogenous zones. In fact, there have been reports that even women with spinal-cord injuries have been able to have orgasms.

But the reality is that many women do not experience orgasm at all, with any kind of stimulation. This is the most common female sexual complaint after low sexual desire. In my view, it is normal to be able to have an orgasm with manual stimulation, a vibrator, oral sex, or intercourse with a partner you care for. If this is not happening for you, I believe that it is a serious enough problem that you should look for solutions. Notice that I qualified my statement by saying "with a partner you care for." I think it would be unrealistic to expect to have orgasms with a partner you don't really care for or trust, or with one who is selfish. I also think it would be unrealistic to expect to have orgasms if you are not receiving adequate levels of stimulation. The fact is that many women are orgasmic with one partner but not with another simply because one partner functions better sexually or because of feelings of love for a certain partner.

Types of Female Orgasm Disorder

In lifelong female orgasm disorder, a woman has never had an orgasm. In *acquired female orgasm disorder,* a woman has had orgasms in the past but is unable to have them now. In generalized female orgasm disorder, a woman cannot have an orgasm with any type of stimulation or with any partner. In situational female orgasm disorder, a woman can have an orgasm with some types of stimulation but not others, or with some partners but not others.

Some women have never experienced orgasm. Others may be able to reach orgasm—even multiple orgasms—through masturbation but not through intercourse. Some may have been able to reach orgasm through intercourse in the past but can no longer do so, or are orgasmic with one partner but not another. Some women who are able to reach orgasm feel they are trying too hard or taking too long. Still others realize that as they approach orgasm they consciously shut down.

Dr. Ruth Westheimer conceptualizes female orgasms in a slightly different way. Here is a list of the various definitions she uses:

* *Primary anorgasmia* occurs when a woman has never had an orgasm by any means.

* *Situational anorgasmia* is a condition in which a woman can only have an orgasm by means of very limited patterns of stimulation. The situation must be perfect or the orgasm won't happen.

* *Random anorgasmia* occurs when orgasms do not happen regularly or in any predictable pattern. Sometimes they happen and sometimes they don't, and there's no way to predict it.

✳ *Secondary anorgasmia* occurs when a woman had a previously reliable orgasm ability, but now enters the plateau phase of the sexual response cycle and can't go any higher.

In my experience, there are two very common types of female orgasm problems. The first is lifelong or primary female orgasm disorder. A woman who has this problem believes that she has never had an orgasm in her life with any kind of stimulation. The fact is that most women who believe they have this problem had orgasms when they were children or adolescents. These orgasms probably occurred either during sleep or as a result of unintentional clitoral stimulation. It's difficult to remember whether you had orgasms as a child because children feel pleasure when they touch their genitals but they don't equate the pleasurable sensations with sexuality in any adult sense.

A second very common type of problem is *secondary,* or *situational, female orgasm disorder,* in which a woman can have an orgasm (or several) with masturbation, manual stimulation, a vibrator, or oral sex, but is unable to have an orgasm with intercourse. Surveys on human sexual response indicate that many women either do not have orgasms at all, or do not have them during intercourse. In some cases, studies they have read or heard about may have convinced some women that they are unable to have orgasms. Certain temporary physiological states can also interfere with the ability to reach orgasm. For example, alcohol and certain prescription drugs can interfere with orgasm.

I believe that, in the absence of nerve damage or other physiological injury or defect, any woman can have an orgasm. If you can reach orgasm through masturbation, you can also do so through intercourse, because this means your body is physically capable. If you can have one orgasm through intercourse, you can have as many as you want through intercourse.

Inability to have an orgasm during certain activities probably has more to do with the nature of the activities than with any deficiency on a woman's part. There are many sites in the female genital region in which an orgasmic response can be triggered. I discussed these sites in Chapter 2, and in Chapters 26 and 27 I describe exercises that provide strong stimulation to these areas.

Physical Causes of
Female Orgasm Disorder

It's rather rare for female orgasm problems to stem from a physical cause. However, brain damage, spinal cord damage, or other nerve damage could cause an inability to reach orgasm. So could diseases of the nervous system, such as multiple sclerosis, or complications due to pelvic surgery.

The most common physical cause of female orgasm disorder is drug use. Alcohol slows down a woman's reflexes and makes it difficult for her to have an orgasm, but by far, the most common culprits are the SSRIs—antianxiety agents like Prozac, Paxil, and Zoloft.

Psychological Barriers to
Orgasm

Given that women have many different sites in their genitals that can trigger orgasm, and given that women on average have a more diffuse orgasm ability than men, why is it that so many women have difficulties with orgasm, especially during intercourse? Here are some of the most common reasons.

The number-one reason why some women have difficulty with orgasm is lack of experience with self-touch. In order to learn to be orgasmic—predictably orgasmic whenever you want to be—it is essential that you learn to touch your genitals and learn which genital areas arouse you the most.

A second reason why some women have difficulty with orgasm is expectations. Expectations can short-circuit your orgasm ability in one of two ways: They can be either too low or too high. A woman with low expectations usually thinks she won't be able to have an orgasm or that it will be too much trouble, so either she doesn't ask for the stimulation she needs, or she doesn't even try to become aroused. A woman with expectations that are too high has an idealized view of orgasm. She thinks that when she has an orgasm, the heavens will open and she'll hear violin music and live happily ever after. It doesn't happen that way. The first few times you have an orgasm, it may feel like a small shiver in your PC muscle, accompanied by rapid heart rate. It's easy to get a little discouraged and think, "That was it? That was the Big O?" You have to give it some time. The PC muscle spasms and rapid heart rate of orgasm are reflexes, but other enjoyable parts of orgasm (like full-body muscle spasms and making noise) can be learned and practiced. Trust me, it all gets better.

Another aspect of problems in reaching orgasm, as I've said, is that women don't remember the orgasms they had as a child or adolescent and can't connect with those feelings in adulthood. In Chapter 27 I show you how to access those feelings using sleep and fantasy.

Probably the most common reason why women have difficulty with orgasm during intercourse is that their PC muscle isn't strong enough to spasm when they have something inside their vagina. In Chapter 18, on self-touch, and again in Chapter 27 I'll explain how to exercise your PC muscle to make it strong enough so that you can have an orgasm when something is inside your vagina.

Another common reason why women have difficulty with orgasm during intercourse has to do with the difference between typical male and female arousal responses. The average man typically gets sexually aroused more quickly than the average woman. If you adhere to a very common sexual script in this culture, when you have sex, your male partner typically does oral sex with you first, then you do oral sex with him, then you have intercourse. This means that when you start to have intercourse, your arousal level has probably decreased. If you think of arousal on a 1-to-10 scale, with a 10 being orgasm, this means that when you start intercourse your male partner is probably up around arousal level 8, while you're probably closer to a level 2. Unless your partner has an excellent ability to last during intercourse without ejaculating, it's going to be very difficult for you to have enough time to become aroused to the point of orgasm.

If you have experienced a problem reaching orgasm, here are some questions you should ask yourself:

∗ Do you feel that your partner is pressuring you to have an orgasm? (It may be more than just a feeling—he may actually be pressuring you.)

∗ Do you feel defensive if your partner asks, "Did you have an orgasm?"

∗ Do you feel there is something wrong with your body and the way it responds sexually?

∗ Do you feel you may not be built like other women?

∗ Are you distracted during intercourse by thoughts such as, "I wonder if I'm going to have one this time?"

✳ Do you engage in frenzied activity during intercourse such as vigorously rubbing your clitoris rather than slowly and sensuously enjoying the feelings of intercourse?

✳ Do you get close to an orgasm with a partner and then feel yourself shut down?

✳ Do you let your partner define whether or not you have had an orgasm without correcting him if he is wrong?

✳ Do you allow your partner to continue activities that bother you or that you do not enjoy?

✳ Do you fake orgasm?

In order to reach orgasm through intercourse whenever you want to, you will have to make some changes! You must take responsibility for the fact that you are not reaching orgasm now. (At the sex therapy clinic where I worked for many years, we said, "Everybody is ultimately responsible for his or her own orgasm.") You will need to learn to stimulate yourself to orgasm before you can show your partner how to do it. If your partner has been pressuring you, you may need to bring this issue out into the open. You may need to discard stereotypes about women's roles during sexual activity and adopt sexual positions that are stimulating rather than "ladylike." You can learn how to communicate with your partner explicitly during sexual activity, even if the idea of doing so seems embarrassing for you now.

Making these changes may be less difficult than you think. Many problems with orgasm are not caused by deep-seated psychological conflicts but rather by simply not knowing how your body works and not doing activities that are stimulating enough. Many women do not explore their own bodies until after they have been with sexual partners. If you do not know how your own body works, you may be unable to withstand real or imagined sexual pressure from a partner. You may believe that you are incapable of having an orgasm, or just feel uncomfortable with the sexual interaction in general. Remember that biological or physical causes for the inability to reach orgasm are very rare.

How long should it take to reach orgasm during intercourse? This is for you to decide. I will teach you techniques in Chapter 27 that are so effective that you can reach orgasm right at penetration if you want to.

Carol

Here's a case that illustrates a situational problem with orgasm that was due to deep-seated psychological problems. Carol, age forty-two, the client of a male surrogate partner who was a colleague of mine, experienced problems in becoming aroused to orgasm. She had experienced orgasms in the past and could reach orgasm through masturbation. Carol's problem was that as she approached orgasm during intercourse she felt herself shutting down and becoming distracted. In working with a surrogate partner she revealed that she had severe psychological conflicts related to a recent incestuous episode. Every episode of intercourse brought back the anxieties associated with that relationship. When she approached orgasm, she literally had flashbacks of being with her relative. For Carol, successfully dealing with her orgasm problem required a combination of talk therapy to deal with the incest and working with a surrogate partner on the distractions and anxiety as they occurred in sexual situations.

Carol also began to understand that she had spent so much time worrying about other people's enjoyment and doing what other people wanted that she had forgotten it was all right to accept her own sexual desires and enjoy herself. Today, Carol regularly experiences orgasms during intercourse.

An Alternative View of Female Sexual Problems

It's very common for a woman to have more than one sexual problem. For example, if a woman has arousal problems, it's obvious that she also has orgasm problems. Low sexual desire often accompanies the other female sexual problems. Because of this, there was a movement several years ago to combine three of the female sexual problems into one diagnosis called *female sexual disorder (FSD)*. FSD includes a constellation of low sexual desire, female sexual arousal disorder, and female orgasm disorder. As of the writing of the most recent DSM, however, it was decided to keep these disorders separate.

A composite diagnosis of female sexual disorder is a good idea in the sense that it reflects the reality that it's fairly common to have more than one sexual problem. Also, female sexual functioning is more psychologically oriented and diffuse than male sexual functioning, as well as more dependent on the interpersonal context of a sexual relationship. I believe that the reason why a diagnosis of female sexual disorder was unacceptable to the compilers of the DSM is that it was being pushed by pharmaceutical companies for their own interests and did not reflect the specific symptom presentations that sex therapists, psychologists, and psychiatrists treat every day. One diagnosis would have made it easier for pharmaceutical companies to put a large amount of money behind one drug rather than behind three or four.

chapter 12

Vaginismus

This chapter and the next are about sexual pain and are organized a little differently from the chapters on the other sexual dysfunctions. Not much is known about sexual pain, especially dyspareunia (psychological pain during intercourse), even though sexual pain may affect as many as 10 percent of women in some demographic groups.

Vaginismus is currently defined in the DSM-IV as a "recurrent or persistent involuntary spasm of the musculature of the outer third of the vagina that interferes with sexual intercourse." The PC muscle that surrounds the vaginal opening goes into a spasm and prevents penetration because the vagina is so tight.

What's Normal?

The majority of women in the world are able to experience sexual intercourse without their PC muscle going into an uncontrollable spasm. The majority of women are also able to have sexual intercourse without pain. Therefore, I would say that having those two abilities is the norm.

Types of Vaginismus

In lifelong vaginismus, a woman has never experienced sexual intercourse. In acquired vaginismus, a woman has successfully experienced sexual intercourse in the past but is unable to do so now. In generalized vaginismus, a woman cannot experience any type of penetration, including by a penis. In situational vaginismus, a woman can experience vaginal penetration with some objects but not with others, or with some partners but not with others.

The two most common forms of vaginismus are lifelong generalized vaginismus and situational acquired vaginismus. In lifelong generalized vaginismus, a woman has never experienced successful vaginal penetration with any object. This usually occurs in young women, although there have been cases of lifelong generalized vaginismus in women in their fifties and sixties. Common causes of this form of vaginismus are a lack of sexual education, and a childhood and adolescent climate of sexual guilt and fear. This type of vaginismus usually includes a history of unsuccessful experimentation with finger penetration or tampon use.

In acquired situational vaginismus, a woman develops the condition as a reaction to a sexual trauma such as rape. The vaginal spasms are usually restricted to attempts at intercourse.

Sometimes it's difficult to make the distinction between vaginismus, dyspareunia, and sexual aversion disorder. If you are dealing with sexual pain, you may find that elements of all of these conditions apply to you. To heal your problems, you may decide to do the sensate-focus programs for all three disorders, beginning with the easiest one first, which is the treatment for sexual aversion disorder.

I know of only one book on vaginismus. It's entitled *Private Pain: It's about Life, Not Just Sex: Understanding Vaginismus and Dyspareunia,* by Ditza Katz and Ross Lynn Tabisel (see Recommended Reading). The authors run a clinic in New York that specializes in treating vaginismus. The book was privately published by their clinic. *Private Pain* is not a self-help book. That is, it does not include exercises to help women and their partners deal with vaginismus. The authors believe that the majority of cases of vaginismus can only be dealt with using professional help. Obviously, I disagree. I mention *Private Pain* because its value lies in the many case histories quoted throughout the book. I think the book would be valuable to women who want to convince themselves that they are not alone with this problem.

Here are some observations I made after reading *Private Pain*. The authors believe that women need to experience what they call the "five penetrations of life" to be able to maintain their vaginal and reproductive health and hygiene, and to enjoy sexual intimacy. These five penetrations include: penetration by a speculum, so a woman can receive a yearly pelvic exam; penetration by an applicator, to administer medicine in the case of a vaginal infection; penetration by a tampon, for feminine hygiene; penetration by a finger, for solitary sexual pleasure; and penetration by a penis, for sexual intimacy with a partner.

Based on these five types of penetration, let me revisit the most common forms of vaginismus and place them in a slightly different framework. Some women are unable to experience any of the five types of penetration. Some women are able to experience some of the five but not others. Finally, some women are able to insert a tampon, a speculum, a medicine applicator, and a finger, but are unable to have sexual intercourse.

Symptoms and Causes of Vaginismus

The authors of *Private Pain* describe vaginismus as a panic attack in the PC muscle. The woman with vaginismus typically has a history of bad experiences with tampons, fear of her own genitals, lack of masturbation, and no knowledge of the PC muscle.

Women with vaginismus often report a ticklish sensation in the inner thighs and vaginal area. In some extreme cases, women have needed to be sedated in order to receive a pelvic examination. Women with long-term cases of vaginismus often become accepting of the idea that they may never have children because of their inability to have sexual intercourse. In some cases, women can have oral sex or even anal intercourse, but not vaginal sex. Having vaginismus can make you feel like a freak. Some women have even gone so far as to undergo painful and unnecessary surgery (a hymenectomy or a procedure to supposedly widen the vaginal opening). Vaginismus is one of the most common reasons for unconsummated marriages. (Erection problems are another.)

Immediate symptoms that occur when penetration is attempted are symptoms of anxiety or extreme arousal of the sympathetic nervous system (the part of the nervous system responsible for the fight-or-flight reaction). These include sweating, shaking, urinary urgency, nervousness, nausea, stomachache, closing the legs tight, general body tension, holding one's breath, grasping onto the bed or a wall, closing one's fists, and scooting up on the bed or examination table to get away from a penis or speculum.

Vaginismus is often accompanied by an inability to look at one's own genitals, touch one's own genitals, masturbate, receive manual or oral sex from a partner, or have an orgasm. It is also sometimes accompanied by weird beliefs about the vagina: misconceptions about its length, structure, and what it looks like inside.

If you have vaginismus, you may have experienced it in various ways. You may think that your partner has an exceptionally large penis or that you are very tight. You may think, "I just can't do it," or, "It just won't go in, no matter how hard I try," or even, "I want to do it, but I'm just not big enough." In fact, vaginismus is unrelated to the actual size of the vagina. It is rare for a vagina to be so small that it will not accommodate a penis of any size. An exception would be in cases of congenital problems with the vagina. For example, there are girls who are born with a vaginal opening but no vaginal canal. Their vagina is only an inch or so deep. But this is very rare.

Obviously, the cause of vaginismus in a sexual situation is fear—fear of one's own genitals and fear of penetration. Causes from the past could include a restrictive religious upbringing, an upbringing in which sexual intercourse was consistently described as painful, failed penetration attempts, actual painful intercourse, sexual inexperience, and not feeling that one has the power to say no to an unwanted sexual situation. Vaginismus is also likely to develop in response to sexual trauma, for example, rape or molestation. It is common for women who develop vaginismus to do so as a defense against pain, especially pain that was never properly diagnosed or treated.

Vaginismus may also develop in response to a partner who thrusts too hard or for too long, causing discomfort or pain. Women sometimes develop vaginismus in response to a partner's sexual problem—for example, problems with erections or ejaculation. Vaginismus can also lead to sexual problems in the partner; for example, a man may develop premature ejaculation in response to a partner whose vagina is always tightly shut.

Treatment Outlook

The authors of *Private Pain* believe that only what they call "marginal" cases of vaginismus can be treated with self-help strategies. I would describe what they call marginal cases as short-term, acquired cases of vaginismus (cases in which the woman was able to have successful penetration in the past), or cases in which a woman can accept all of the types of penetration except the type that occurs during intercourse.

If you have an overwhelming, incapacitating fear that prevents you from looking at or touching your own genitals, or that prevents you from receiving a pelvic exam, you will probably need professional help to deal with your problem. Although vaginismus can be extremely frustrating and scary, it is the sexual dysfunction that has the highest cure rate. I encourage you to give the program in this book a try. The sensate-focus exercises can't hurt you, and if you're still afraid after trying them, you can always decide to see a sex therapist.

With vaginismus, it may be more important than with other sexual problems to determine the underlying psychological causes of the condition. If your vaginismus was caused by a sexual trauma, you will need to deal with that trauma, and you may need to seek a qualified therapist. Let me assure you: Your fear and anxiety stemming from past trauma and pain can be overcome, and the sexual exercises in Chapter 30 can help with the vaginal muscle spasms.

To overcome vaginismus, you can learn to exercise and control the muscles around your vagina, to relax your stomach and thigh muscles, to focus on the sensations in your genitals, to touch your own genitals, and to masturbate to orgasm with or without objects in your vagina. You and your partner can learn to communicate honestly with each other about the fear and frustration you have both been experiencing, and you can develop trust in each other.

Sally

Here's a case history that illustrates generalized lifelong vaginismus. Sally, age forty-eight, developed a typical case of vaginismus in response to molestation as a child, and she had never received any help or treatment. Before marriage she feigned a number of illnesses in order to avoid intercourse with her future spouse. In twenty-five years of marriage, she had fewer than ten successful episodes of sexual intercourse. (I define successful here as including penetration; she found no enjoyment in any of these instances and in fact felt them to be quite painful.) Her husband developed a severe case of premature ejaculation and sought extramarital relationships in which he eventually had successful and satisfying intercourse.

Unlike most of the other case histories in this book, Sally's case does not have a happy ending. Her husband begged her to accompany him to therapy, but she refused to admit there was anything wrong with her. Her life continued to be frustrating and depressing. Unfortunately there are many women like Sally. But many other women in Sally's situation have obtained help and have overcome vaginismus, and they now enjoy pain-free and satisfying sexual expression. In fact, of all of the sexual dysfunctions that I talk about in Sexual Healing, *vaginismus has the highest treatment success rate. In most cases, all it takes is one episode of being able to relax the PC muscle and engage in pain-free intercourse to set the stage for further enjoyment.*

Chapter 13

Dyspareunia

Dyspareunia is currently defined in the DSM-IV as "recurrent or persistent genital pain associated with sexual intercourse in either a male or a female." In reality, most cases of dyspareunia involve women. More specifically, dyspareunia is psychological pain with sexual intercourse. This means that in order to diagnose dyspareunia, you have to rule out all potential *physical* causes for the pain. When men experience pain during intercourse, it is usually much easier to rule out physical causes than it is for a woman, because with men there are fewer medical conditions that are known to cause pain during intercourse.

Patterns of Dyspareunia

In lifelong dyspareunia, a person has had pain with intercourse ever since she or he started having intercourse. In acquired dyspareunia, a person experienced pain-free intercourse in the past but has pain now. In generalized dyspareunia, a person has pain during intercourse with any person or upon penetration with any object. In situational dyspareunia, a person has pain with some partners but not others or upon penetration with some objects but not others.

I have never heard of a case of situational dyspareunia. The most common forms of the disorder are lifelong, in which a person has never been able to experience pain-free intercourse, and acquired, in which a person develops psychological pain during intercourse secondary to a traumatic event.

What's Normal?

It's normal to be able to have sexual intercourse without pain. The majority of people report that they feel pleasure from sexual intercourse rather than pain. However, I recently read some research suggesting that about 15 percent of women in their late teens and early twenties expect sexual intercourse to be painful, and for them it is.

It's also normal to experience occasional pain in the vagina or penis. Most likely this is temporary and is caused by one of the physical problems I describe in the next few pages. I have tried to provide an exhaustive list of all the conditions that might cause sexual pain, but it's certainly possible that I have overlooked something.

Physical Causes of Sexual Pain in Men

When men have pain during sexual intercourse, it usually results from a medical cause that's not too difficult to identify. The following sections identify some of the categories of medical problems that need to be ruled out. These are all common causes of pain during erection, intercourse, or ejaculation.

Sexually Transmitted Diseases

The following is not intended as a comprehensive look at sexually transmitted diseases or safe sex. I discuss these medical conditions only in the sense in which they are related to sexual pain.

Bacterial sexually transmitted diseases like gonorrhea and chlamydia can cause sexual pain, including intense itching and burning during both urination and intercourse. Gonorrhea and chlamydia are diagnosed by analyzing the discharge from the penis under a microscope. Another bacterial sexually transmitted disease, syphilis, usually does not cause genital pain. A syphilitic sore, or chancre, looks nasty but is usually painless. Bacterial STDs respond to antibiotics.

Herpes, which is a viral sexually transmitted disease, can definitely cause genital pain. Herpes sores develop into groups of blisters that are extremely painful when they burst. When a person has a herpes outbreak, it is very obvious due to the existence of the blisters. When herpes is dormant and blisters are not present, there is no pain. Another viral sexually transmitted disease, human papilloma virus, or HPV, is the virus that is thought to cause genital warts. Although the warts may be unsightly, they usually are not painful. Removing them, however, either through cauterization, cryosurgery, medication, or surgery, can be painful. As you probably know, viral STDs cannot be cured, although many people who have them go for years between painful outbreaks.

Infections of the urethra, such as nonspecific urethritis, can be sexually transmitted and can cause a burning sensation during urination and pain during intercourse, as can bladder infections.

Infections

The epididymis (ducts within the testes) and the prostate gland are both susceptible to acute infections. In the case of epididymitis (inflammation/infection of the epididymis), a testicle swells up, making ejaculation painful. Acute infection of the prostate gland, called *prostatitis,* can also cause painful urination and ejaculation. Both of these conditions respond to antibiotics.

Cancer

Prostate cancer is a common condition among older men. A conservative estimate is that one in eleven men in the United States will develop prostate cancer at some time in their lives. Prostate cancer can cause difficulty urinating and ejaculating, as well as pain upon doing so. The development of prostate cancer is often preceded by benign enlargement of the prostate. Even if the prostate gland has not developed cancer, enlargement can still cause pain during urination and ejaculation.

Another common form of male genital cancer is testicular cancer, which tends to affect younger men (Lance Armstrong is a famous example of an otherwise healthy man who developed testicular cancer in the prime of life). Symptoms include a lump on a testicle, swelling of a testicle, or a sense of heaviness or dragging in a testicle. Pain with erection or ejaculation is also a symptom of testicular cancer.

Other forms of male genital cancers exist—for example, cancer of the penis—but they are extremely rare in the United States.

Other Medical Conditions

Hernias can cause genital pain. In a common form of hernia, part of the intestine sags into the scrotum, causing the scrotum to swell up, often to the size of a grapefruit. Such a condition could obviously cause a lot of pain during intercourse.

Another condition called *phimosis* can cause painful erections. In phimosis, which affects uncircumcised men, the foreskin of the penis is too tight, preventing the man from having a full erection. The solution is to have the foreskin cut or stretched. In cases in which it is really tight, a full circumcision may have to be performed.

A less-understood condition is called *Peyronie's disease,* in which hardened areas or plaques form in the erectile tissue, causing the penis to curve to one side. In very severe cases of Peyronie's disease, the erectile tissue forms multiple plaques and takes on a corkscrew-like appearance. This can be very painful and can eventually prevent erection. If the plaques are identified at an early-enough stage, they can be removed surgically. Peyronie's disease can be caused by injury to the penis, which is sometimes called *penile fracture.* What generally causes this condition is that a man is having intercourse with a really hard erection, pulls all the way out of the vagina, and misses the vaginal opening on the next stroke. The trauma causes injury to the erectile tissue, forming a long-lasting bruise and possibly a plaque that creates a permanent curve. It kind of goes without saying that the condition is extremely painful.

Being located outside the body, the testicles are susceptible to injury, often during sports. Another type of injury is testicular torsion, in which the cord that supports a testis inside the scrotum gets twisted.

Physical Causes of Sexual Pain in Women

Many women, especially young women, expect sexual intercourse to be painful, and for about 15 percent of young women it is. This is not right. Sexual intercourse should never cause pain. The sections that follow describe some of the most common medical and behavioral causes of sexual pain for women. You'll note that the list is longer for women than it is for men.

When talking about women's sexual pain, I usually distinguish between what's called *outer pain* and *inner pain,* or pain that's felt at the vulva or vaginal opening versus pain that occurs with deep penetration. Some authors call this *insertional* or *superficial dyspareunia* versus *deep dyspareunia.* Superficial dyspareunia is similar to vaginismus.

Sexually Transmitted Diseases

The bacterial sexually transmitted diseases gonorrhea and chlamydia can cause itching and burning either with urination or with sexual intercourse.

Vaginal infections, which are caused by imbalances in the vagina's normal pH, can also be a source of pain. They include conditions such as bacterial vaginosis, trichomoniasis (also called trichomonas or trich), or yeast infections. All of these cause itching. They can be transmitted sexually, or they can occur as a result of stress or other problems that cause a lowered immune system. They are generally felt at the vaginal opening.

Yeast infections are especially known for causing pain during intercourse. The most obvious symptom of a yeast infection is a thick, white discharge. When the discharge comes into contact with the vulva, it can cause the skin to become inflamed and become so irritated that it cracks. This can cause the vaginal opening to be intensely painful during the first few strokes of intercourse. Women who take birth control pills are more vulnerable to yeast infections. So are women who have diabetes. Wearing clothing that is too tight or sitting around in wet clothing after swimming can also trigger yeast infections.

The viral sexually transmitted disease genital herpes causes blisters that can be intensely painful when they rupture. This is because the herpes virus typically inflames one particular nerve and causes it to fire repeatedly. If you have herpes sores on your inner or outer vaginal lips or in your vaginal opening, even the thought of sexual intercourse would probably cause you to cringe. In fact, some women experience outbreaks of genital herpes that are so painful they can't wear clothes. In order to urinate they have to sit in a bathtub full of either cold or hot water. Herpes sores higher up in the vaginal canal or on the cervix would probably not be as painful.

Acute Infections

Other infections in the pelvic area can cause sexual pain. Acute infections of the urethra or the bladder can result in pain at the vaginal opening. The vulva or the opening to the vagina can sometimes become temporarily inflamed.

Sexual Habits

Sometimes sexual pain is caused by doing certain things during intercourse. For example, if a woman's partner attempts to penetrate her vagina before she has lubricated and without using any externally applied lubrication, it can cause pain at the opening and along the walls of the vagina. Sometimes all that is needed to free a woman from sexual pain is to use lubricant, proceed to intercourse more slowly, and shift positions if the woman is uncomfortable.

Another thing that can cause sexual pain is a night of rough sex. Having sexual intercourse in a rough manner can cause abrasions or even tears in the vaginal walls. These will heal up quickly, but if you attempt to have sex again soon after the rough sex, you will probably feel some pain, both at the vaginal opening and along the vaginal walls.

Childbirth

The aftermath of childbirth can cause sexual pain because it is traumatic to the vagina and cervix. On average, most women resume sexual intercourse by about seven weeks after childbirth. However, an incompletely healed or incorrectly performed episiotomy can be painful for some time.

Surgery

Certain types of pelvic surgery can result in painful intercourse. Sometimes hysterectomy or other pelvic surgery can inadvertently cause nerve damage that produces not only pelvic pain but also difficulty with arousal and orgasm. Scar tissue left over from surgery can be painful.

Menstruation

Menstrual problems can cause pain during intercourse. The most common menstrual problem is cramps during a woman's period. These can cause deep pain during sexual intercourse. On the other hand, some women report that having sexual intercourse during menstruation helps menstrual cramps, because the contractions and spasms associated with orgasm often relieve the cramps.

Menopause

Menopause brings changes to the vagina due to the decrease in estrogen. This can cause what's called *atrophic vaginitis,* or *vaginal atrophy.* A decrease in estrogen causes a lack of lubrication and causes the walls of the vagina to become thinner. This can make intercourse very painful. A solution is to use an estrogen cream or suppository that is applied directly to the vagina.

Growths

Various nonmalignant growths in the pelvic area can also cause pain. Some of these include uterine polyps, uterine fibroids, or ovarian cysts. All of these conditions can cause a sense of deep pain, as can endometriosis, which is a condition in which the inner lining of the uterus (the endometrium) spreads beyond the uterus to other pelvic structures.

Cancer

There are many forms of female reproductive cancers that can cause sexual pain. Cervical cancer does not usually cause pain in its early stages, although the main symptom of cervical cancer is bleeding after intercourse. The cervix itself does not have the type of cells that can sense discrete pain information. In fact, biopsies can be done from the cervix and upper vaginal walls without anesthetic. However, the area around the cervix is extremely sensitive to pressure, and some women find it painful if their partner's penis hits this area during intercourse.

Uterine cancer could cause pain and abnormal cramping and bleeding. Ovarian cancer could cause pain if there is a large tumor present. Cancers of the vulva or vaginal walls are very rare but could also cause pain.

Other Conditions

Gastrointestinal problems such as irritable bowel syndrome, cramps, a full intestine, or gas can cause intercourse to be painful. Women with orthopedic problems, such as back problems or hip problems, often experience pain during intercourse. The PC muscle can cramp up, especially if a woman is anxious, and this can be very painful.

Vulvar Vestibulitis

Vulvar vestibulitis is a sort of "mystery condition" that can cause pain during intercourse. I call it a mystery condition because there is no agreement about whether it's physical or psychological; there is no agreement about what causes it; and there is no agreement as to whether it's primarily an immune system problem, a muscle problem, a skin problem, a blood flow problem, a nervous system problem, or a psychological problem. It is a condition that involves a sensation of burning and/or itching at the opening of the vagina (the vulva). Sometimes it is accompanied by obvious redness or inflammation, but often it is not. It is sometimes called *burning vagina syndrome.* Another synonym for it is *vulvodynia.*

To understand what this condition feels like, you have to understand the difference between what it feels like to have a penis and what it feels like to have a vagina. Men are much more aware of their penises on a minute-by-minute basis than women are of their vaginas. One man described to me the sensation of having a penis in the following way: "Having a penis is kind of like having a live fish in your pants. You can always feel it in there, but sometimes it starts flopping around." (He was an avid fisherman; can you tell?) In contrast, having a vagina is more like having a nose. Unless you're aroused or it's causing you pain, you're just not aware of it. For the woman who has vulvar vestibulitis, this is not true. Her vagina suffers a constant burning sensation that often makes it difficult to wear clothes, let alone masturbate or enjoy oral sex or sexual intercourse.

Health experts have different hypotheses about what causes vulvar vestibulitis. Some doctors believe it's a chronic cramp in the PC muscle as a result of long-term vaginismus. Others believe it's primarily a skin inflammation, although in many cases even though the skin feels like it's inflamed, there's no obvious redness. Some doctors believe it results from highly increased activity in a particular nerve to the genitals. Still others believe it's an autoimmune disorder in which a woman literally becomes allergic to the skin of her own vulva. The prospect that this condition is psychological also exists. Problems that tend to go along with it include somatizing disorder, irritable bowel syndrome, fibromyalgia, chronic fatigue syndrome, depression, and interstitial cystitis (chronic bladder infections).

Obviously, doctors attempt to treat this condition differently depending on what they think the cause is, and depending on whether they think the cause is a medical one or a psychological one. Some of the psychologically based treatments that have been used include hypnotherapy, sex therapy, cognitive-behavioral therapy, and biofeedback. Acupuncture has also been used.

Two types of surgery have also been used to treat this condition: laser surgery to remove the outer layers of skin of the vulva, and vestibulectomy, a surgical procedure in which the shiny tissue surrounding the opening of the vagina, the vestibule, is removed in order to remove the sensitive nerve endings located there. Although a vestibulectomy sounds like an extremely radical procedure, one recent study showed that it worked better than cognitive-behavioral therapy and biofeedback. This result is in line with several medical articles I read years ago on the topic, which indicated that most women who had surgery for vulvar vestibulitis reported an improvement in their condition.

In the past, vulvar vestibulitis was diagnosed with a cotton swab, which was used to poke at various areas of the vulva with increasing pressure. During the probing, a measuring device called a *vulvagesiometer* was also used to detect vulvar sensitivity.

Although experts agree that vulvar vestibulitis is a very serious problem, they currently don't know exactly what to do about it. If you have these symptoms, it would probably be best to consult with both a medical doctor and a psychologist, as well as with any available support groups. I honestly don't know whether the self-help program I outline for dyspareunia in Chapter 31 can be used to treat vulvar vestibulitis because I've never attempted to treat a case of it. Sometimes the symptoms last for a while and then go away on their own. If you would like to read a first-person account written by a woman who has dealt with this problem, I recommend a book called *The Camera My Mother Gave Me,* by Susanna Kaysen (see Recommended Reading).

Symptoms of
Sexual Pain in Women

The specific symptoms of sexual pain will vary with each woman. The following are some examples from *Private Pain,* the book I mentioned in the last chapter:

* Superficial vulval pain or tenderness

* Vulvar itching, burning, or stinging

* Pain or pressure behind the pubic bone

* Pain at the vaginal opening upon initial entry

* The sensation of being torn at the vaginal entry

* Mid-vaginal pain such as burning, sharp searing, or cramping

* Vaginal dryness, friction, and irritation

* Deep pain with thrusting, as if something is being bumped into

* Urinary burning and urgency

* Pain with orgasm (if the woman was aroused to completion of the sexual act)

Physical or Psychological Pain?

As I stated at the beginning of the chapter, dyspareunia is psychologically based pain experienced during sexual intercourse. This means that all of the medical conditions listed above must be ruled out before a diagnosis of dyspareunia can be made. It also means that in order for dyspareunia to be diagnosed, a man or woman must undergo a very thorough medical evaluation. For a woman, this will obviously include a pelvic examination, which can be incredibly painful for a woman with dyspareunia.

There are other ways to determine whether a woman's pain is psychological. Everybody experiences pain differently, but some types of pain simply aren't possible physically. For example, some women describe their pain as a sharp, piercing pain at the entrance to the vagina. From an anatomical standpoint, this is physically possible. Other women describe their pain as a sharp piercing pain about halfway up the side of the vagina or higher. From a physical standpoint, this is highly unlikely because most areas of the vaginal wall lack the nerve receptors to feel that type of discrete sensation, although the whole length of the vagina can feel a sensation of stretching.

Deep throbbing pain on one side of the abdomen or the other with intercourse is definitely possible, especially if the pain only happens once a month or every other month. In my experience this is usually caused by nonmalignant ovarian cysts.

Psychological Issues Related to Dyspareunia

Psychological causes of lifelong dyspareunia are similar to those that cause vaginismus: lack of sex education, fear of the genitals, or being taught that sex is painful. Psychological causes of acquired dyspareunia are somewhat more complicated. Acquired dyspareunia could be caused by sexual trauma such as rape. It is also commonly caused by sexual guilt or remorse over perceived sexual transgressions. I've read of many cases in which a woman developed dyspareunia after having an extramarital affair. Relationship issues can also cause dyspareunia. Some women develop sexual pain after their partner has been sexually unfaithful or has caused them other problems.

Some controversy exists about whether dyspareunia and vaginismus should be considered two different problems or whether they should be considered the same problem, because they both involve sexual pain during intercourse. I believe they should be thought of as different problems and treated differently. Vaginismus has only to do with the PC muscle, whereas superficial dyspareunia may cause pain at the vaginal opening, but it's usually caused by vulvar vestibulitis.

The program I describe in Chapter 31 of this book is for women. That's because I have never seen a case of psychologically based sexual pain in a man, and in my reading I have not come across any treatments for it. The program in this book also treats only deep, psychologically based dyspareunia. I honestly don't know whether the exercises I describe in Chapter 31 will help superficial dyspareunia. If you have superficial dyspareunia, you will be better off using the exercises described in Chapter 30 for vaginismus.

In most cases of women's sexual pain, a physical problem can be found and treated. Vulvar vestibulitis is much more complicated, because it could be either psychological or the result of an autoimmune condition.

Lydia

Lydia, age thirty, came to a sex clinic complaining of sexual pain. She experienced pain at the opening of her vagina when she attempted to have intercourse. By the time she came to our clinic, she was desperate. When she was in her early twenties, a gynecologist told her that her vaginal opening was abnormally small and recommended a surgical procedure to widen it. She underwent the surgery, but the recovery was extremely painful for her. When she attempted to have intercourse again eight weeks after the surgery, it was even more painful than before.

Lydia's sex history revealed that she had never masturbated and had a shocking level of ignorance about the female genitals, especially considering the surgery she had been through. To solve her problem with sexual pain, she went through a treatment program that began with extensive education about self-touch and the female anatomy, as well as many weeks of relaxation exercises. It took a while, but eventually she was able to experience pain-free intercourse.

Part III

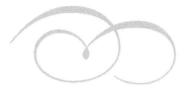

BEGINNING SEXUAL HEALING

In this section you'll find chapters on the importance of touch and on how to do the touching exercises. Next come chapters on relaxation, sexual fitness, and self-touch. These three chapters include exercises you can do by yourself. The last four chapters of the section contain basic sensate-focus exercises you can do with your partner.

chapter 14

The Healing Touch

The essence of touch begins inside our skin rather than on its surface. We may not realize it, but many of us need to heal some aspect of our relationship with our own body. Beginning in our early childhood, society bombards us with unrealistic messages about what our bodies should look like. At the very least, most of us grow up to be out of touch with our bodies.

Sexual healing reconnects our mind and our body, and it uses the power of that unity for our health and well-being. If whole-body (holistic) health is what we are after, how our body feels is more important than what it does or how it looks. The key to knowing our bodies' feelings lies in the simple ability to give and receive touch.

Touch Is Vital

Touching has been a traditional treatment for illness throughout human history. Religious figures such as Jesus and some saints used the laying on of hands to heal people. Later, in Europe, those who were ill or infirm were brought before the king, whose touch supposedly could cure them. Today, *curanderos* in Latin American communities often use touch as part of their treatment.

Touch can communicate a number of things, such as comfort and positive expectations. As a result, touch influences our physical well-being. In fact, quite a bit of research has been done on the positive health effects of touch. Much of it was brought together by Ashley Montagu in his classic book *Touching*. Although *Touching* was first published in the early 1970s, it is still in my opinion the best book available on the healing powers of touch. Montagu describes how skin contact affects both mental and physical health throughout all stages of our lives, beginning with birth. Studies show that infants who are touched have much higher survival rates than those who are deprived of human contact. Infants who are stroked and caressed develop more healthily, and in later life they experience fewer emotional and mental problems. Studies with adults have found that being touched can lower heart rate and blood pressure and promote physical relaxation in general. Even simply stroking a pet can lower a person's blood pressure and heart rate.

There is no doubt that infants and children need touch to survive, and although research hasn't been conducted to study whether adults need touch to survive, why would our need to be touched end with childhood? The countless ways that touch benefits us—heals us—may be the reason why we feel so good when we are touched. While I hope this book introduces you to the wonders of sexual healing, I believe the greatest thing it will do is deepen your appreciation for the power of touch.

The Nonverbal Power of Touch

In the language of the study of nonverbal communication, touch is known as an "intensifier." This means that whatever mood already exists in a given social situation, touch will make the mood stronger. Remember the first time your partner reached out to touch you before you became lovers? Or when you were a little child and bumped your head, do you remember how having your mother hold you and hug you made the pain go away much faster than if she'd simply said, "There, there ... now go and play."

Not all touch intensifies good feelings. Here is a common example. Let's say you have just met someone who for whatever reason gives you the creeps. If this person touches you while the two of you are talking, your mood toward him or her will become even more negative. In the same way, not all sexual touch is healing. Sexual touch can be used coercively, especially the use of inappropriate sexual touches between adults and children. This kind of touch is highly destructive and exploits power dynamics. Sexual molestation and abuse are especially sad because they pervert something good. People who experience harmful touch in childhood often have difficulty with sexual touch later in life.

Touch also conveys power, especially in the workplace. If an employer touches a subordinate during an interaction, it intensifies the individuals' awareness of the difference in power between them. Whether consciously or not, many people use touch to communicate their feelings and intentions.

In *Sexual Healing* you will learn to use the intensifying power of touch for positive purposes: to bring healing energy to your mind, body, and intimate relationships. If a healing attitude already exists between you and your partner, sexual touching will intensify the healing intent the two of you already share.

The Healing Powers of Touch

Touch has been shown to have various positive healing effects. I believe this is because touch addresses both the body and the mind. For example, touching in a pleasant situation has a positive effect on the immune system. Touching also makes it easier to share feelings. Studies show that touch encourages self-disclosure. Patients touched in the genital region by doctors and nurses during physical examinations often reveal personal sexual information. It appears that being touched in intimate areas taps into intimate thoughts and feelings.

Not surprisingly, touch has positive effects on people facing medical recovery. Patients who are touched by nurses recover from surgery faster than those who are not touched. It is unknown precisely how touching in this situation helps people get better. It could be that touch directly promotes relaxation, or that it stimulates a person's pain-killing and healing mechanisms. Or it could be that the act of touching communicates caring and imparts to the patient a sense of self-worth and the expectation of becoming well. I suspect it is a combination of these things.

Sensate Focus:
The Touch that Heals

An intimate sexual relationship offers an excellent context in which we can experience the healing powers of touch. Sadly, the social norms for adults in North American culture do not encourage or allow much physical contact. For many of us, especially men, sexual encounters are the only situations in which we are allowed to touch other people and to enjoy being touched by them.

There is a particular kind of sensual touch—and a particular way to do this kind of touching—that promotes healing. It is called *sensate focus*. The exercises that appear later in this book are built around the sensate-focus approach. As mentioned, sensate focus was developed by Masters and Johnson and has been refined over the years by others. The term *sensate focus* may sound technical, but it is actually quite simple—and self-explanatory. It is a technique in which you focus your attention as closely as you can on the sensations that you are feeling. This is the essence of all of the sexual healing exercises: Direct all of your attention to where you touch your skin or your partner's skin, or to where your partner touches you.

The specific type of touch we will use is a caress. A caress involves a delicate touch on the skin rather than a massage-type stroke. Other books may refer to this kind of touch as "sensual massage," but strictly speaking, it is not massage. A massage generally involves manipulation of the large muscles of the body and is performed for the benefit of the person being massaged. A sensate-focus caress benefits both the person touching and the person being touched.

A healing sensate-focus caress has the following characteristics:

✳ It is very slow.

✳ It is done for the toucher's own pleasure.

✳ It is free of psychological pressure, including pressure to perform.

✳ It is focused.

✳ It happens in the here and now.

✳ It is sensuous.

There are no specific techniques for caressing in the "right" way. Whether you are caressing yourself or your partner as part of an exercise, caress in the way that feels best for you, within the general guidelines outlined in this section.

First, your caress should be light and very, very slow. Remember that touching and being touched in a slow, sensuous, or comforting way relaxes both touchee and toucher. A rapid or heavy touch triggers the sympathetic nervous system rather than the parasympathetic nervous system and conveys a sense of psychological pressure that is not relaxing for either person.

When you touch your partner, explore his or her body for your own pleasure. You may use either long, sweeping strokes or short ones, as long as you touch slowly. This is up to you. Try both long and short strokes and use the style that feels best to you.

I cannot overemphasize the importance of a slow caress! If you think you are moving your hand slowly enough, consciously cut your speed in half and see how this affects your ability to stay focused. Both you and your partner will feel more free to relax if the exercises are done very slowly, with eyes closed and without talking. You cannot caress too slowly.

The exercises don't require getting into certain physical positions for doing particular caresses. I find that the best position for any caress is the one that enables you to touch with the least amount of physical exertion. For example, if you want to caress your partner's back, rather than straddling his or her body, try lying in full body contact with your partner while you touch his or her back with one hand. You can also use other body parts, such as your hair or chest, to do a caress, as long as you stay comfortable.

When doing any sensate-focus caress, always maintain contact with your partner. Avoid surprising your partner with a sudden touch when you switch hands. If you use lotion or body oil for a caress, warm the lotion or oil in your hand before you apply it, and maintain contact with your partner's body when you put more lotion on your hand.

Several elements of the sensate-focus caresses can help to take the pressure off of you and your partner. Most sensate-focus exercises are broken down into two roles: active and passive. One person caresses while the other person receives the caress, and then you switch roles so that both partners have a chance to experience both roles. Making a clear agreement about when it is each partner's turn to be the active partner and when it is time to trade roles can eliminate the pressure caused by wondering whether you're "giving enough" in response to your partner's caresses. When it's your turn to be the passive partner, that's your job: to simply enjoy the sensuous attentions of your partner.

When you are the active partner, touch your partner for your own pleasure, not your partner's pleasure. That's right—your own pleasure! This is another reason why the sensate-focus exercises are so good at taking the pressure off. One of the biggest sources of anxiety and pressure in sexual encounters is wondering if you are pleasing your partner or if you are doing a good job. By touching for your own pleasure you remove that source of pressure and take a sexual encounter back to its most basic elements.

Does this seem like a "selfish" way to engage in a sensual encounter with another person? It's true that many of us have negative feelings about the word *selfish*. We may have been told as children that we were selfish when we wanted to do things that gave us pleasure. However, many people with sexual problems are actually too "unselfish." As a result of trying to give too much, they have lost the ability to enjoy their own feelings. Think of your behavior in sexual encounters as lying on a continuum from "selfish" to "unselfish." Some of you may be on the unselfish side—a little more concerned about your partner's enjoyment and satisfaction than about your own. In the early sensate-focus exercises I will ask you to move closer to the "selfish" end of the continuum by concentrating on your own feelings without worrying about your partner. When you are touching your partner in any exercise, touch for your own pleasure and for no other reason. Touch and caress strictly for your own enjoyment without considering at this point what types of touches or caresses your partner might prefer. Find what pleases you.

You may notice that this advice goes counter to what is recommended by the authors of many highly regarded books on sexuality. They recommend that sensate-focus caresses be done with the goal of pleasing one's partner. Where I use the phrases "active partner" and "passive partner," some authors refer to the roles as "pleasurer" and "pleasuree," or "giver" and "receiver." I have found that this orientation toward the exercises increases anxiety and performance pressure. In my experience, encouraging clients to touch for their own pleasure has brought nothing but positive results, while allowing a client to attempt to give me pleasure generally results in increased pressure to perform, increased anxiety in a sexual situation, and a shutdown of arousal.

It is normal and loving to want to please your partner and to want to know that your partner is enjoying himself or herself. Learning to focus on your own sensations and your own enjoyment will actually make you more sensitive to your partner's needs and feelings in the long run. Knowing what you enjoy will make it easier to communicate those things to your partner. Learning to concentrate on and enjoy your own sensual and sexual feelings when you are the passive partner in a sensate-focus exercise will give you the confidence that your partner enjoys the same freedom when you take the active role.

When you are the active partner, do a caress as instructed and try to keep your attention on the exact spot where your skin touches your partner's skin. There is no need to speak to your partner during an exercise or ask for any feedback. Assume that the caress feels good or at least neutral to your partner. Do not worry about whether or not your partner is enjoying the caress. It is his or her responsibility to let you know whether you are doing something that causes discomfort.

When you are the passive partner, lie in a relaxed position. Relax any of your muscles that feel tense. Pay attention to exactly where your partner touches your skin. Mentally follow your partner's hand as it caresses your body. Do not respond to your partner in any way. Do not tell him or her what to do, and do not moan and wriggle around. The only time you should give your partner any feedback while you are passive is if he or she does something that hurts you or makes you feel uncomfortable (for example, rubbing too hard or scraping a nipple by accident). Remaining passive will allow your body to fully experience your sensual arousal.

As you read the instructions for the active and passive roles for each exercise, you may be concerned that this is not the way in which sexual encounters proceed in real life. In real-life sexual encounters, both partners do various activities, often simultaneously. But in real-life sexual encounters, partners often intentionally or unintentionally pressure each other to perform sexually, and in real-life sexual encounters partners often worry about what the other person is thinking or what the other person would like. People spend a lot of time in real-life sexual encounters being distracted.

The program I describe here is innovative. It teaches you to free yourself of intrusive thoughts like, "I wonder if she's really enjoying this." By concentrating totally on where your skin touches your partner's skin, you will be fully involved and present in what you are doing. And although only one person is active at a time, there is an aspect of mutuality, because both partners are focusing on the same thing at the same time. You will find that this is actually more sensually arousing than when you and your partner are doing different activities at the same time.

The reason for artificially breaking down the sexual encounter into clearly defined active and passive roles is very simple: You need to experience nondemand interaction. You avoid giving feedback to your partner when you take the passive role so that your partner can touch you for his or her own pleasure without having to worry about what you like or want. Similarly, when you are in the active role, you can touch for your own pleasure without worrying about whether or not you are pleasing your partner.

You may feel some resistance to the labels "active" and "passive." Some people feel uncomfortable about being labeled passive. It is important, however, for each partner to fully experience both roles. If you are a woman having problems becoming aroused or reaching orgasm, learning to feel comfortable with the active role will help you. If you are a man having problems with getting erections or reaching orgasm, being in the passive role will be a valuable experience for you. Try not to limit yourself to "traditional" male and female roles—you may find that being in an unfamiliar role can be quite enjoyable and liberating.

Let's talk a bit more about the guideline to direct all of your attention to the spot where skin touches skin. This is the essence of the sensate-focus process. Throughout all of the exercises in this book, you are to focus your awareness as closely as you can on your own sensations. Always focus all of your attention on your skin where it comes into contact with your partner's skin. If your mind wanders off to something else at any point during any exercise, consciously bring it back to the point of contact between your skin and your partner's skin.

When you first begin doing sensate-focus exercises, you may feel that you are focusing on the sensations in your skin only part of the time—perhaps half the time or even less. It is normal to become distracted now and then. Simply recognize that your mind is suddenly elsewhere and bring it back to the place where your skin makes contact with your partner's skin. If you do an exercise and find that you were not really able to focus on the touch, repeat the exercise at a later time until you are able to focus on the touch at least 50 percent of the time.

Suppose you are a man whose face is being caressed. Your partner is caressing your face in a way that feels good for her. She is not taking into account what you like or what might feel best to you. Suppose she caresses your whole face once or twice and then lingers on your forehead for what you perceive to be a long time. If you have thoughts such as, "I wish she'd go back to my chin," or, "I wish she would hurry up and touch my ear—that would really turn me on," or even, "When are we going to have sex?" then you are failing to concentrate fully on your experience of the present moment. Once you realize this is happening, you must consciously will your attention back to the point of contact between your skin and your partner's skin. This is what we call staying in the here and now. Dwelling on thoughts about sexual problems you had in the past will distract and depress you. Speculating about what will happen in the future (even a few seconds into the future) will make you anxious. Stay in the here and now!

Let's say that you are caressing or being caressed and you are thinking, "This feels good, but it's just not turning me on. Something must be wrong." Relax. It's not supposed to be turning you on. Sensate-focus touch is sensual rather than sexual. Men, you are not expected to get an erection during the sensate-focus exercises. Many men do not get an erection during a face caress, back caress, front caress, or even a genital caress. Women, you are not expected to experience vaginal lubrication during these caresses. If you do experience sexual arousal, that's fine. You may notice a momentary twinge in the groin area, a feeling of wetness, or the presence of a half or full erection. Notice if that happens, but then return your attention to the area that your partner is touching or that you are touching on your partner. Do not focus on your genital area unless that is the area being touched.

If you feel sexually aroused during any caress, do not try to make it "better" by squirming around or rubbing up against your partner. On the other hand, do not do anything to push your arousal away or to contain it. It is perfectly acceptable to feel sexually turned on during any of the exercises, but it is not necessary to be turned on in order to learn from the exercises.

The Healing Mindset

In addition to the physical exercises you and your partner will do, *Sexual Healing* encourages you to develop a healing mindset. This is the first step to being healed of sexual problems or becoming a sexual healer. In anything having to do with health, your expectations and intentions are crucial in determining whether healing will take place.

Here are some thoughts about how to develop a healing mindset. Whenever you do a sensate-focus exercise, take care to gather your energies and attention into a positive, healthful frame of mind. Try to feel the many facets of a loving relationship—unconditional love, acceptance, unselfish goodwill, complete involvement, positive energy, and lack of pressure or goal orientation. Then, transmit these attitudes to your partner nonverbally through your touch.

Don't expect to be able to feel and convey all of these feelings right away. We are all on a journey toward this mindset. Try the best you can during any exercise to embody and convey the expectation that you and your partner will be healed. Over time, as you work with the exercises, you will find that your healing mindset is growing stronger and deeper.

Now that you've been introduced to the "what" of sensate-focus exercises, the next chapter offers a few more concrete guidelines for "how" to do them.

chapter 15

How to Do
Sensate-Focus
Exercises

In the previous chapter you read about characteristics of the sensate-focus touch. In addition to knowing how to touch, there are other philosophical and practical issues that you also need to know in order to do the exercises described in this book. The first issue is the importance of being able to trust your partner.

Trust

For people with long-standing sexual problems, sex can become something they avoid in thought and conversation as well as in behavior. People with sexual problems often find it difficult to trust a partner, especially if the sexual problem (such as vaginismus) originated in a trauma such as incest or rape by someone who was trusted. Often, a person who experienced a sexual trauma at an early age went on, naïvely, to attempt to deal with the problem by initiating sexual activity too soon or persisting in unhealthy sexual experiences that only increased their lack of trust.

The sensate-focus exercises can help to build trust between partners, because each exercise has limits and ground rules to which both partners should adhere. For example, the face caress calls for touching only the region from the top of the head to the base of the neck. It is not uncommon in my experience for men to exceed the boundaries of this exercise by touching their partner's breasts. When this happened in my practice as a surrogate partner, I asked the client to please stay within the bounds of the exercise. Why, you might ask? Obviously, I like to have my breasts touched as much as anyone else, so why not just let him do it? After all, it might give him an erection, which is where we're heading in the long run.

It is important to understand that staying within the limits of an exercise and holding your partner to those limits helps to develop an atmosphere of trust in which both partners know what to expect and know that the other is trying to help create a good experience. If my partner pushes the limits of an exercise, I know that he is not totally focused on the touch, and this also distracts me from being able to focus 100 percent on the touch.

Say that a couple agrees to do a face caress for twenty minutes each. As the man is caressing the woman's face, he moves his hand down to touch her breast and soon she reaches back to stroke his genitals, and before you know it, they are having intercourse. Going beyond the exercise in this way is not a major issue if both people are free of sexual problems and are using the sensate-focus exercises primarily to increase the pleasure in their sex lives. But here is what will happen for couples with sexual problems: They will not learn what the exercise is designed to teach them—that is, how to touch and be touched in a sensual manner. They will learn instead that every touch leads to sexual activity. This will reinforce the anxiety or performance orientation that caused their problems to start with.

To get the most from the sensate-focus exercises, stay within the limits of the exercises. For the first few exercises (unless otherwise specified), do not go on to genital contact or sexual intercourse either during or after the exercise. You will only undo what you have learned in the exercise.

Sex therapists differ about whether you should continue having intercourse or doing the other sexual activities you were used to doing while you go through a sex therapy program. Most sex therapists put a temporary ban on sexual intercourse for their clients during sex therapy until an exercise actually calls for it. I don't, necessarily, depending on the nature of the problems. You will have to make your own decision. On the other hand, I *do* recommend that you avoid following a nonsexual exercise with sexual activity. Take a break first, or you will reinforce in your mind the idea that sensual touching is always followed by sexual activity.

Use your feelings as a guide. If you feel any doubt about doing a sexual activity that you have not yet reached in the sensate-focus exercises, it is best to hold off. However, if both you and your partner feel totally comfortable with continuing to do sexual activities even without, for example, orgasms, go ahead.

Whether you have intercourse during the sexual healing program will depend on the nature of your problems. Obviously, a man who cannot maintain an erection would not be able to have intercourse, but a man with inhibited ejaculation would. A woman with vaginismus would not be able to have sexual intercourse, but a woman with orgasm problems would.

Finally, if you feel that you cannot stay within the limits of the exercises, you should not do them. To add more sexual contact than instructed during an exercise will do you and your partner more harm than good if you are trying to heal a sexual problem. Not only will you fail to benefit from the exercise; you will have taught your partner that you are untrustworthy, whereas if you adhere to the limits of an exercise, you will build trust. Building trust can help you rid yourself of a performance orientation toward sexual activity.

Feedback after the Exercises

Each sensate-focus exercise concludes with a feedback discussion, during which you should speak openly and honestly with your partner. Many couples with sexual problems have learned to be dishonest with each other about their sex lives. An example would be a woman who continually fakes orgasms. You may feel embarrassed to admit that you have lied to your partner or withheld the truth, perhaps for many years, but your joint decision to finally do something about your problems should give you the confidence to start responding to one another honestly.

The exercises will not do you any good if you lie about your feelings. For example, please do not tell your partner you enjoyed an exercise if you really didn't. Please do not tell your partner you were able to concentrate if you weren't, just so you appear to be doing things correctly.

Here are the questions you and your partner should ask yourselves and each other after each sensate-focus exercise:

1. How comfortable was each partner with the active role? With the passive role? Were you able to remain completely passive while in the passive role? If you felt uncomfortable with either role in an exercise, you should repeat the exercise until that role becomes comfortable and natural for you.

2. For how much of the time were each of you able to fully concentrate on sensations while you took the active role? Ideally, you should feel you are concentrating on the sensations of touch most of the time, but the actual amount of time you are focusing is not as important as learning to recognize when you are distracted and

bringing your mind back to the touch. If you have trouble focusing in either role during an exercise, you need to practice that role in the exercise until you are able to concentrate more fully.

In order to move on to the next exercise, I believe you should be able to concentrate on the touch at least 50 percent of the time in the previous exercise. To help yourself figure out if your concentration is improving from exercise to exercise, you could make yourself a chart of your progress in concentration. Think of your ability to concentrate on either a 1-to-10 scale or a percentage basis. For example, on the 1-to-10 scale, perfect concentration would be a 10, and concentrating about half the time would be a 5. Use a notebook and record the name of the exercise, the date and time you did it, and the degree of your ability to concentrate in both the active and passive roles.

Some people raise objections at this point. "These exercises are too boring and repetitious. There's no way I can focus on touching for twenty minutes." What can I say? Learning a new behavior requires three things: actually doing the behavior, finding the behavior in some way rewarding, and repeating the behavior. If you feel bored, you are not focusing on the point of contact between your skin and your partner's skin. The way to relieve your boredom is to consciously will yourself to pay attention to your practice of the exercises.

It is natural for extraneous thoughts to intrude during a sensate-focus exercise. Out of nowhere you may start to think about your kids or your job. This type of distraction is different from boredom and is nothing to worry about. Simply catch yourself and bring your mind back to the touch. You will know that you were totally focused on the touch if after an exercise you feel that it was too short or that the time passed much more quickly than you expected.

Christa Schulte, the author of *Tantric Sex for Women,* suggests a technique for getting rid of intrusive thoughts. She recommends visualizing a trash can and a deep freeze. When a thought pops into your head, decide whether it should be discarded as unhelpful or stored for later retrieval. For example, if it's a performance-related thought, such as, "I wonder if I'm getting an erection," it probably belongs in the trash. If so, visualize it going into the trash can, then return your focus to the touch. If it's a thought about something that needs to be addressed later, such as a problem with your kids, visualize it going into the deep freeze, where it will be waiting for you to retrieve it later, after the sensual encounter, so you can deal with it then. Then, once again, return your awareness to the sensations.

3. When you were active, how much of the time did you do the exercise for your own pleasure? How much of the time were you thinking about your partner or trying to please your partner? Did you worry about whether your passive partner was enjoying the caress, or did you wonder about what he or she was thinking about? If you really focus during the active role, thoughts about your partner should not enter your mind, other than thoughts about what your partner's body feels like to you. An exception would be if you can see by outward physical signs that your passive partner is anxious and is not relaxing. You can also record what percentage of time you spent doing the exercise for your own pleasure versus the amount of time you spent worrying about your partner.

4. When you were in the passive role, did the touch feel like a caress or like a massage? Did it feel mechanical at all? Did you feel pressured to respond? If the active partner's touch is perceived by the passive partner as being rough, fast, or mechanical, the active partner may need to adjust his or her caressing technique.

5. Did either partner experience sexual arousal during the exercise? If so, did you try to get rid of it, try to make it better, or just leave it alone? It will make it easier to talk about arousal levels if you use a 1-to-10 scale. Remember, there is never any pressure on you to reach a certain level of arousal during any exercise. But if you do feel arousal, it's good to keep track of it so you learn which sensual and sexual activities you find more or less arousing.

6. Did each partner follow the instructions for the exercise, or did one or both partners attempt to go beyond the limits? Did each person feel that the exercise was in general a positive experience? Was either partner working at it (that is, by trying to please, or trying to become aroused)?

7. After each exercise, both partners should report on their anxiety level during the exercise, as well as on their perception of their partner's anxiety level. Again, you can use a 1-to-10 scale, with 1 being no anxiety and 10 being extreme anxiety. Feedback about anxiety is especially important for people who are dealing with sexual aversion disorder, vaginismus, dyspareunia, or premature ejaculation.

You should repeat an exercise if either partner experienced high anxiety that did not go away, if either partner felt unable to concentrate most of the time in either role, if either partner felt pressured to respond, or if either partner didn't adhere to the limits of the exercise.

A good way to give feedback is for each partner to keep a notebook record of his or her reactions to the exercises and then share the notebooks with each other. It's also helpful to keep a journal while you are going through the sexual healing process in order to record your experiences and feelings.

Setting a Schedule

Improving your sex life, healing your sexual problems, enhancing your relationship, and overcoming sexual fears all require a commitment of time. Some sex therapy programs ask both partners to make a contract to do certain exercises at certain times. You and your partner will decide how often you are able to do an exercise. If you tend to disagree about time management or have difficulty remembering schedules, a written agreement may help. It is my experience that it is better to do the exercises at prearranged times rather than to wait until you "feel like it."

I recommend setting a schedule at the beginning of each week and then sticking to it as much as possible. Some of the exercises that you do by yourself (like the PC muscle exercises and breathing exercises) should be done every day. Other than that, the ideal time frame for doing exercises with your partner would probably be two to three partner exercises a week. One exercise a day is too much. Your mind and your body need time to internalize changes. You should do at least one partner exercise a week in order to maintain continuity. In Chapters 23 through 31, which discuss healing specific sexual problems, I recommend exercises in a particular order.

Most of the exercises take about an hour to an hour and a half and use the following format: You and your partner lie together and breathe for five minutes. Then one partner is active and does a focusing caress (a relaxing face or back caress) for five to ten minutes. Then you switch roles and the other partner does a focusing caress. Then you do the main exercise, usually for about twenty to thirty minutes. If the main exercise has both an active and passive role (some do not), lie together and breathe for five minutes between roles. Also, lie together and breathe for a few minutes at the end of an exercise.

Multiple Problems

What if both partners have a sexual problem or one of you has more than one problem? How do you know which exercises to do first? In general, I make the following recommendations.

If you have more than one problem, do the exercises first for the problem that comes first in the sexual response cycle. For example, if you are a woman with both arousal and orgasm problems, do the exercises for the arousal problem before you do exercises for orgasm. If you have an anxiety problem as well as other sexual problems, deal with the anxiety first.

The exception to this would be desire problems. If you have both desire problems and arousal problems, deal with the arousal problem first. The desire problem will most likely take care of itself once you are confident you can become aroused.

If both a man and a woman are having problems, I generally recommend dealing with the man's problem first, because a woman is more likely to become aroused and have an orgasm if her partner is functioning well. For example, if the man has premature ejaculation and the woman has problems with orgasms, it's best if he learns at least some degree of ejaculatory control before she tries to solve her problems with orgasm.

If both of you are having problems, another option is to alternate and do one exercise for the man's problem and then one exercise for the woman's problem. This way no one feels left out.

If you are the fully functioning partner of someone with problems, there will still be plenty for you to do. The relaxation exercises, sexual fitness exercises, and self-touch exercises will all benefit you.

I hope the suggestions I've made in this chapter encourage you to go on. Even if you and your partner both have problems or if you have more than one area of concern, the sensate-focus exercises are powerful and have the potential to positively affect your sex life. Although there are certain guidelines to follow, as outlined in this chapter, try to keep sight of the fact that the exercises will be relaxing and enjoyable.

chapter 16

Relaxation

This is the first chapter that contains exercises. I purposely made it short to ease you into the sexual healing process. All of these exercises will help you relax, which will provide you with a first step toward a solution for the anxiety that is causing your sexual problems.

The first three exercises are simple breathing exercises that you can do every day.

Proper breathing is the basis of life—and of feeling alive. The oxygen we take in with every breath is our lifeline, but a lot of us don't breathe properly, and improper breathing can create anxiety and make sexual problems worse. The more anxious and pent up we feel, the more constricted our breathing becomes and the less oxygen we take in.

❧ Exercise 1. BASIC BREATHING

Before you do anything else, you need to make sure that the way you are breathing is relaxing you and not making your sexual problems worse. You should pay attention to two aspects of breathing. The first is slowness. Slowing your breathing will relax your whole body. The second aspect is evenness. Keep your breathing consistent and even in order to allow sexual energy to flow throughout your body. Holding your breath when you become sexually aroused will diminish your arousal.

To start this first breathing exercise, lie comfortably on your bed with your clothing loosened. Place your hand over your heart to get a sense of how fast it is beating. You do not need to time your heart rate.

Now place your hand on your abdomen. Blow all the air in your lungs out through your mouth. Slowly breathe in through your mouth, and then, immediately but slowly, exhale. Pause several seconds between exhaling and inhaling. Do not pause between an inhalation and an exhalation—in other words, don't hold your breath. The inhale/exhale cycle should be one continuous process. Lie quietly and breathe like this, slowly and evenly, for a few minutes.

❧ *Exercise 2.* ADVANCED BREATHING

If you are especially anxious or have a lot of stress in your life, try the following breathing exercise. Lie down in a relaxed position. Rapidly blow all of the air out of your lungs through your nose. Now, inhaling slowly, take all the air you can back in through your nose. Think of this as caressing the inside of your lungs with air. As soon as all the air is in your lungs, start breathing it back out, slowly. Don't hold your breath at all, and don't pause between exhaling and inhaling. Your breathing is now under your conscious control.

Do this form of breathing five or six times in a row. It will slow down your heart rate and lower your blood pressure. This simple breathing exercise, done regularly, can relax you enough for you to be able do the exercises in this book.

❧ *Exercise 3.* BELLY BREATHING

Lie comfortably on your back. Loosen any tight clothing. Place one hand on your stomach or abdomen and the other on your heart. Now take a deep, slow breath that you can feel all the way down to your abdomen. Breathe as if you are drawing breath down through your body, into your legs and toes. This type of breathing, called *belly breathing,* will cause your abdomen to expand and rise; when you exhale, it will contract.

As you breathe, inhaling and exhaling should be one continuous process. Don't hold your breath at all after you inhale. Feel the air flowing all the way into your lungs and all the way out. Visualize the air as a white light flowing into and out of you, both relaxing you and energizing you. If you want to, rest after each exhalation. Take two deep belly breaths and then breathe normally for about a minute. Take two more belly breaths and breathe normally for another minute. Repeat this pattern of breathing for about ten minutes.

❧ *Exercise 4.* DEEP MUSCLE RELAXATION

Sexual healing relies on deeply relaxed muscles. Deep muscle relaxation is a well-known antidote for anxiety, with special benefits for lovemaking. When you have mastered it, you will know your own body so well that if a muscle group becomes tense during lovemaking, you will immediately notice it. You can then consciously and immediately relax so that muscle tension won't interfere with your lovemaking.

Lie down on your bed, on your back, in a comfortable position. The object is to tighten each group of muscles in your body, hold it as tight as you can for a few seconds, and then relax it. Starting with your right foot and then moving to your left foot, systematically work your way up your entire body, tensing and relaxing each muscle group in sequence: feet, calves, thighs, entire legs, buttocks, abdomen, stomach, chest, neck, hands, lower arms, upper arms, entire arms, and face. Remember to keep breathing normally as you do the exercise.

chapter 17

Sexual Fitness

S exual fitness is a big component of sexual healing. It's a good idea for your genitals and the rest of your body to be in at least reasonable shape, although you don't have to be an athlete to make great love. That's what is so wonderful about lovemaking. Anybody, at almost any level of fitness, can enjoy satisfying sexual intimacy. If you have physical problems or limitations, you can still make love by adjusting your position, limiting the amount of time you spend, or eliminating certain activities that cause you physical problems. All it takes is some creativity and the ability to listen to your body.

There are a few simple things you can do to get in better shape for making love. I call these "sexual fitness" exercises, but don't worry—they don't work up a sweat. By strengthening the muscles in your pelvic area and learning how to relax the rest of your body, you can spend more delicious time in intimate, arousing lovemaking.

General Fitness

Before we get into specific pelvic exercises, let's talk for a minute about general aerobic fitness. Are you in great physical condition—a triathlete or marathon runner? Or are you a fitness disaster area—a true couch potato? Most of us are somewhere in between these extremes. To receive the most healing from this program, you need to have a basic level of general fitness. What does this mean?

If you smoke, please do your best to stop now or begin tapering off. It is a proven fact that cigarette smoking is one of the worst things you can do for your sex life (not to mention your lungs). Nicotine is a stimulant that restricts blood flow to the small blood vessels in the skin. It erodes your ability to feel skin sensations and impairs circulation to the point that many smokers have difficulty becoming aroused and having orgasms.

If you don't exercise on a regular basis, start walking. Try to take a brisk walk for fifteen or twenty minutes every day. Any exercise you can get will energize you and prepare you for lovemaking. As always, consult your physician before you begin any exercise program.

Nutrition

I believe that eating and drinking, like making love, are two of the greatest pleasures in life. Simple pleasures like these are the things you can share with your partner that make your daily life richer. I also believe that most people can enjoy delicious foods and drink superb wines without becoming obese or alcoholic. Have you ever heard of the so-called French paradox? The French are renowned for eating fatty foods and drinking wine, and yet for the most part they are healthier, thinner, and in better shape than most Americans. There are a lot of possible explanations for this phenomenon, one being that the French tend not to snack between meals, and, while growing up, tend to exercise more. And don't forget, the French are famous for their abilities as lovers as well. Could it be that they know something we don't about how pleasurable eating, drinking, and lovemaking fit into a healthy, cohesive lifestyle?

There is no doubt that nutrition is critical to maintaining a healthy body and overall well-being, so it is important that your nutritional needs are being met. Learn and follow the basics of good nutrition. Lots of resources are available in bookstores and online to help you do this. One extremely important dietary guideline that many Americans fail to follow is the necessity of eating plenty of fresh fruits and vegetables every day. Experts recommend getting at least five servings daily of veggies and fruits. Next time you're about to order a side of fries to go with your sandwich, quickly check in with yourself: Have you had your daily five? If not, why not order a fresh green salad instead? (And ask for about half as much salad dressing as usual—that's a good way to cut down on one source of fat in your diet.)

The popularity of the weight-loss segments on the *Dr. Phil* show illustrate the fact that so many people in the United States need to lose weight for health reasons. Are you severely overweight? I don't mean "pleasingly plump," which is normal and not unhealthy. If you are clinically overweight (20 to 40 percent or higher above the ideal weight for your height), it may put a damper on a satisfying sex life. That much excess weight can directly impair your ability not only to move around during lovemaking, but also to feel sensations in the genital area and to have erections and orgasms. Men who are severely overweight often find that the fat layer over their pelvic area reduces their penis length by several inches, which becomes a direct cause of problems in making love. (This condition is called *concealed,* or *hidden, penis.*)

Drugs

Drugs are nonnutritive substances that are intended to affect the structure or function of the body. They can be man-made or derived from plants. Drugs can be taken orally, injected, or administered in a number of other ways.

Many people believe that certain drugs are aphrodisiacs—substances that stimulate sexual desire. But aphrodisiacs do not exist. Sharing an occasional glass or two of wine or champagne with your partner may help the two of you loosen up and let go of the week's stressful events, as well as enhance feelings of pleasure in general, but excessive use of alcohol can cause problems with erections, ejaculation, and orgasm.

Some people report that they feel more sexual desire if they smoke marijuana or snort cocaine. Any positive effects from these drugs are short-term. The long-term effects of all illegal drugs is to impair your ability to make love, on top of compromising your physical and mental health.

What about prescription drugs? I've already gone into the effects of these on the specific sexual problems described in Chapters 5 through 13. Impaired sexual response is a side effect of many prescription drugs, including ulcer medications, high blood pressure medications, and even antihistamines. The selective serotonin reuptake inhibitors (SSRIs), such as Prozac, Paxil, and Zoloft, can impair both sexual desire and orgasm. If you are concerned about a current prescription you take, consult your physician to discuss your options.

I am not a health nut or fitness buff, and I generally prefer to spend my time talking about the positive effects of lovemaking; still, this is advice I must give: If you want your lovemaking to be better so that you share a powerful, healing bond with your partner, stop smoking; moderate your eating, drinking, and use of prescription medications; get some exercise; and don't use illegal drugs.

Sex-Muscle Exercises

The first stage of sexual fitness is getting yourself in reasonable physical shape, as discussed above. The second stage is getting your "sex muscles" in good shape. The *PC,* or *pubococcygeus, muscle group,* often called the *PC muscle* for short, runs from the pubic bone in the front of your body to the tailbone in the rear. It supports the floor of your pelvic cavity and your pelvic organs, and, more intriguingly, is the key to a longer-lasting, healing sexual union. Both men and women can do special exercises to strengthen, tone, and gain expert control over the PC muscle group.

➤ *Exercise 5.* PC MUSCLE EXERCISE FOR WOMEN

Before you can begin to exercise your PC muscle, you must locate it. Place one of your fingers lightly against your vaginal lips or inside your vagina up to the first knuckle. Pretend you are urinating and want to stop the flow. The muscle that tightens around your finger when you do this is the PC muscle. Internally, you should feel a drawing together or a drawing upward in your vaginal and pelvic area.

When you squeeze the PC muscle, make sure you are not also tensing your abdomen or thigh muscles at the same time. Also, remember to keep breathing regularly as you squeeze and relax. You should be able to tighten your PC muscle without its being obvious to anyone looking at you. Once you have located the PC muscle, there's no need to keep your hand on it as you tighten and relax it.

Three times a day, spend a few minutes flexing and relaxing your PC muscle twenty-five times. Squeeze the muscle, hold it for two seconds, and relax it for two seconds. Breathe deeply and steadily throughout. You can do these flexes anytime, anywhere—driving your car, waiting in line, brushing your teeth.

If you are older, overweight, or have had children, you may want to start with as few as five or ten repetitions, then work your way up to twenty-five. The PC muscle tires easily and may not relax fully each time when you first start to do the exercises, but it will tone up quickly. It is important to do this exercise every day for the rest of your life as a vital part of maintaining your sexual fitness.

A strong PC muscle offers many benefits for women. It tightens and tones the vagina, and gives you better bladder control. It also helps tone the vagina after giving birth. (These exercises were first developed by an obstetrician, Dr. A. H. Kegel, to help control incontinence in pregnant women and women who had just given birth, and they are often referred to as Kegel exercises.)

A strong PC muscle also makes it easier to have orgasms. In both men and women, flexing the PC muscle at the moment of orgasm intensifies the orgasm. This is because when your PC muscle is in shape, more blood can flow to the genital area, and more blood can be expelled from the genital area during orgasm. A toned PC muscle is essential if you are seeking sexual healing. And aside from all of the reasons listed above, doing the PC muscle exercises is fun and feels good.

    ~~ *Exercise 6.* PC MUSCLE EXERCISE FOR MEN

To locate your **PC** muscle, lightly place two fingers behind your testicles. Now imagine that you are urinating and want to stop the flow. The muscle that you squeeze internally to stop the flow is the PC muscle. Practice stopping and starting your urination a few times so that you know where this muscle group is located.

Every day, three times a day, flex and relax this muscle group twenty-five times. Now that you know where the muscle is, you won't have to touch it to exercise it. Make sure that you have isolated the muscle and that you are not tightening your abdomen, buttocks, or facial muscles during the exercise. Keep every other muscle in your body as relaxed as you can, and remember to breathe evenly as you squeeze and relax. It is easy to do this exercise. Tightening and relaxing the PC muscle should feel good; you may even feel slightly aroused, because when you exercise this muscle you are temporarily increasing blood flow into the genital area.

It may take you a while to work up to twenty-five repetitions. If you are older or overweight, you may want to start with only five or ten repetitions and then gradually work your way up. Don't do more than twenty-five repetitions at a time, or your PC muscle may get sore. It will take about three weeks for the muscle to get in shape, and then you really need to do this exercise every day for the rest of your life. It is an important part of maintaining your sexual fitness. Men whose PC muscle is in good shape can enjoy better erections, more sensation in the genital area, better ejaculation control, stronger orgasms, and even multiple orgasms.

Another important benefit of the PC muscle exercises for men is improved prostate health. The stronger your PC muscle is, the stronger your ejaculation will be, which means that your prostate gland is more likely to expel all of its contents during ejaculation. Men who have consistent, complete ejaculations tend to have fewer problems with prostate enlargement as they age.

If you are using the program outlined in this book to solve a specific sexual problem, the PC muscle exercises are essential for you. In therapy, the clients who learned most quickly to have orgasms, control their ejaculations, and have better erections were those who were diligent about exercising their PC muscle. Have I sold you on this exercise? I hope so.

ᥫᩬ *Exercise 7.* ADVANCED PC MUSCLE EXERCISE FOR MEN AND WOMEN

After you have done the basic PC muscle exercises for three or four weeks, try this more advanced version. In addition to twenty-five quick repetitions, add ten slow repetitions. Try to gradually tense the muscle for a count of five, hold it for a count of five, and then push it back out for a count of five. The first time you try this exercise you may only be able to do it once or twice. Eventually, you can work up to ten repetitions. Then try a version of the exercise where you tighten the PC muscle for a count of ten, hold it for a count of ten, and release it for a count of ten. It may take you days or weeks to accomplish this. How much time it takes doesn't matter; the improved muscle tone does.

ᥫᩬ *Exercise 8.* PELVIC THRUSTS

Another aspect of sexual fitness is to have strength in and control of the voluntary muscles in your pelvic area. People who experience sexual problems often unconsciously tighten the muscles in their pelvic area, which prevents blood from flowing in and prevents them from becoming as aroused as they could. The next three exercises—pelvic thrusts, rolls, and tilts—are for your abdomen, buttocks, and thigh muscles. They will help you loosen up and release the tension from those areas. They are good for both men and women.

Pelvic thrusts can be done either lying down or standing. The idea is to rock your pelvis from back to front without moving any other parts of your body. It is especially important to keep from tensing your stomach or leg muscles.

If you are lying down, bend your knees and put your feet flat on the floor, and rock your buttocks slowly up and down so that they are the only part of your body that moves off the floor or bed. Your lower back may also rise off the floor or bed a little bit. Do this as quickly or as slowly as you like and as many times as you like. You can thrust to music if you wish, or vary the speed of your thrusting.

The important thing is to keep all your other muscles relaxed and to keep your breathing regular. Do not hold your breath. To make sure you are breathing correctly, it may be helpful to grunt or make some other noise with each thrust.

If you want to do the pelvic thrusts while standing or walking, simply stand and rock your pelvis back and forth, or, as you walk, consciously thrust your pelvis forward with each step.

⤳ Exercise 9. PELVIC ROLLS

Pelvic rolls are similar to thrusts. Either lying down or standing, roll your hips backward-sideways-forward in a continuous motion. Think of Elvis Presley. If you have difficulty getting the hang of this movement, buy a hula hoop and practice with it. Practice pelvic rolls at different speeds, including doing them as slowly as you possibly can. And remember to breathe normally.

Combine thrusts and rolls, and do them to music if it feels good. Try to do a series of thrusts and rolls for ten minutes every day. Close your eyes while you do the exercises so you can really feel your body. The secret to doing these exercises is to thrust and roll your pelvis while still staying loose. Men, especially, tend to have tight hip muscles. Loosening them up can often increase your ability to become sexually aroused and have erections.

⤳ Exercise 10. PELVIC TILTS

The third pelvic exercise is the pelvic tilt. Lie on your back with your knees up. Keep your lower back on the floor, and practice tilting your pelvis up and down. This is similar to the pelvic thrust but your lower back stays on the floor and you use a smaller range of movement.

Pelvic tilts can also be done standing up. Simply hold your lower back in one position and tilt your pelvis back and forth.

Concerned about back problems? In my experience, most people can do pelvic thrusts, rolls, and tilts without risk, especially if they do them

slowly. If you have back problems, especially in your lower back, consult your physician before attempting them, and go easy.

⚬⚭⚬

A number of other exercises can be beneficial to lovemaking, particularly those that involve stretching, squatting, and spreading your legs. In general, any sport or physical exercise benefits your love life because it improves your cardiovascular conditioning, flexibility, body image, and general physical health and well-being. So if you already have a fitness program you are comfortable with, incorporate the PC muscle exercises and the pelvic exercises into it, and continue having fun.

An exception to this general guideline is cycling. Although cycling is good for aerobic conditioning, a lot of times it's not good for your sex life. Long sessions of cycling can put pressure on the nerves in your groin area and potentially interfere with erection and arousal. If you regularly cycle for long distances, and if you're experiencing sexual problems, you might want to consider switching to another fitness activity.

chapter 18

Self-Touch

Y ou are now ready for some exercises that will teach you more about your body and its natural sexual response. The sensual and sexual exercises presented in this chapter all involve learning to touch using the sensate-focus technique. You can practice these exercises by yourself before going on to the exercises you will do with your partner. You should do these exercises no matter what area of your sexuality you want to heal.

Before you start the exercises, let's review the sensate-focus principles from Chapter 14:

❋ Sensate-focus touch is slow.

❋ It is done for your own pleasure.

❋ It is free of psychological pressure or pressure to perform.

❋ It happens in the here and now.

❋ It is sensuous.

〰 *Exercise 11.* TOUCHING AN INANIMATE OBJECT

In this first exercise, you will touch an inanimate object. Doing so introduces you to sensate-focus touch and prepares you to work first with yourself and later with a partner. It may seem a little silly at first, but I have asked you to begin with an object, rather than your lover, so that when you progress to touching your partner you are not self-conscious. By the time you come together with your partner, touching in this healing way will be second nature.

Set aside about fifteen minutes during which you will not be disturbed. Pick two or three things to touch that look like they would feel good (a piece of velvet or a fur rug, for example). Place one of the objects on your lap. Let's say it's a piece of velvet. Lightly touch it with rhythmic strokes, as slowly as you can. Focus all of your attention on how your fingers feel on the velvet. Close your eyes. Don't think about what just happened or what is to come; simply be in the present.

Caress the velvet in as many different ways as you can think of—stroking with the nap, against the nap, up and down, in a circular motion. If your mind drifts, bring it back to what you are doing. Get in touch with sensuality—how this object feels good against your skin. You cannot caress too slowly. If you think you are moving your hand slowly enough, try cutting your speed in half and see how this affects your ability to focus on the touch.

Stop the exercise after fifteen minutes. Can you feel how relaxed you became from the simple act of touching? Your breathing and heart rate have slowed. This simple touching exercise has the same effect as meditation.

Instead of touching something soft like velvet or fur, you could try touching an object that is cold and hard, such as a small statue. I used to keep a small marble statue of a seal for clients to use. It was smooth, with a cool temperature that was pleasing to the touch, and it had lots of curves. Everyone who picked it up ended up naturally caressing their face with it because the cool temperature and smooth texture felt so good.

ᐱ *Exercise 12.* TOUCHING YOURSELF

To learn how you would like to be touched, and in preparation for the sensual exercises you will do later with your partner, it is important to practice sensate-focus caresses on yourself. Remember that the emphasis is sensual rather than sexual. By learning to touch yourself in a relaxing, gentle way, you will lay the foundation for all the exercises that follow.

Do you feel a little self-conscious caressing yourself? Many people do, especially when they move to their genitals and especially if they have never touched themselves in this way. This feeling is natural. Practicing the self-caress will make you more comfortable. It is very important to learn about your own bodily response so that you can increase your ability to become aroused and awaken your ability to heal yourself and your partner. Of course, as with any exercise, don't do anything that makes you uncomfortable.

Choose a setting where you will not be disturbed. Pick a small area of your body, such as your arm, your chest, or your thigh, for your first self-caress. For this exercise, don't touch your genitals. We'll get to them later. Put some lotion or massage oil on your fingertips, and slowly begin to touch yourself. Focus on the exact point of contact between your hand and your body. If your mind wanders off to something else, bring it back to exactly how your skin feels, both your fingertips and the skin being touched. Stroke yourself slowly and lightly. Touch only the skin—do not massage any muscles. Is your touch sensitive enough to feel your individual hairs? Think about what you feel right now, rather than anything you have been taught or remember from the past.

If you have trouble concentrating, slow down your touch. Use more lotion if your skin feels rough or dry. Spend fifteen minutes on this caress, learning the feeling of your own hand against your skin.

⌒ *Exercise 13.* TOUCHING YOUR GENITALS

In this exercise you will caress your genital area, but the touch you will use is different from masturbation. Many adults use masturbation as a comforting way to receive touch, but the genital caress is somewhat different. The goal is not to feel sexual, turn yourself on, or have an orgasm. The goal is to learn what kind of touch you like. What feels good to you? If you do this exercise with the healing mindset I talked about in Chapter 14, you will also learn that it is healthy—not selfish—to touch yourself.

Sit or lie naked in a comfortable position, in a comfortable space. Remember that caressing is not the same as masturbating. The purpose of this exercise is not to have an orgasm but to learn the different, pleasurable sensations of your body.

If you are a woman, warm some baby oil or other lubricant on your fingers and begin to slowly touch your inner thighs and your vaginal lips. If any part of your body feels tense, make a conscious effort to relax it. This caress may include only your outer genitals, or it may include stroking inside your vagina as well. You could do one caress on your vulva and a separate one on the inside of your vagina, and another one that includes both. Do whatever you are comfortable with and enjoy.

Concentrate on the touch exactly the way you did when you caressed the nongenital part of your body in the previous exercise. If your mind starts to wander off, slow down the movement of your hand and consciously bring your mind back to the point where skin touches skin. Try different touches. Touch yourself the way your partner usually touches you, then the way you usually touch yourself. Then touch yourself in a completely new way. Caress your outer and inner lips, your clitoris, and the opening of your vagina. Do not spend any more time on your clitoris than you do on other parts of your genitals.

Using plenty of lubrication, insert a finger into your vagina. See if you can feel some of the inner vaginal areas I described in Chapter 2, such as the A-spot and the G-spot. (You probably won't be able to feel your cervix or your cul de sac with your finger because they're deep inside.) Stroke the walls of your vagina and see if you can feel the muscle structure—the rugae I described in Chapter 2. Relax all your muscles and keep your breathing even. Concentrate on the landscape of your body—the changes in texture, temperature, and arousal as you touch different areas.

If you become sexually aroused, that is perfectly okay, but remember that this is not the goal. The only goals are to enjoy yourself and to learn about your body. If you become aroused, take a deep breath and make a conscious effort to relax your muscles. Gently, slowly, stroke yourself to feel maximum sensual awareness and sensual enjoyment. If you have an orgasm, that is okay. Do not try to make it happen, do not try to make it better or stronger, and do not try to push it away. Try not to tense up against it—just experience it. Continue the genital caress for about fifteen minutes.

If you are a man, use some baby oil or lotion on your fingers if you like. Slowly begin to caress your penis and scrotum, concentrating on the temperature and texture of your skin. Don't worry about whether you have an erection—you don't need one to do the exercise. You are just exploring the sensations your penis and scrotum are capable of feeling and which types of touch feel good.

Slowly stroke the head and shaft of your penis. Stroke the frenulum, the sensitive area on the underside of your penis where the head meets the shaft. Keep your attention on the exact point of contact between your fingers and your genitals. If your mind wanders off, slow the movement of your hand and bring your mind back to the touch. Experiment with different types of touch. Touch yourself the way you usually do, the way your partner does, and in as many different ways as you can.

Keep all of the muscles in your body relaxed, and breathe evenly. If you feel yourself approaching orgasm, that is okay. Don't try to make it happen, don't try to make it better, and don't push it away. Just allow orgasm to wash over you. Continue this caress for fifteen minutes.

Congratulations! You've taken the first step toward sexual healing. Pretty easy, wasn't it? After completing these exercises, most people experience heightened sexual awareness. A lot of people feel better about themselves immediately. Still others see themselves as more sensual and sexual. A few people have very intense experiences with these exercises. The genital caress may bring up feelings of sadness or tearfulness. If so, just feel the feelings and let them pass through you. And don't worry: This is part of the sexual healing process.

Developing Arousal Awareness

You are now ready to learn a process called *peaking*. Arousal awareness is the first step in the peaking process. Peaking is the basis for treating many of the sexual dysfunctions, including desire problems, arousal problems, and problems with orgasm. Peaking is really the foundation for the sexual healing program. In Chapters 23 through 31, which deal with healing specific sexual dysfunctions, I'll talk about how to use arousal awareness and peaking to heal each specific sexual problem.

Peaking is a process in which you allow your sexual arousal to go up and down in a predictable and controllable wavelike pattern. Before you can learn to peak, you must be able to recognize how sexually aroused you are. Furthermore, it's easiest to learn the peaking process by yourself using self-touch. Then you can use it with any kind of stimulation from your partner—manual caressing, oral sex, or intercourse.

To develop arousal awareness, think of your sexual arousal on a scale from 1 to 10, with a 1 being no arousal and a 10 being orgasm. For men, it is important that you notice how aroused you feel, regardless of how strong your erection is. You can learn to recognize feelings of arousal internally or emotionally without having to look at your erection.

The following guidelines will help you recognize how aroused you are: At levels 2 and 3 you feel mild twinges of arousal, but arousal is not really constant. Levels 4 and 5 are constant, low levels of arousal, and levels 6 and 7 are steady, moderate arousal. At levels 6 and 7 you really feel that you don't want the stimulation to stop. At level 8, if you had to talk, you would sound somewhat out of breath. You are aware of your heartbeat and you feel the blood roaring in your ears. Level 8 corresponds to Masters and Johnson's plateau phase of the sexual response cycle. Level 9 is the feeling that you are very close to orgasm. Anything beyond level 9 is the feeling that orgasm is inevitable.

It doesn't matter which number you reach on the arousal scale either the first time or any time you do the arousal awareness exercise. What is important is that you start to get a sense of how close you are to orgasm or how far you are from orgasm. If you only reach level 2 or 3, that is fine. If you immediately go straight to level 10, that's fine also. The important thing is that you concentrate on the touch at the moment and let arousal happen as it will, without trying to make it better or push it away.

The fact that I am asking you to describe your sensual and sexual arousal on a 1-to-10 scale may sound contradictory to what I said earlier in the book about not putting pressure on yourself. Please don't get the impression that I am asking you to grade or evaluate yourself or your performance in any way. The numbers are to help you *describe* your sexual response, not rate it. For example, reaching a level 9 during any exercise is not better than reaching a level 3. The idea is not to see how high you can go, but rather to become aware of the difference in how you feel at the different levels. I use numbers because most people understand the concept of a 1-to-10 scale and find it easy to use.

∿ *Exercise 14.* AROUSAL AWARENESS DURING SELF-TOUCH

To do the arousal awareness exercise, repeat the genital caress by yourself, extending the time to twenty minutes. As you caress yourself, give numbers to the different states of arousal you feel. Every five minutes or so, ask yourself, "Where am I now? What is my arousal level?" Use the sensate-focus method for your caresses. Keep your attention focused on how your skin feels, and allow your awareness of how aroused you are to come and go as it will. Focus on the touch. Relax. Breathe. Keep your body as still as possible. If you go all the way to orgasm, try to experience it without moving your body or tensing up.

∿ *Exercise 15.* PEAKING

During peaking, you manipulate your arousal levels to go up and down predictably in a wavelike pattern. To begin, relax, breathe, and caress yourself the way you did for the arousal awareness exercise. When you feel you are at level 3, stop caressing and note that your arousal drops back down a couple of levels. Caress yourself again until you feel you are at arousal level 4. Again, stop the caress and allow your arousal to go back down a couple of levels. Continue through all the levels if you can, stopping at each one to allow the arousal to drop a level or two—5, 6, 7, 8, 9, and 10 (orgasm). Remember to keep your caress as slow as possible and to focus on the touch. Spend about five minutes on each peak, including both the up and down phases.

In the peaking process, the phase in which you allow your arousal level to go down is as important as the phase in which it goes up. Feelings or emotions of all kinds can be defined as changes in bodily states and mental states. We perceive feelings to a large degree in terms of contrast. Letting your arousal decrease and then allowing it to come back up provide the contrast you need in order to be able to recognize how aroused you are.

Allow plenty of time for your arousal to go down, even though you may be tempted to forget about the exercise and go all the way to orgasm. When you begin to caress yourself for each new peak, be sure to start slowly.

⌒ Exercise 16. PLATEAUING

Plateauing is an advanced form of peaking in which you recognize an arousal level and try to stay at that level for a few seconds or even a minute or two. Like peaking, plateauing begins with a genital self-caress. As you did in the peaking exercise, focus on the touch, relax, and breathe.

Do a couple of low-level peaks (levels 3 and 4). When you reach level 5, stop the caress and let your arousal go down, but only to level 4. Then start the caress again and allow your arousal to go up to level 6. Keep hovering between levels 4 and 6 by stopping and starting the caress. After a while, see if you can recognize the finer distinctions, such as level 4½ or 5½.

See if you can plateau at higher levels like 6, 7, 8, and 9 just by stopping and starting your caress. Do the plateauing exercise for twenty to thirty minutes. If you want, let yourself go all the way up to orgasm at the end of the exercise.

Now is a good time to remind you to make sure you don't pressure yourself during any exercise. It's easy to feel a sense of pressure during plateauing because of all of the stopping and starting and thinking about numbers. Remember that your only goal here is healing. It doesn't matter which levels you reach during any peaking or plateauing session. The important things are taking the pressure off yourself and learning to recognize your arousal levels. Depending on what sexual problem or problems you are dealing with, the sexual healing program will call for you to repeat the peaking and plateauing exercises many times with different types of stimulation.

Besides starting and stopping your caress, there are several other ways to teach yourself to maintain a desired level of arousal. You can plateau by changing your breathing, squeezing your PC muscle, or switching your focus from the area you are caressing to another part of your body. I'll explain these techniques in more detail in the chapters on dealing with particular problems, but here are a few simple versions you can start practicing now.

When you reach a level at which you would like to plateau, take a couple of slow, deep breaths. This will cause your arousal to go down about half a level. When your arousal has gone down half a level, speed up your breathing so you are almost panting. See if you can maintain your arousal at a particular level by alternating between breathing slowly and more quickly.

You can also plateau by squeezing your PC muscle. When you reach a level at which you would like to plateau, give your PC muscle a couple of quick squeezes. This will take your arousal down about half a level. When your arousal is down about half a level, continue the stimulation and allow your arousal to go back up. When you get beyond the desired level, squeeze your PC muscle again. See if you can plateau at a particular level by squeezing your PC muscle and then relaxing it. (Note: The PC muscle plateauing technique should not be used by men who have difficulty ejaculating.)

A final way to plateau is to switch your focus from the area of your body you are caressing to an area you are not currently caressing. Let's say you are a woman and you are caressing your clitoris. When you reach a level at which you would like to plateau, keep stroking your clitoris, but mentally shift your focus to an area you are not touching, such as your inner vaginal lips. See if you can keep your focus on one area as you touch another area. This will take your arousal down about half a level. When that happens, resume focusing on the area you are touching. See if you can maintain your arousal at a desired level by switching your focus back and forth between an area you are touching and an area you are not touching.

Nontouching Suggestions to Promote Sexual Healing

In addition to learning to touch yourself, you can use journaling and affirmations in your sexual healing process. Remember from Chapter 1 that sex therapy as Masters and Johnson pioneered it is cognitive-behavioral therapy. This means that sex therapy includes ways to change both your behavior and your thinking. The sensate-focus touching exercises are obviously the behavioral part of the therapy. And because our minds and bodies can't be separated, changing your behavior also changes the way you think about yourself.

But you can also change your thoughts in a more direct way. One technique for doing so is journaling. This simply means keeping a diary of the exercises you do and the thoughts you have as you move through the process. Another cognitive-therapy technique is using affirmations, or positive self-talk. In this technique you make lists of positive statements about your progress in the sexual healing program as well as about goals for the future.

Examples of affirmations are statements such as, "I feel good about myself," or, "I enjoy touching myself." These would be appropriate statements to use at this point in your sexual healing journey. As you move farther into the book and begin to work on your specific sexual problems, the statements could become much more specific and sexual, such as, "I feel good when I have an erection," "I can last as long as I want to during intercourse," or, "When my partner touches me, I get really aroused." The way to use these statements is to write them down in a list, look in a mirror, and say the statements out loud to yourself several times a day. I won't give you a list of specific statements to use, because they're much more powerful if you make them up yourself based on your individual needs. It's a good idea to write new statements every time you complete a new exercise or step in your process.

chapter 19

Basic Partner Exercises: Spoon Breathing and the Face Caress

The next four chapters contain the basic sensate-focus exercises you will do with your partner. I've purposely broken this section into smaller chapters so you don't get overwhelmed. Each basic sensate-focus partner exercise introduces some new elements. All of them will help you gradually learn to reduce your anxiety in sensual and sexual situations.

When these exercises are assigned to couples in sex therapy, the therapist uses them not only for treatment purposes but also for additional diagnosis. Often, just doing these basic exercises can pinpoint issues that you and your partner may not have been aware of.

All of the descriptions of the exercises in these four chapters include a lot of detail about what you might experience from a psychological standpoint. They also include detailed information about feedback that you and your partner can give each other after the exercises. No matter what specific sexual problem you are healing, use the structure of these exercises as a model for doing the later sensate-focus exercises.

⌒ *Exercise 17.* SPOON BREATHING

Lie together with your partner on a comfortable bed or couch with one person's back snuggled up against the other person's front. Lie with your legs bent so that you fit together, like two spoons in a drawer. The person who is in back places his or her hand on the stomach of the person in front. Lie perfectly still and do not talk or squirm around, even if you feel yourself becoming aroused. The purpose of this exercise is relaxation. Pay attention to either your own breathing or your partner's breathing. Slow your breathing down by taking three or four deep breaths and exhaling forcefully.

Make sure that all of your muscles are relaxed by concentrating on each leg and imagining that it is sinking into the bed. Also picture your shoulders sinking into the bed.

This exercise is a prelude to sensate focus in that you should keep your attention on the overall sensations of warmth and closeness that come from lying next to your partner. The breathing you do in this exercise is the same type you learned to do in Chapter 16, on relaxation, only now you are doing it with a partner. Can you become as relaxed with your partner as you did when you breathed by yourself?

In general, spoon breathing may be done clothed or in the nude, but for the first partner session, in which you do the face caress (Exercise 18), you should spoon breathe with your clothes on. Spoon breathing will help you make the transition from any activities you were doing to a relaxed, neutral state. Spoon breathe before doing any partner exercise, between switching active and passive roles in any exercise, and again after the exercise. Alternate being the person in back and the person in front. Do not do this exercise while watching television or doing anything else. Devote your full attention to relaxation and listening to your body. Spoon breathe for five to ten minutes. After you have spoon breathed for about five minutes, you'll notice that your breathing will tend to synchronize with that of your partner.

◠◡ *Exercise 18.* THE FACE CARESS

The first partner sensate-focus exercise is called the face caress. To do this caress, you will need some type of skin lotion that both you and your partner like. You will also need to find a quiet, comfortable room in which to do the exercise. Take the phone off the hook and send the kids to the babysitter. You need a room in which you will not be disturbed for forty-five minutes to an hour. You will also need a clock or watch so that you can time the exercise.

The person who will be active first should sit with his or her head against a headboard or wall, with a pillow on his or her lap. The passive partner should lie between the active partner's legs, head on the pillow, face up. It is important to have the passive partner's face within easy reach of the active partner. The exercise is done fully clothed, but you will want to take off your shoes and belt so that it is comfortable to lie down.

The face caress includes everything from the top of the head to the base of the neck. The active person should begin by taking some of the lotion and warming it up in her hand (let's assume the woman is the active partner first). Then caress your partner's face. Remember, to caress means to use an extremely slow and sensuous touch. Simply touch the skin rather than trying to feel or massage the muscles underneath the skin.

You are already familiar with the general instructions for sensate-focus exercises from Chapter 14, but I'll repeat them here:

* ✳ Sensate-focus touch is slow.

* ✳ It is done for your own pleasure.

* ✳ It is free of psychological pressure of any sort.

* ✳ It is focused.

* ✳ It happens in the here and now.

* ✳ It is sensuous.

To begin the face caress as the active partner, slowly move one or both hands across your partner's forehead and down his cheeks. Move across his chin and down to his neck. Don't neglect his ears. Many people find touching or stroking another person's ears to be a very sensual experience. Caress the bridge of your partner's nose, his eyelids, and underneath his eyes. Remember to caress as slowly as you can. Continue the face caress for fifteen to twenty minutes, stop and spoon breathe again, and then switch roles. Spend fifteen to twenty minutes in each role.

What you are learning to do here is to focus as completely as you can on the sensations in your skin, both when you are active and when you are passive. Pay attention to the exact point of contact between your skin and your partner's skin.

When you are the active partner, caress for your own pleasure. Caress your partner's face in a way that feels good to you. Do not worry about what your partner is thinking or try to make your partner feel good. Your partner will tell you if you do anything that is unpleasant. If your partner does not say anything during the exercise, you may assume that your caress feels good or at least neutral.

Because you are probably not used to this type of activity, you may find it hard to focus at first. Your mind may wander off to work or household tasks. If this happens, it is not a problem. Just recognize that you have become distracted and bring your focus back to the touch. When you are active, one way to relieve boredom or distraction is to consciously slow the speed of your caress by half. One thing your mind should not be wandering off to is whether you will be disturbed during the exercise. Make sure that the place you choose in which to do the exercise is free of distractions. You should feel completely free to lie back and enjoy the exercise.

In order to learn to focus as fully as you can on the touch, it is best to cut down on stimulation to the other senses. For example, do not play music while you are doing the caress. Most people find it pleasant to listen to music, but for now we are trying to remove any sensory input that will compete with the caress. You will also want to close your eyes during at least part of the caress in order to concentrate more fully on the touch.

Talking is almost always a distraction during a sensate-focus exercise. If you are the passive partner, the only time you should talk during the caress is if your partner does something that hurts or bothers you. If you are the active partner, you should not talk at all, except to say, "I'm done now." Don't ask your partner, "Is this okay?" or, "Do you want me to use lotion?" Do what you want to do and don't worry about your partner. Trust that your partner will tell you if something is bothering him or her. Touch in the way that feels best for you.

When you are the passive partner, your only assignment is to relax and enjoy the caress. It is not necessary to tell your partner what a great job he or she is doing. Telling your partner how wonderful you feel during the caress or finding some nonverbal way to say it (such as moaning or moving around) will only put performance pressure on your partner.

Here are some issues that commonly come up for couples as early in the program as the face caress. The first, as I have mentioned, is distracting thoughts. It is natural to have thoughts about other things during a caress. The important thing is to recognize that this is happening and bring your attention back to the touch. Sometimes the thoughts will be about the exercise, for example, "I wonder if he's thinking about touching my breasts," or, "I wonder if this will really help my sex life." If you are having thoughts of this type, it means you are not enjoying what is happening with the caress in the here and now. Rather, you are looking into the future, or, perhaps, worrying about the past ("Gee, it felt really good when she stroked my ears. I wonder if she'll do that again"). The solution for distracting thoughts is to bring your mind back to the touch.

It is also natural to feel some anxiety when beginning a caress. Do not expect to immediately relax completely, even if you did a few minutes of spoon breathing beforehand. It may take several minutes for you to become relaxed enough so that you can enjoy the caress. This is why each partner will normally take each role for at least fifteen to twenty minutes.

When you are the active partner, take just a moment to notice whether your partner seems to be relaxed at the beginning of the caress. Later, notice whether there are any changes in your partner during the caress; for example, has your partner's breathing become slower and more regular? This is a sign that he or she is relaxing. Many people become so relaxed during the face caress that they start to fall asleep. You might find it restful and enjoyable to sleep, but by doing so you will not learn anything from the exercise. If you are active and your partner begins to fall asleep, gently tap him or her on the shoulder.

If you find that the opposite is true and you just cannot relax during the exercise, tell your partner. Switch roles and see if this helps you to relax, or go back to some more spoon breathing. There is no point in continuing an exercise if you are wound up so tightly that you can't relax, even when you slow down your breathing, loosen your muscles, and focus on the touch. Stop for now and come back to the exercise later.

The face caress is an exercise in sensuality, not sexuality. If you become sexually aroused during the face caress, this is fine. If you have severe premature ejaculation and you ejaculate during the face caress or any other exercise, this is also fine. Be aware of your arousal, but do not try to make it better and do not try to get rid of it or contain it in some way. Focus on the part of your body that is being touched at that moment, rather than on your genitals.

Feedback

After each exercise, you and your partner will give each other feedback about how you felt. The feedback questions for all of the exercises are discussed in detail in Chapter 15, but I'll review them here. Don't forget to write the questions and answers in your journal. Use the following guidelines to discuss the face caress, the back caress, the front caress, and the genital caress.

1. When you were passive, were you able to relax totally and to refrain from moving around? Or did you feel compelled to do something to convince your partner that he or she was doing a good job?

2. When you were active, did you take pleasure for yourself rather than worrying about whether your partner was enjoying the caress? When you are active, you should be able to take pleasure for yourself most of the time.

3. Which role were you more comfortable with, the active or the passive role? Was it easier for you to focus in one role than the other?

4. What percentage of the time were you able to focus on the touch when you were active? When you were passive? Ideally, you should be able to focus on the touch over 50 percent of the time. If you are not able to focus this much, repeat the exercise as many times as you need to until your concentration improves.

It may be helpful to examine the types of thoughts that are interfering with your concentration. If mundane things intrude, such as the laundry or the shopping list, you probably just haven't had enough practice focusing. It may take a few sessions. If you are having thoughts or anxiety about your sexual problems or about future exercises, this is normal. Tell yourself you can worry about these things at some other time, so they don't interfere with your focusing. Use the trash can/deep freeze technique you read about in Chapter 15 to help rid yourself of intrusive thoughts. Some people who have anxiety disorders related to their sexual problems (see Chapter 6) may actually need antianxiety medication in order to focus at the level necessary to do the sexual exercises.

Finally, many of us have trouble focusing on one thing because we are so used to multitasking—talking on the phone while eating or driving, or using a computer and a personal organizer at the same time. The sexual healing program is the exact opposite of multitasking. The most important thing you learn to do in this program is to give your full attention to only one thing at a time. Being able to return to this ability will improve the quality of your life in general.

5. Did you feel anxious during the caress? Were you able to deal with the anxiety by focusing, breathing, and relaxing? (See number 9, below, for more guidelines about dealing with various issues, including anxiety.) Could you feel yourself becoming less anxious as the caress went on? The important thing is not how high or low your anxiety level was at any point during the caress. The important thing is that you are less anxious after the caress than before.

6. If you felt sexually aroused during the caress, did you just accept it and keep your attention on where you were being touched, or did you try either to make the arousal better or to get rid of it?

7. Did you enjoy the caress? Did you feel pressured to perform when you were active, or did you touch your partner the way you wanted to touch him or her? When you were passive, did you feel pressured to respond and tell your partner how great it was, or did you feel free to just relax and accept pleasure for yourself?

8. Was it easy for you to stay within the bounds of the exercise, or did you want to touch areas other than the face? Did you stay within the limits? It is natural to want to continue and do something more sexual, but in order to build trust, it is important to do what you both agree to do in the beginning.

9. Did you have a problem with feeling anxious? If so, you need to focus on your breathing. Did you have a problem remaining passive? If so, you need to relax the muscles in your stomach, thighs, and buttocks. Did you have a problem with staying in the here and now? Did you want to please your partner? Were you working at doing a good job? If so, you need to practice focusing on the touch. Did you have a problem focusing? You may need to caress more slowly. Most of the problems you encounter during any sensate-focus exercise can be resolved by three familiar words: focus, breathe, relax.

꒭

The face caress will help you identify any problems you may have at a basic level because it is nonsexual and nonthreatening. If you were able to focus and relax, if your anxiety level decreased as a result of the spoon breathing and the face caress, if neither of you felt much performance pressure, and if you stayed within the limits of the exercise, you should go on to the next exercise, in Chapter 20, which is the back caress. If answering these feedback questions pinpointed some problem areas for you, you may want to repeat the face caress until you become completely comfortable with it.

And finally, here is a time sequence to remind you how to do the face caress and most of the subsequent sensate-focus exercises:

* *Spoon breathing:* five to ten minutes

* *Face caress, first partner:* twenty minutes

* *Spoon breathing:* five to ten minutes

* *Face caress, second partner:* twenty minutes

* *Spoon breathing:* five to ten minutes

* *Feedback*

chapter 20

Basic Partner Exercises: The Back Caress

S
o far in this program you have done relaxation exercises, sexual fitness exercises, self-touch exercises, and spoon breathing and the face caress with your partner. Spoon breathing is done to give you a chance to relax and make the transition from the everyday stresses of your life to a mode in which you will be receptive to sensual arousal. During the face caress, you learned to focus on touch and practiced active and passive roles.

The back caress will introduce several new elements. It is the first sensate-focus exercise that you will do in the nude, and it is the first sensate-focus exercise that involves parts of the body you may already associate with sexual arousal, for example, the buttocks.

∾ Exercise 19. THE BACK CARESS

To do the back caress, you need a bed or some other comfortable surface with plenty of room for both of you to stretch out. This whole session will take about an hour. As always, you need a quiet room where you won't be disturbed; you also need a large towel and possibly some talcum powder.

The back caress is done in the nude, and includes the entire back of the body from the neck to the feet, but not the genitals. First, to relax, do some spoon breathing for about five minutes. Decide which partner will be active first. The passive partner should lie comfortably, face down, with a towel underneath his or her body. The passive partner keeps the arms at his or her sides or underneath the head. The active partner should lie on his or her side next to the passive partner and maintain as much body contact as possible during the exercise.

Remember the basics: focus, breathe, relax.

Let's say the man is active first. Begin to stroke your partner's back with one hand. Slowly run your palm or your fingers over your partner's shoulder blades and then down her spine. Remember, this is not a massage. The object is to use your hand to feel as good as you possibly can by touching the back of your partner's body.

The way I usually do the back caress is to snuggle up against my partner and use my hand to reach as many parts of his back as I can. Then I change positions so I can touch his legs and feet. I usually use some type of baby powder or body powder to do the back caress. It increases the sensual arousal for me because my hands tend to perspire, which makes my touch a little rough. You can decide for yourself whether you think powder would feel good.

Some authors recommend doing the back caress with the active partner straddling the partner's back and using both hands. I find that I get much more feeling when I do the caress as I have described—lying up against my partner and exerting a minimum of physical effort. I find that doing a back caress in a traditional massage position (straddling my partner) tends to set the exercise up as a performance situation right at the beginning, and then the expectation is conveyed to your partner that he or she must respond. Also, if you do the caress as I suggest, you will be much more comfortable and you won't get sore leg muscles from sitting or kneeling. This leaves you free to enjoy more sensual arousal.

When you are the active partner, caress your partner's back, buttocks, and legs for your own pleasure. Think of your partner's body as a playground and touch anywhere that feels good to you. You will maximize your ability to focus on sensations if you close your eyes during the caress. Remember to stroke your partner's body slowly. If you have trouble focusing, consciously slow your caressing motion down to half the speed it was before. If thoughts about whether your partner is enjoying the exercise intrude, bring your mind back to the exact point of contact between your skin and your partner's skin.

Pay attention to how your partner's different body parts feel when you slowly stroke them with your palm versus your fingertips. Some areas on the back of your partner's body that may feel especially good to touch include the back of the neck, the spine, and the thighs right underneath the buttocks. You may find that different parts of your partner's back feel especially good to you.

As a variation, you could use your upper body to caress, in addition to just your hand. Use your hair, face, or chest to caress if you can do it for your own enjoyment without worrying about whether your partner likes it.

Pay attention to temperature and texture. Run your fingers around the depression at the base of your partner's spine. Run the tip of one finger slowly up your partner's backbone. You may want to conclude the caress with a final gesture, like a soft pinch on your partner's earlobe, or by running your fingers through your partner's hair.

If you are doing the back caress and you feel or see your partner's body tensing up (for example, as you touch his or her thighs, you see the muscles tighten), lightly pinch or press down on the tense area as a reminder to your partner to relax. You should be able to notice your partner tightening up or moving around. Remind your partner to breathe, and continue with the caress.

When you are the passive partner, enjoy yourself. Allow yourself to soak up the sensations like a sponge. Breathe evenly and relax your muscles. Keep your mind on the exact point of contact where your partner is touching you. Try not to move. Just passively accept stimulation into your body. The only time you need to communicate with your partner is if he or she does something that bothers you or hurts you.

If you become sexually aroused during the back caress, fine. Just enjoy the arousal and bring your mind back to the exact point of contact between you and your partner. We are not concerned with sexual arousal yet. What we are doing is practicing sensate focus so that it becomes natural whenever you touch your partner or whenever you are touched. We are building a foundation so that when you move on to exercises that are more overtly sexual, you will naturally focus on how your body feels when you touch or are touched.

Each partner should do the back caress for about twenty minutes. Spoon breathe for a few minutes both between role changes and again at the end of the exercise. Please continue at this point to observe the instructions for active and passive roles. There should not be any mutual caressing yet. Finish the exercise by discussing the feedback questions with your partner and recording the answers in your journal.

The most common problem when doing the back caress is using a massage technique rather than caressing. The goal is not to manipulate the muscles underneath the skin in order to make the person being massaged feel good. The idea is rather for your skin to become alive with sensations. You should not even be aware of muscles—you should just be aware of skin.

A more serious problem is failure to stay within the limits of the exercise. For example, did either partner reach between the legs and attempt to caress the genitals? The genitals are not part of the back caress, and when you include parts of the body that are not in the exercise, you put performance demands on your partner and interfere with the ability of both of you to focus on sensations, to enjoy the caress, and to learn from the exercise. If you touch your partner's genitals during the back caress, you are jumping ahead to a future exercise, which means you aren't staying in the here and now. You need to learn the basics of sensate focus first. Furthermore, if you go beyond the limits of an exercise, your partner will go into a vigilant, spectatoring mode, instead of being able to enjoy and focus, and will wonder, "Will he keep doing this? Should I say something about this now?" This vigilance response is a sign of anxiety and is physiologically incompatible with the relaxation that is necessary to enjoy sensate-focus exercises.

Underlying this problem of jumping ahead is feeling sexually aroused and thinking that you have to do something about it. If you do experience sexual arousal during the back caress or any other sensate-focus exercise, just enjoy it. As the passive partner, you should not wiggle around or push yourself against your partner's hand or the bed. Men, if you get so aroused during the caress that you get an erection or even ejaculate, just enjoy it. Don't try to push the arousal away or make it better somehow. Women, if you lubricate or feel aroused, just enjoy it and continue the exercise. Contrary to popular belief, nothing bad will happen to you if you become aroused and don't have an orgasm. You don't need to experience sexual arousal in order to learn from the caress, but if it happens you can still complete the exercise.

Another problem you may encounter in doing the back caress is the presence of anxiety. Your partner in the active role will notice if you are tensing the muscles in your thighs or buttocks during the exercise. Other signs of anxiety include rapid breathing that does not slow down or squirming or twitching during the caress. What can you do to get rid of the anxiety? If you are the active partner and you notice your partner tensing up, moving around, or breathing rapidly after the exercise has gone on for a few minutes, stop the caress and talk quietly to your partner about it. If your partner is feeling some anxiety, go back to spoon breathing for a few minutes, or do some deep breathing of the kind you learned in Chapter 16.

To review: Did you have a problem with anxiety? If so, you need to focus on your breathing. Did you have a problem remaining passive? If so, you need to relax your muscles. Did you try to please your partner? Did you have a problem staying in the here and now? Were you trying to do a good job? You need to practice focusing on the touch. Did you become distracted? You need to practice a slower touch. Remember, focus, breathe, and relax.

In the initial sensate-focus exercises such as the back caress, people with specific sexual concerns may find it difficult not to be preoccupied with their issues. For example, if you are having erection problems, your biggest concern may be whether or not you are getting an erection. Remember, we are not concerned with erections yet and it is not necessary to have an erection during the back caress.

If your problem is premature ejaculation, you may be worried that you will ejaculate during an exercise. If you feel any sexual arousal at all during an exercise, don't try to make it better and don't try to push it away. Just accept it. It's all right if you ejaculate during any sensate-focus exercise as long as you don't try to stop it. If your problem is inhibited ejaculation, you may be tempted to go beyond the limits of an exercise to something more sexual. Keep the sensate-focus exercises separate from any sexual activities you may do later.

If you are a woman and your problem is the inability to have an orgasm, your biggest concern during the back caress will probably be whether or not you are aroused. Don't try to become more aroused than you are, but if you feel arousal don't try to push it away. Remain passive when you are in the passive role, and when you are active don't try to turn yourself on. Just enjoy the touch.

If you have vaginismus or a phobia about sexual activity, anxiety may be your biggest concern during this exercise. Your partner can help you monitor your anxiety level and help you make sure that you are breathing evenly and that your muscles stay relaxed.

Here is a time sequence for the back caress and many of the subsequent exercises:

* *Spoon breathing:* five to ten minutes

* *Back caress, first partner:* twenty minutes

* *Spoon breathing:* five to ten minutes

* *Back caress, second partner:* twenty minutes

* *Spoon breathing:* five to ten minutes

* *Feedback*

chapter 21

Basic Partner Exercises: The Front Caress

The next exercise is the front caress, which includes casual genital touching. The new element that is introduced in this exercise is caressing the front of the body. Most people associate areas on the front of the body with sexuality. In addition, most people feel somewhat vulnerable when they are on their back with their breasts and genitals exposed. This exercise may trigger some performance pressure or a perceived need to please your partner.

ᕫ Exercise 20. THE FRONT CARESS

You will need to set aside an hour to an hour and a half for this session. You will need a quiet room, talcum powder, a towel, and some baby oil or mineral oil.

Before you do the front caress, do a few minutes of spoon breathing to relax. Then each partner can do a focusing caress to become even more relaxed. A focusing caress is a shortened version of a nonsexual caress done to make a transition into a new, more sexual exercise. The focusing caress can be either a face caress or a back caress. You may each decide which you would like to do. You should each do a focusing caress for ten minutes prior to the first active partner starting the front caress.

For the front caress, the passive partner should lie on his or her back in a relaxed position. The front caress includes the whole front of the body from head to feet. It also includes the genitals, but only in a "casual" way, which means that you do not spend any more time on the genitals than you do on any other part of the front of the body. If you use baby powder on the front of your partner's body, when you begin to caress the genitals use the towel to wipe the baby powder off your hands, and use baby oil to caress the genitals. The front caress does not include finger penetration of the vagina; it is a sensual exercise and is not done to arouse your partner sexually.

The instructions for the front caress are the same as for the back caress. The active partner should lie next to the passive partner and maintain as much full body contact as possible. Use some talcum powder on your hand and on your partner's body if you tend to perspire. The active partner should slowly stroke the passive partner's body, beginning with the face, neck, shoulders, and arms, and moving down across the chest, stomach, abdomen, and genitals to the thighs, calves, and feet.

Caress as slowly and lightly as possible. It is important to be systematic; don't jump from the feet to the head but rather proceed down the body, caressing one part at a time. It is also important to maintain contact with your partner's body. Keep your hand on your partner as much as possible so as to avoid touches that are surprising or startling. Maintaining contact on your partner's body with your hand also helps him or her to relax.

Touch for your own pleasure. Think of your partner's body as a playground and touch whatever parts feel good, in the way that feels best for you. You may use your palm, fingers, back of your hand, or arm. Toward the end of the caress you may want to kneel and caress your partner's body with your face, hair, or chest. This can be very sensuous. Don't concern yourself with what your partner is thinking or feeling during the caress. Your partner will tell you if you do something that makes him or her uncomfortable.

Your partner will feel pressured to respond if you caress too rapidly or too roughly. Avoid putting pressure on your partner, and maximize your own enjoyment by caressing as slowly and gently as you can. Focus on the exact point of contact between your skin and your partner's skin. If your mind wanders to other things, bring it back to the exact point of contact. If you do the caress for your own enjoyment and focus as well as you can, your partner will enjoy the caress also.

When you are passive, your only task is to relax and enjoy the caress. Focus on the exact point of contact between your skin and your partner's skin. The only time you need to say anything to your partner is if he or she does something that bothers you or hurts you. Otherwise, try to relax and breathe while remaining receptive and still. If you feel yourself tensing up, slow your breathing down and imagine your leg muscles sinking into the bed.

If you are in the active role, you may notice that your partner is not relaxing. Some signs that your partner is anxious include muscle tension, rapid breathing, rapid heart rate, and a quivering stomach. If you see that your partner's body is tense, lightly pinch or press on the body part that is tense to signal your partner to relax. Your partner may not even be aware that he or she is tense.

The front caress has more potential to produce anxiety than the back caress. When we lie on our backs, our chests and genitals are exposed and we feel vulnerable. One thing you can do to promote relaxation in your passive partner is to slow your touch down. Another is to slowly stroke your partner's abdominal area in a circular motion. At the same time, remember that you are not trying to "fix" your partner. Your biggest concern should be touching in a way that feels good for you. Take a few deep breaths yourself—your partner will probably imitate your breathing. If the front caress becomes too anxiety-producing, back up to an earlier exercise, or back up to a body part that is less threatening to touch, such as the face, until your own or your partner's breathing has slowed.

Because the front caress has the potential to be sexual, there will be more temptation to slip back into your old habits of touching. You may find yourself trying to turn your partner on. This will make it more difficult for your partner to stay in the here and now because he or she may think, "I wonder if he will touch my genitals again?" or, "Oh, no, she's heading down toward my penis."

It may also be more difficult to remain passive than it was in previous exercises because you may be used to moving around or moaning when your breasts or genitals are touched. Allow yourself to experience the arousal without trying to do anything about it. If you feel aroused, don't try to make it better by moving around, and don't try to push it away. By remaining passive you are teaching your body to feel as much arousal as it can possibly feel. If you move around at this stage you will lower your arousal level rather than make it stronger.

You will have different concerns during the front caress depending on which sexual problems you experience. If you are a woman who is having orgasm problems, it may be difficult for you to remain passive during this exercise. When active, you may be tempted to arouse yourself by rubbing against your partner. You may also be tempted to try to please your partner. You have the potential during the front caress to learn how much enjoyment you can get from touching your partner in a sensual way. You also have the potential to learn to relax and allow your body to experience maximum stimulation. The front caress can also give you practice in learning to leave yourself alone and respond the way your body wants to, rather than the way you think your partner wants you to.

If you are having erection problems, the front caress is a crucial exercise for you. It may bring up all of the fears you have about not getting an erection. Do not expect the front caress to give you an erection. It probably will not. It doesn't for most people. If you do have an erection just allow it to happen. Don't move around, and don't squeeze your PC muscle, as doing so will make your erection go down. If you do get an erection, you may feel you want to use it. Instead, see this as your first opportunity to practice relaxing with an erection rather than doing something with it.

If you are concerned about premature ejaculation, you may be worried that you will become too aroused and ejaculate. If you ejaculate during the caress, don't worry about it. Let your partner know that you are going to ejaculate so that it is not a surprise. Relax as much as you can and allow yourself to experience the ejaculation. The important thing in the front caress is not how long you last but whether you can leave yourself alone and allow yourself to experience arousal, enjoyment, and ejaculation. At this stage it is important for you to relax your body as much as possible. Your partner can help you recognize when your body is showing signs of anxiety.

If you are having problems with inhibited ejaculation, it may be difficult for you to leave yourself alone and proceed slowly in this exercise. Be especially attuned to whether you may be subtly pressuring your partner with your touch.

If you have vaginismus or are experiencing general sexual anxiety, the front caress is a very important exercise for you, and you may have to repeat it several times in order to learn to relax fully. You may feel severe anxiety and muscle tightening as your partner's hand approaches your genitals. At all times keep your attention focused on where your partner is touching rather than looking ahead to where he may touch you next. Your partner can help you by giving you a gentle touch on your thigh if your muscles are tensing up and you seem to be unaware of it.

There are a number of ways that you can do the front caress, depending on what your problem is and how you feel. If you are very relaxed, use your face, chest, or hair to caress your partner. If you are a little bit anxious, it may be best to do only part of the front caress; for example, you may want to start with just the top half of the body. Or you may want to do the front caress without touching the genitals.

If you are very, very anxious, you may want to do a preliminary exercise in which you take your partner's hand and guide it over your body. You may do any of these variations, as long as you discuss it with your partner first and agree ahead of time on exactly what to do. Being able to successfully predict your partner's touch will do wonders in helping you learn how to relax and trust.

Here is a time sequence for the front caress and many of the subsequent exercises:

* *Spoon breathing:* five to ten minutes

* *Focusing caress, first partner:* five to ten minutes

* *Focusing caress, second partner:* five to ten minutes

* *Front caress, first partner:* twenty minutes

* *Spoon breathing:* five to ten minutes

* *Front caress, second partner:* twenty minutes

* *Spoon breathing:* five to ten minutes

* *Feedback*

chapter 22

Basic Partner Exercises: The Genital Caress and Oral Sex

The new elements that are added in this chapter are extended caressing of the genitals using both your hands and your mouth. Before you begin a genital caress, take some time to review the locations of both the male and female genital structures that are described in Chapter 2.

The Genital Caress

Our knowledge of female anatomy has increased since the first edition of this book. To find your partner's G-spot, insert your longest finger straight into her vagina, hook it over her pubic bone, and try to point your finger back at yourself. The G-spot will feel a little rough, and as you continue to touch it, it will swell up.

To find your partner's A-spot, insert your longest finger straight into her vagina and gently rub it along the top wall. This area will feel smooth, and it may start to lubricate as you continue to touch it.

To find your partner's cervix, insert your longest finger all the way into her vagina and point it first up and to the left and then up and to the right. On either the left or right side, you will feel a lump. This is the cervix.

If you run a finger along the side walls of your partner's vagina, you'll notice that they feel kind of ridged or corrugated. These are the rugae, the striated muscles that run along the walls of the vagina.

Remember not to force your finger into your partner's vagina or to stroke it too roughly. If you can't easily reach a deep vaginal area such as the cervix, save contact with that area for intercourse. Also, remember to use plenty of lubrication.

❧ Exercise 21. THE GENITAL CARESS

The genital caress will take about an hour to an hour and a half. You will need a quiet room, a towel, some talcum powder, and some kind of lubricant that both partners like and is safe on the genitals. Some suggestions are K-Y jelly, mineral oil, baby oil, or massage oil. I tend to use an oil-based product rather than a water-based product, because oils seem to warm up more rapidly on the body. But feel free to use a water-based product if you prefer. Adult stores sell a number of products that mimic vaginal lubrication.

Begin your genital caress session with some spoon breathing. Then each partner may choose a focusing caress (either a back caress or a face caress). Don't slack off or become mechanical about these initial, focusing caresses. Do them for at least ten minutes each, and pay attention to what you are feeling.

When you are the active partner, begin by caressing your partner's body with powder as you did during the front caress. This time you will spend at least half of the caress on the genitals. After about ten minutes of the front caress, wipe the powder off your hand and warm up some baby oil in your hand. Slowly begin to caress your partner's genitals with your fingers.

If your passive partner is a woman, use lots of lubrication and slowly move your fingers over her outer vaginal lips, inner vaginal lips, and clitoris. Then slowly insert your finger into her vagina. Pay attention to how the inner and outer lips feel and how the different areas inside her vagina feel. Feel the vaginal walls and the muscles around the vaginal opening. Think of the inside of your partner's vagina as a clock, and move your fingers from twelve o'clock all the way around in a circle.

If your female partner has dyspareunia or sexual pain, do the genital caress only on her outer genitals. Don't attempt finger penetration at this stage. We'll include penetration as part of the progression of exercises in either Chapter 30 or Chapter 31.

The genital caress is the same as the other caresses in that you are touching for your own pleasure. If you slip into rubbing your partner's clitoris or trying to turn her on in some way, she will be able to feel this shift in your intention. She has agreed to be passive and not to respond no matter what you do, so stay with the exercise. Take this opportunity to really learn how your partner's genitals feel without any interference or distractions.

As part of the genital caress, lie between your partner's legs as you are caressing and learn what her genitals look like. Many sexual problems are caused by ignorance about the genitals. Take this opportunity to learn every hair and every fold of skin. If you feel yourself becoming mechanical or bored with the caress, slow down. Caress your partner's genitals for ten to fifteen minutes. Do it for your own pleasure. If you can see your partner's body tensing up, lightly pat her legs as a signal to relax.

If your passive partner is a man, caress the front of his body for about ten minutes and then warm some lubricant in your hand. Slowly caress his penis and scrotum with your fingers. Don't try to turn your partner on. Do the caress so that it feels as good for you as possible. If you slip into wishing your partner would get an erection, bring yourself back to your enjoyment of the caress. Your partner has agreed not to move around or respond verbally, so take this opportunity to learn what your partner's genitals feel and look like. Slowly move your fingers around the shaft and head of the penis, and then slowly run your fingers around each testicle.

It doesn't matter whether your partner has an erection during the genital caress. A soft penis feels just as good to touch as an erect one. The sensations are not better or worse, just different. Experience exactly what the skin feels like on the different areas of your partner's genitals. If you see your partner's body becoming tense, signal him to relax with a light tap on the leg. Make sure your partner is not holding his breath. If he becomes aroused and ejaculates, gently wipe him off and continue the caress. Do the genital caress for ten to fifteen minutes.

When you are the passive partner during the genital caress, lie on your back with your legs slightly spread. Place your arms at your sides or underneath your head. Close your eyes. As you receive the genital caress, all you need to do is focus, breathe, and relax. The only time you need to talk to your partner is if he or she does something that hurts or bothers you. Allow yourself to soak up all of the sensations like a sponge.

It may be difficult to remain passive, but remember, if you try to make your arousal better by moving around, you are in fact working against yourself by diminishing your arousal. Also, be sure to keep your PC muscle relaxed during this exercise. If you become aroused, that's fine. If you don't, that's fine, too. If you get an erection, have an orgasm, or ejaculate, fine. What matters is whether you can leave yourself alone and enjoy

yourself. Don't force anything. Just passively experience the feelings and enjoy them.

The biggest barriers to the genital caress are anxiety and performance pressure. Focusing should not be a problem. By now you should have enough practice with sensate focus that it is second nature. You should be able to focus as long as you reduce your anxiety and get rid of performance pressure.

Anxiety will manifest itself in your body. Is your breathing irregular, or are your muscles tensing up? Your partner can help you recognize and correct this. Performance pressure will manifest itself in distracting thoughts such as, "I wonder if I'm starting to get hard," or, "I wonder if I'm going to have an orgasm." If you catch yourself thinking instead of feeling, bring your mind back to the touch.

Your partner will probably be able to tell if you are having distracting thoughts just by watching your body. If you are focusing on your genitals, blood will flow to that area and your genitals will warm up, whereas if you are spectatoring, blood will flow away from the genital area and it will feel kind of clammy.

Finish with spoon breathing and feedback.

Oral Sex

After you have done the genital caress often enough to become comfortable with it, you are ready to try oral sex. Oral sex is a variation on the genital caress. Before I describe the exercise, let me say a few words about oral sex in general.

Many couples have either never experienced oral sex or find the practice negative or even revolting. For that matter, many people "perform" oral sex but either don't enjoy it, feel coerced into it, or do it just to please the other person and get it over with. Oral sex is a sexual practice that is probably associated with more performance anxiety than any other practice, possibly even more than intercourse.

Having said that, I also have to tell you that oral sex has the potential to be one of the most enjoyable and healing sexual practices that you can do. Most women report that they reach orgasm more easily with oral sex than with intercourse, and that the orgasms they have with oral sex are really intense.

Many sexual self-help books talk about oral sex as though there are techniques that will guarantee orgasm in every sexual partner, or techniques that every man or every woman will enjoy all of the time. This is misleading. Being able to enjoy oral sex depends more on how relaxed and focused you are than it does on what techniques are used.

If you recognize that you have a negative attitude toward oral sex, relax. Be reassured that there is nothing inherently dirty about genitals. As long as your partner has washed his or her genitals and is free from infection, you have nothing to worry about.

Responsibility, Part 1

The following exercise is the first one that involves the possibility of exchanging bodily fluids. It is your responsibility to make sure you don't transmit or expose yourself to a sexually transmitted disease. This means that for any exercise involving oral sex or intercourse, if you and your partner are not in a monogamous relationship, you should use a condom. Sensate-focus exercises *can* be done with condoms, but doing so somewhat decreases the sensations. (See also "Responsibility, Part 2," in Chapter 23.)

⟪ *Exercise 22.* ORAL SEX

The oral sex exercise is optional in this program. I encourage you to experience oral sex in the context of a sensate-focus exercise because there are few things as enjoyable as doing or receiving a sensuous, nondemand oral genital caress. Your tongue is an organ with a lot of nerve endings. Why deny yourself the pleasure you could receive by using it to caress your partner? You may be surprised to find that when the performance aspect is removed from oral sex, you will like it.

What if the genitals do taste funny or smell funny to you? We acclimate rather rapidly to odors; that is, after a few seconds, we find that we don't notice them. Also, you will find that licking with certain parts of the tongue produces taste, whereas licking with other parts, such as the tip, does not produce taste. That's because taste buds are present on some parts of the tongue but not on others. Allow yourself to discover which parts of your tongue are more sensitive and which you enjoy licking with.

If you have little experience with oral sex, don't expect to enjoy it right away. It may take some time. But the best way to learn to enjoy oral sex is to do it often and to receive it often—both in a nondemand way.

If you are afraid that your partner's genitals will not smell good, ask your partner to shower or wash before the exercise. In fact, it might be a good idea to shower together and wash each other's genitals, or wash them as part of this exercise.

There are other things you can do to make oral sex much more enjoyable. One is to either partly or completely shave your genitals. It's much more enjoyable to both give and receive oral sex if the hair on the genital area is shaved or trimmed.

You can caress the genitals with baby oil or mineral oil before you do an oral-genital caress. Getting baby oil or mineral oil on your mouth won't hurt you. However, some people prefer to use flavored gels or lotions on the genitals. All adult stores sell these, and they come in a huge number of flavors. If you decide to buy flavored lubricants, make sure the packaging says that the product is safe for oral sex.

Think of sensate-focus oral sex with your partner as simply using your tongue instead of your hand to do the genital caress. The same instructions apply, and, if you have been doing the sensate-focus exercises and learning from them, you are probably already anticipating what I am going to say next. (Remember that behavior therapy is all about repetition.)

* Do the caress for your own pleasure.

* Do the caress slowly and to explore.

* When you are the passive partner, remain totally passive.

* When you are active, do the caress for your own pleasure.

* When you are active, do not pressure your partner to respond.

* Do the caress in a sensuous manner, to make your tongue feel good rather than to turn your partner on.

Begin this exercise with spoon breathing and focusing caresses. Then decide who will be active first. The active partner should do a front caress for five minutes or so. Then use some lubricant and caress your partner's genitals with your fingers for a few minutes.

To begin the oral part of the caress, if your passive partner is a woman, be sure both of you are in comfortable positions. Your partner should either lie down on her back with your face between her legs or sit leaning back against a wall or headboard with her legs spread comfortably apart.

Now, slowly move your lips and tongue along her inner thighs, outer vaginal lips, inner vaginal lips, clitoris, and in and out of her vagina. Do this for ten or fifteen minutes. Focus on the exact point of contact and explore how the different parts of your partner's genitals feel and taste to the different parts of your mouth.

If your tongue, chin, or neck starts to get tired or sore, change positions and relax. You may be holding your tongue too stiffly in an effort to please your partner. Your tongue should be relaxed.

Do not stiffen your tongue and rub it forcefully against your partner's clitoris. Do not forcefully suck or slurp at your partner's inner or outer lips. Do not insert a finger into your partner's vagina or rub her clitoris with your finger while you lick her vaginal opening. Your partner will be likely to interpret any of these actions as a demand to respond, which will cause her to remain anxious and be unable to relax. The point of the oral sex exercise is for you to enjoy sensations in your mouth and for your partner to be able to enjoy herself with no demands on her to show how much she likes it.

If your passive partner is a man, spend about five minutes on a front caress. Then caress your partner's genitals with some lubricant on your hand for a few minutes until you are both focused and relaxed. Next, slowly use your tongue and lips to lick all over his penis and scrotum and thighs. You may want to take his whole penis into your mouth and slowly let it back out again. Explore freely, and do what makes your tongue feel good. Lick the area behind his testicles. Insert your tongue into the creases between his thighs and scrotum. Experience how each different area feels or tastes to your lips and tongue.

Do not suck on your partner's penis in such a way that your head moves up and down. Only your tongue and lips should move during this exercise. If your neck or tongue becomes tired or sore, move to a different position. Your tongue should remain relaxed and not stiff. If you feel pressured to perform, stop and caress some other part of your partner's body until you feel that you are focused enough to enjoy the oral sex again. It is best if you respond to what you want rather than to what you think your partner wants.

If your partner indicates that he is about to ejaculate, decide whether to take the semen in your mouth or whether to temporarily stop the caress while your partner ejaculates. If you have not done the caress for the full fifteen minutes, wipe off the semen and continue the caress.

Do not use your hand to masturbate your partner during this caress. Remember, you are doing this caress only for your own pleasure. It doesn't matter whether your partner gets aroused or not or whether he gets an erection or not or whether he ejaculates or not. What does matter is that you do what feels good for you and that you focus on the feelings in your mouth during the caress.

As with all of the other sensate-focus partner exercises, finish with spoon breathing, and be sure to both give feedback after the exercise.

Part IV

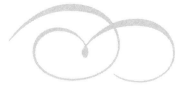

HEALING
SPECIFIC SEXUAL
PROBLEMS

In this section you'll find chapters containing healing exercises for each of the nine sexual dysfunctions described in Part II. It is important to read the background material in Parts I and II and to do the preliminary exercises in Part III before plunging into this portion of the program.

chapter 23

Healing Premature Ejaculation

*P*remature ejaculation, also called *rapid ejaculation,* is not defined by how long you last (whether in seconds or minutes), how many strokes you can take before ejaculation, or whether your partner has an orgasm. Rather, premature ejaculation occurs when you ejaculate before you want to, and when you don't feel you are in control of your ejaculation.

Some experts believe that it should not matter how long a man's erection lasts. They believe how long a man is able to have intercourse before he ejaculates is not important—if he ejaculates before he wants to, he can simply continue to have intercourse with a flaccid penis. After spending many years treating men with premature ejaculation, I get upset when I read these ideas. I have seen too many men psychologically devastated by this problem. They find the condition intolerable because they want to last longer when making love—both to more fully please their partner and to spend a longer time enjoying lovemaking without worry and without pressure. In addition, I find that the length of time a man lasts during lovemaking can affect his opportunity to experience the healing touch of his partner. Premature ejaculation can be a serious sexual problem if it detracts from the ability to heal and be healed sexually.

You don't have to be a marathon man, but you should have enough ejaculation control that you can last as long as you wish about 75 percent of the time. If you have a high sex drive, it is normal to ejaculate before you want to some of the time, especially if you are young, if you don't have sex regularly, or if you are with a new partner. This is not a cause for alarm and it is nothing to be ashamed of. If you have ever had control, you have the ability to gain it back, and for life.

It is also important to remember that the quality of lovemaking is not dependent on the amount of time or amount of activity. I believe in teaching ejaculation control for life rather than encouraging men to make love for a certain period of time. Sometimes you and your lover may want to spend long periods of time in intercourse, and at other times you may just want a quickie. Both ways of making love celebrate your intimacy, so you should have the pleasure of these options, but with premature ejaculation, you don't.

Premature ejaculation is a straightforward problem to treat, especially when your partner is willing to help you. You will need to make a time commitment of about three hours a week to tap into the sexual power that the exercises in this chapter develop. By the end of about six weeks your control should be much better.

In order for a man to be healed of premature ejaculation problems, three things are necessary:

1. He must learn full-body relaxation. Body tension is a direct contributor to premature ejaculation.

2. He must learn to gain voluntary control of his PC muscle. Premature ejaculation happens when your anxiety level goes so high that your PC muscle spasms out of control. The PC muscle exercises you learned in Chapter 18 will prove to be very important here. Pay special attention to the relaxation phase of each PC muscle squeeze. You will need to learn how to recognize when your PC muscle is tense and how to voluntarily relax it.

3. Finally, and most importantly, in order to heal premature ejaculation, a man must learn to accept and recognize the sensations he is feeling in his genitals at every step of a sexual encounter. You can only control that which you own and accept.

The sensate-focus exercises in this chapter will help you accomplish all three of these goals.

Outdated Treatments for Premature Ejaculation

Before I give you some exercises to help premature ejaculation, I want to tell you a little bit about the development of behavioral techniques to treat this problem. In the 1950s, a physician named James Semans developed what he called the *stop-start technique.* In this technique, which was primarily designed to be used during intercourse, the woman would be on top. She would thrust until the man reached a point when he felt he was close to ejaculation. He would then say, "Stop," and his partner would stop thrusting until he felt his arousal go down to a comfortable level, and then he would say "Start" and she would start thrusting again. They would repeat this process for several minutes until he decided to ejaculate. I think you can see some of the problems with this technique. It doesn't fit my criterion of teaching you to be aware of your arousal. The only two arousal levels this technique teaches are level 1 and level 9, or level 1 and, "Oops, too late!"

One of the main things to remember about premature ejaculation is that, by definition, the man with premature ejaculation does not know when he is close to ejaculation. If you think about it in terms of the 1-to-10 arousal scale, he does not have any awareness of the lower levels like 2, 3, 4, and 5. So the Semans technique really only works with men who have some awareness of their arousal scale, and most men with premature ejaculation do not.

Then, in the 1960s, Masters and Johnson developed treatment for premature ejaculation based on their research on the human sexual response cycle (which I described in Chapter 2). They noticed that when a man was close to ejaculation, his testicles and scrotum would rise up close to his body. They reasoned that if they could figure out a way to keep a man's testicles away from his body, this would delay ejaculation. So they invented a technique called *testicle tugging*. The technique is meant to be used during sexual intercourse in the missionary position. When the man feels that he is close to ejaculation, he tells his partner, and she reaches underneath him, grabs his scrotum, and pulls it down and holds it. You can see that this technique has the same problem as the stop-start technique: It doesn't teach you the difference in feelings at each arousal level. In addition, it has the added downside of potentially being very painful.

Masters and Johnson also developed the "squeeze technique." This can be used with intercourse or with manual or oral stimulation. The woman stimulates her partner, and when he says he is close to ejaculation, she puts her thumbs and the first two fingers of both hands under the head of his penis and squeezes as hard as she can. This supposedly decreases a man's urge to ejaculate (no kidding!). Obviously this technique doesn't help you learn arousal levels. In addition, it can be painful and is difficult to use, because by the time the man becomes aware that he is close to ejaculation, the woman really doesn't have time to visually locate the penis, position her hands, and squeeze, especially if they have been having intercourse with her on top. Nevertheless, I have included a description of the squeeze technique at the end of this chapter in case you want to try it. Some men have responded well to it, especially after they have gained some degree of ejaculatory control.

What Else Doesn't Work

There are some other techniques that men have used to try to last longer. I call them "quick-fix" techniques. Please don't think you can take a shortcut by using any of them. They don't work (although they might help you last longer during one episode of intercourse), and they tend to make the problem worse in the long run.

One of the oldest suggestions for lasting longer is to think about something else when you are having intercourse. Some of the suggested topics I've read about include thinking about having sex with an ugly woman, doing math problems in your head, reciting baseball statistics, thinking about mowing the lawn, thinking about a bloody car accident, and thinking about having sex with your grandmother. Please don't fall for any of these. The only way to get ejaculation control is to learn awareness of what you are feeling, not try to ignore it.

Some adult-product stores sell creams that purport to numb the penis and therefore delay ejaculation. They numb your penis all right, but the result is that you still ejaculate quickly without feeling it. Also, these creams can be transferred to your partner's vagina during intercourse and interfere with her sexual response.

Some men use alcohol to slow down their ejaculatory reflex. This works, because alcohol slows down *all* of your reflexes (and does so quite well). However, engaging in this practice can easily cause you to develop tolerance to alcohol. If you start out drinking two beers to slow yourself down, before you know it you need a whole six-pack (or twelve-pack) to accomplish the same thing. The end result is that you go into a coma before you have a chance to have sex. (I'm exaggerating here, but don't use alcohol strictly for ejaculation-control purposes.)

I've also read advice that suggested that a man use a condom in order to last longer because the condom desensitizes the penis so he doesn't feel as much. That's a problem, because the point is to develop control while still feeling as much as possible. In addition, condoms have a tolerance effect, in the sense that you may become so accustomed to using one that pretty soon you need two to gain the same degree of control.

Some men masturbate to "take the edge off" before they believe they will have an opportunity to have sexual intercourse. This works against you in the long run, because masturbating quickly for the sole purpose of ejaculating—rather than enjoying the sensations—will make your problem worse.

A Medical Solution

There is one medical solution that's been shown to work for premature ejaculation. That's the use of Prozac, Paxil, Zoloft, or any of the other medications called *selective serotonin reuptake inhibitors (SSRIs)*. If you take one of these drugs for ejaculation control, you don't take it every day. You take it on the day you are planning to have sex. I've seen some clients use this technique successfully, but it does nothing to help your arousal awareness. In addition, you have to watch out for this practice as you get older, because the SSRIs can negatively affect your libido—believe it or not, even in a man who's had long-term premature ejaculation.

Some men have taken Viagra or other, similar drugs in order to last longer. The theory behind this practice is that if you take Viagra when you really don't need it for erections (that is, you already have strong erections), even if you ejaculate quickly you'll stay hard and be able to continue intercourse after you ejaculate. This works for some men.

Sensate-Focus Exercises
for Premature Ejaculation

The mainstays of the ejaculation-control program I describe in this chapter are the peaking process and variations on it. Remember to end each exercise with five to ten minutes of spoon breathing followed by each partner giving feedback based on the questions provided in Chapter 15.

    ∿ *Exercise 23.* AROUSAL AWARENESS WITH A PARTNER

The first step in ejaculation control is arousal awareness, which you learned to do in the chapter on self-touch. Now you will do it with your partner.

    As you did in Chapter 18, think of your sexual arousal on a scale from 1 to 10, with a 1 meaning you are not aroused at all and a 10 meaning you are ejaculating. Remember, this 1-to-10 scale refers to how you feel, not to your *physical* response, i.e., your erection level. (For a review of how you

may expect to feel at each level, see Exercise 14, Arousal Awareness During Self-Touch, in Chapter 18.)

Begin the session with focusing caresses (back caresses are recommended) for five to ten minutes each. Then you may do a front or genital caress with your partner before you begin the arousal awareness process.

Take the passive role and lie on your back. Your partner will begin a front caress and move into a genital caress, as well as oral sex if she desires. She should do these caresses for her own pleasure, as in all of the early sensate-focus exercises. Every five minutes or so, your partner should ask you about your arousal level. She should vary the stimulation so that sometimes your arousal level is low and sometimes it is relatively high. Try to give your partner feedback that is as honest as possible, even though it may be more difficult to recognize your arousal level than it was when you did the exercise by yourself.

The first time you monitor your arousal level with your partner, you may be unable to distinguish all of the different levels between 1 and 10, or they may go by very quickly. Remember to breathe and to keep all of your muscles relaxed. Make sure you are not tightening your PC muscle. Try not to panic or fight off ejaculation. Breathe instead.

The purpose of this exercise is to learn to recognize all of your different arousal levels, even if they don't go up in order. It doesn't matter if you go up steadily or go up and down several times. If you go all of the way up through ejaculation, that's fine. If you are only able to reach what you consider to be a level 2 or 3, that's fine too.

Women, as the active partner, do the caress for your own pleasure. When you ask your partner what his arousal level is and he tells you, slow the caress and then begin again. Do the caress very slowly, especially the genital caress and oral sex, and especially if your partner has a severe problem with premature ejaculation. It is important for your partner that the stimulation be slow and predictable. In addition, touching slowly will help you focus on the sensations. If your partner holds his breath at some point during the caress or tenses his thigh muscles, stop the caress and remind him to relax.

Men, if you are really concerned about premature ejaculation, remember to stay completely passive. Keep your breathing even. Don't hold your breath when your partner touches your abdomen and genitals—focus on the touch. Ask your partner to touch you more slowly if you are having trouble focusing. Try not to tense your thigh muscles. It doesn't matter if

your partner is able to touch you for two seconds or twenty minutes before you ejaculate.

After you do the arousal awareness exercise with your partner for the first time, give your partner feedback about whether she needs to go more slowly so that you can focus more easily. Remember, we are not yet trying to control an ejaculation, so whatever happens, happens.

During this exercise, do not attempt to control your ejaculation at all. Your first impulse when your partner touches your genitals will be to tense up, hold your breath, and think about something else. Tell yourself to relax, and focus on your genital sensations the way you did when you did the arousal awareness exercise by yourself.

If you do ejaculate quickly during this exercise, your partner should give you a front caress for a few minutes and then start over with the arousal awareness exercise. Any time you ejaculate quickly during any exercise, you can always start the exercise over after a few minutes.

If you have had a problem with premature ejaculation for some time, you may have begun to feel that ejaculating is not pleasurable. You may be having ejaculations but not orgasms. When you feel that you are at the point of inevitability, you may experience an "Oh no!" feeling rather than a strong feeling of pleasure and impending release. Use this arousal awareness exercise to train yourself to start enjoying your ejaculations again rather than dreading them. From now on, whenever you have an ejaculation as a result of exercises you do from this book, I want you to passively allow yourself to experience it without tensing up and without moving. Enjoy it whenever it happens. It is fine for you to ejaculate at any time during this program if it's going to happen. Your eventual ability to learn to ejaculate when you want to will depend on never trying to control an ejaculation. Ejaculating during an exercise does not mean that you have somehow "failed" the exercise. In fact, the opposite is true. If you enjoy an ejaculation whenever it happens, you have done the exercise well. Every time you have an experience in which you have an ejaculation and enjoy it rather than fight it, you are training yourself to last longer.

There are two things we want to reinforce here and one thing we don't. The two things we want to reinforce are having an ejaculation and enjoying it, and staying aroused for some period of time with stimulation but without ejaculating. The thing we don't want to reinforce is trying to control an ejaculation once it is going to happen.

If you are the partner of a man having problems with premature ejaculation, you may become frustrated when your partner ejaculates quickly. The best thing you can do to help at this stage, however, is to encourage him to enjoy the ejaculation whenever it happens. If your partner ejaculates quickly during any exercise, remember that you can always begin the exercise again after a few minutes.

On the flip side, it doesn't matter if you *don't* have an ejaculation during these exercises. What matters is that you leave yourself alone and allow yourself to experience various levels of arousal without interfering with your own pleasure.

Do the arousal awareness exercise as many times as you need to with manual and oral stimulation until you can reliably reach and recognize levels 7 and 8. It may take two or three or more repetitions until you are confident that you can distinguish how aroused you are. Repeat the exercise until you can receive manual and/or oral stimulation for fifteen minutes and experience various arousal levels.

⤳ *Exercise 24.* PEAKING WITH MANUAL STIMULATION

Remember that a peak is a wavelike increase in arousal. You know how to do a peaking exercise by yourself from Chapter 18. Now you'll do it with your partner's help. I'll describe three versions of a peaking exercise: one with manual stimulation, one with oral stimulation, and one with intercourse. The intercourse exercises call for you to be the passive partner first and then the active partner.

Before you begin, you and your partner should do focusing caresses with each other. Pleasure your partner with a front caress, genital caress, or some oral sex. To start the peaking exercise, lie on your back in the passive role. Your partner will begin a slow front caress and gradually move to your genitals. She should use plenty of lubrication.

When you reach level 3, let her know by saying either "Three" or "Stop." Your partner will then move her hand to your belly, thighs, or some other part of your body until your arousal has dropped one or two levels. Then she will caress your genitals again until you report level 4. She will stop and let your arousal go down again.

As you reach each peak, say the number level out loud, take a deep breath, and relax your PC muscle and other pelvic muscles. Throughout the exercise, remember to focus on the point of contact between your skin and your partner's skin. Do the exercise for about twenty-five minutes. Continue peaking up through levels 5, 6, 7, 8, and 9, and all the way to ejaculation and orgasm at the final peak if you want to. Try to do at least five or six separate peaks during this exercise.

If you have a severe problem with premature ejaculation, you may be unable to go all the way up the scale the first time you do the exercise, and that's okay. Worst-case scenario: You have such a serious case of premature ejaculation that the second your partner touches your genitals, you ejaculate. This probably won't happen, but if it does, wait a few minutes and start the exercise over. Do more focusing caresses between the first and second peaking exercises. During your second attempt at the exercise, you should be relaxed enough after an ejaculation to be able to recognize several arousal levels.

Alternatively, if you have trouble with this exercise, do a peaking exercise in which your partner touches some part of your body other than your genitals. Repeat the manual peaking exercise as many times as you need to until you can recognize all of the levels on the arousal scale. Then move on to a peaking exercise with oral stimulation.

Here are some additional options for the manual peaking exercise. Remember that if you have a problem with premature ejaculation, you don't know how to recognize the low levels on your arousal scale. You could do one manual peaking exercise just practicing the lower arousal levels of 3, 4, and 5, and stop there. Then, the next time you do the exercise, you could add another, higher level. Or, if you can recognize the lower levels but have trouble with the higher levels, you could always do a manual peaking exercise in which you only practice the higher levels of 6, 7, 8, and even 9. Sometimes it can take quite a bit of practice to be able to recognize level 9 and back away from it. Remember, at this stage, never consciously try to hold back an ejaculation. If you don't ask your partner to stop in time, don't panic. Just let the ejaculation happen and enjoy it. You can always try again later.

If you have trouble recognizing a particular level, do an entire manual peaking exercise in which you only practice one level. For example, if you can recognize levels 1 through 7 but have trouble asking your partner to stop at level 8 in time to avoid the certainty of ejaculation, do one exercise in which you practice several peaks at level 8 and allow your arousal level to go down almost all the way back to level 1 between peaks. Or, better still, if you have trouble recognizing level 8 and asking your partner to stop in time, do a manual peaking exercise in which you do several peaks at the level right before 8 (level 7). Then, the next time you do the exercise, you will have a better grasp of level 8.

When you become more confident in your ability to recognize all of the levels on the arousal scale passively with manual stimulation, start to become active by adding some movement. As your partner caresses you, do some pelvic rolls and thrusts. Move only your pelvis; don't tighten your stomach, thigh, or PC muscles.

When you're peaking at higher levels during this exercise, your partner can stop and "detumesce" you for a few seconds after each peak is reached. Tumescence is the flow of blood to the genitals. With each successive peak, more blood enters the genitals and you become more aroused (provided that you remember to take deep breaths and that your muscles are relaxed). When you reach each peak, your partner can detumesce you by stopping the stimulation of your genitals and stroking your abdomen and thighs in the direction away from your genitals. This will cause blood to leave your genitals temporarily and your arousal level to go down.

The first time you do the peaking process with manual stimulation, remember to stay passive. Take a deep breath and relax your leg muscles whenever you feel a surge of arousal. The peaking process will not benefit you if you are tense or try to control your ejaculation. Breathe deeply as you reach each new level. Your partner may notice if you are tense or holding your breath at any point during the peaking process, and she can help you by reminding you to breathe and relax.

Stop between peaks long enough for your arousal to go down about two levels. It is just as important for you to get a sense that your arousal is going down as it is for you to get a sense of your arousal going up. The "down curves" of each peak are just as important as the "up curves," because the down curves give you the sense that your arousal level is controllable if you breathe deeply and your partner stops the stimulation.

Peaking will result in ejaculation control through self-awareness and relaxation, rather than through working at controlling your ejaculation or worrying about it. If you have a problem with premature ejaculation, at no time during any exercise should you attempt to control your ejaculation by tensing up your muscles. If you feel that you want to control your ejaculation, repeat the arousal awareness exercise or other, earlier exercises until you are more confident of your ability to relax.

If you do ejaculate fairly quickly during any exercise in the peaking process, your partner can do a front caress with you for a few minutes and then start the peaking exercise over. Chances are good that you will experience some level of arousal again.

❧ Exercise 25. PEAKING WITH ORAL SEX

Begin with each partner doing focusing caresses on the other. Then give your partner a sensate-focus front caress or genital caress, or do oral sex with her. Then lie on your back. Your partner will begin a front and genital caress with her hand. Then she'll start to caress your penis and scrotum with her lips and tongue. Take about twenty-five minutes and peak up to levels 3, 4, 5, 6, 7, 8, and 9 if you can. Remember to keep breathing regularly during the stimulation, breathe at each peak, keep your muscles relaxed, and focus on the sensations.

Oral sex can be really stimulating for a man who has a problem with premature ejaculation. If you want to, you can break this exercise down into several steps. The first time you do the exercise, you could just do levels 3, 4, and 5 and stop there. You could then repeat the exercise, adding a new level each time. Or you could repeat the exercise, peaking several times at one level. Once you have more confidence in your ability to last during oral sex, you could start to make yourself active by doing some pelvic rolls or thrusts.

Another technique that can help you last longer is to have your partner adjust the ways she does oral sex. A lot of men have trouble gaining awareness of their arousal level if their partner takes the penis all the way into her mouth and sucks really hard. Your partner needs to use a little finesse here. She needs to begin the genital portion of the exercise by just slowly licking your penis and scrotum. Then, if you are comfortable with it, she can slowly take your penis into her mouth and let it back out. Another alternative to some of the peaking techniques I discussed above is to do a whole peaking exercise with your partner just licking rather than sucking your penis. Then, when you feel more comfortable, gradually have her introduce sucking into a future repetition of the exercise.

Peaking with Intercourse

Before I describe how to peak inside your partner's vagina, I would like to say another thing about premature ejaculation in general. Many men feel they ejaculate too quickly, when in fact the time they spend inside their partner's vagina is probably equal to or longer than average. According to a survey conducted by the University of Chicago in the 1990s, the average amount of time an American man spends during actual intercourse is somewhere between four and eight minutes. By using the exercises in this book you will be able to have intercourse for a longer period of time. However, after you have done all of the exercises for premature ejaculation, you may feel that the level of arousal you reach is much more important than how long you can last.

Responsibility, Part 2

The following exercise is the first one that includes intercourse. Many of the exercises described later also include the possibility of intercourse. When doing any exercises involving the possibility of intercourse you will need to make sure you use reliable contraception if you don't want to become pregnant.

If you haven't already done so, you will need to choose your method of contraception carefully, as some methods could potentially interfere with the sexual healing program. For example, spermicides cannot be used if you are going to do an exercise that includes both oral sex and intercourse, as they should not be ingested. Oral contraceptives don't interfere with actual sex acts, but their long-term use can decrease a woman's sex drive. Bottom line: No method of contraception is perfect, but, again, you must use a reliable method if you don't want to become pregnant.

ᑫ *Exercise 26.* FIRST INTERCOURSE FOR PREMATURE EJACULATION

The peaking process continues from hand and oral stimulation through intercourse. Before you begin peaking with intercourse, however, I would like for you to experience an episode of nondemand intercourse. There are two forms of nondemand intercourse: flaccid insertion and the "quick dip." Use the quick dip if you tend to have strong erections. Use flaccid insertion if you tend to have less strong erections.

The Quick Dip

For the quick-dip version of the exercise, the couple adds a quick episode of intercourse to the end of a manual or oral peaking exercise. Do not use the quick dip until the man has experience with peaking during hand or oral stimulation at levels 8 and 9. The reason for the quick dip is not to practice lasting longer during intercourse. The purpose of the quick dip is to allow you to enjoy your ejaculation as much as you can.

If you are aroused after a manual or oral peaking session and have peaked up to level 8 or 9, go ahead and have your partner get on top of your penis while you continue to lie on your back. Try to stay as passive as possible and let your partner do the thrusting. Use the sensate-focus method; that is, focus on the feel of your penis inside her vagina, breathe, and relax your leg muscles. It doesn't matter how long you last before ejaculating. This isn't a test to see how long you can hold out. It is a form of nondemand intercourse—a way for you and your partner to experience heightened arousal. Peaking prior to ejaculation will make your ejaculation stronger and more enjoyable when it happens.

Flaccid Insertion

If you choose the flaccid-insertion version of nondemand penetration, start with focusing caresses, such as back caresses. Then give your partner a genital caress or oral sex. Lie on your back and have your partner stimulate you to levels 4, 5, and 6 with manual and oral stimulation. Then lie on your side facing your partner as she lies on her back. This is the side-to-side scissors position. Interweave your legs so that your genitals are up against each other.

Stroke a lot of lubrication onto your penis and around your partner's vaginal opening. Now slowly insert your penis, whether it is flaccid, erect, or somewhere in between. Relax all of your muscles, breathe, and note your arousal level. If it is a 6 or under, begin slow pelvic rolls and thrusts and start peaking. Peak at levels 5, 6, 7, and 8, stopping between peaks for as long as you need to. See if you can do several peaks for about fifteen minutes, then ejaculate if you desire.

If your arousal level is higher than 6 when you first insert your penis, stay still and allow your arousal level to decrease. Or you can withdraw and allow your arousal level to go down. Then re-enter, even if you are flaccid. If all you are able to do this first time is to lie inside your partner without moving, that's fine—it is progress. Enjoy the sexual intimacy it brings. You should keep repeating this exercise until you can both recognize your arousal levels and you can move inside your partner. Breathe, relax, and focus on the sensations. You will do fine.

For this version of the exercise, it doesn't matter how much of your penis goes into your partner's vagina, how long it stays there, whether it stays erect, whether you have an ejaculation, or whether your partner has an orgasm. Just relax and experience the feelings, whether they last a few seconds or a few minutes. What is important in this exercise is that you don't pressure yourself, and that you allow yourself to experience the feelings of your penis inside your partner's vagina while remaining comfortable. If you do ejaculate, leave your penis inside your partner's vagina and continue to experience the sensations for a few more minutes.

After you can do the side-to-side position for fifteen minutes, try the peaking exercise in different intercourse positions, in the following order: butterfly, woman on top, rear entry, and man on top. Your best position will probably be the butterfly position. Men tend to have more control in this position because their center of gravity is in their hips and legs rather than their chest. Start each new position in the passive role and let your partner do all of the moving at first. Then, when you get more confident, you, too, can start moving.

General Pointers for Peaking with Intercourse

Remember that in peaking with intercourse, just like in peaking with any other kind of stimulation, you can break the exercises into smaller exercises. You could do one exercise with only low-level peaks and one with only higher-level peaks. You could do an exercise in any intercourse position in which you do repeated peaks at a particular level.

Do each version of the exercise as many times as you need to until you can easily reach level 7 or 8 or until you can passively allow stimulation for fifteen to twenty minutes. Allow roughly five minutes for each complete peak, including both the up curve and the down curve. In any peaking session, it doesn't matter whether or not you have an orgasm, ejaculate, or have an erection. Continue all the way to orgasm if you can do so without working at it. The only difference between you and someone who is not concerned with ejaculation is that you may have to move a little slower or repeat some exercises more than once.

     Exercise 27. PLATEAUING FOR PREMATURE
                  EJACULATION

Plateauing is similar to peaking, as you learned in Chapter 18 on self-touch. When you peak, you allow your arousal to rise to a certain level and then you stop the stimulation so that your arousal level goes down. With plateauing, you allow your arousal to go to a certain level, and you try to stay at that level for anywhere from a few seconds to a couple of minutes. Plateauing is a great skill to have for ejaculation control. In fact, the way most adolescents or young men initially learn to control their ejaculation is through a rudimentary form of plateauing, in which they learn to recognize the arousal levels right before ejaculation and stay clear of the "danger zone" by changing their position or movements.

There are four strategies you can learn to use to plateau: changing your breathing, changing your movements, changing your focus, and squeezing your PC muscle.

Begin your first plateauing session with focusing caresses. Then give your partner a genital caress and oral sex. Lie on your back and relax. Your partner will give you a manual front and genital caress. When you reach a level 4, instead of telling your partner your level, take a couple of deep breaths. This should cause your arousal to go down a half level or so. When you feel that you are below a level 4, speed up your breathing. This should cause your arousal to go up about a half level. As your partner continues to caress you, see if you can maintain a level 4 for several seconds by adjusting your breathing.

Now relax and allow yourself to go up to a level 5. Thrust against your partner's hand. Then slow down your movement and your arousal should go down about a half level. See if you can maintain a level 5 by starting and stopping your movement.

Now relax and allow yourself to go up to level 6. When you reach a level 6, shift your focus to some part of your body that your partner is not currently touching. See if you can maintain a level 6 for a few seconds by switching your focus back and forth from the part of your body that your partner is touching to some other part she is not touching.

The final plateauing technique is using your PC muscle to decrease your arousal level. Allow your arousal to go up to level 7. When you reach level 7, gently squeeze your PC muscle a couple of times. This should cause your arousal to go down about a half level. Relax your PC muscle and allow your arousal to go back up. See if you can maintain a level 7 for a few seconds or more by squeezing and relaxing your PC muscle. It's not necessary to squeeze it very hard. One very gentle squeeze may be enough to take your arousal down a half level. You may need to experiment a little bit to find out exactly how hard you need to squeeze your PC muscle for this technique to be effective.

Continue the exercise, plateauing at levels 8 and 9 if you can. Use whichever technique seems to work best for you or is most comfortable for you. You can use just one technique for each plateau, or you can try combining them.

Once you have learned to plateau with manual stimulation from your partner, you can then practice the different plateauing techniques with oral sex and with intercourse in several different positions. I would recommend doing the positions in the following order: side-to-side, butterfly, woman on top, rear entry, and man on top (missionary).

As with peaking, you can do the plateauing exercise several different ways. You could do an exercise where you practice only the lower levels. Or you could do an exercise where you practice only the higher levels. Or you could do an exercise in which you plateau several times at the same level.

∾ *Exercise 28.* REPETITIVE PENETRATION FOR PREMATURE EJACULATION

This exercise also appears in the next chapter, on healing erection problems, because it works well for both problems.

Many men with premature ejaculation have a form of anxiety that is called *point-of-penetration anxiety.* This means that the most anxiety-provoking moment of a sexual encounter is when they first insert their penis to have sexual intercourse. Many men with premature ejaculation find this point to be such an overwhelming source of stimulation that they literally ejaculate immediately upon penetration. If they can get past that high-anxiety point of penetration, often they're okay with the continued stimulation of intercourse.

If you have point-of-penetration anxiety, here is an exercise you can do to overpractice the act of penetration itself. Before you begin, exchange back caresses for about ten minutes each, and then do a front caress or genital caress with your partner. Make sure you have lubrication handy.

Lie on your back and take the passive role. Do a couple of comfortable lower-level peaks as your partner caresses you with her hands and lips. Then change positions and have your partner lie on her back. Have her tilt her pelvis and put her legs up in the air (the butterfly position). Now apply lubrication to both of your hands, kneel between your partner's legs and slowly begin to caress your penis with one hand, using a lot of lubrication.

With your other hand, caress your partner's genitals, also with a lot of lubrication. Then start to caress her genitals with your lubricated penis. Caress her outer genitals first, and then slowly insert just the head of your penis into her vagina.

Remove your penis from your partner's vagina and caress her genitals with it again. Then insert your penis again, this time going a little deeper.

Remember to breathe and to keep your muscles as relaxed as you can. Focus on the sensations. Practice several insertions within a twenty-minute time frame, using peaking to allow yourself to go a little higher on the arousal scale each time. Try to stay within the 4-to-8 arousal range for most of the exercise.

If you have very severe premature ejaculation, you may need to start this exercise when you are at a very low arousal level, even a 1 or 2. You can do the exercise without an erection, which helps some men get comfortable with penetration. Just use more lubrication if you don't have an erection.

❧ Exercise 29. THE PC MUSCLE SQUEEZE

The PC squeeze exercise will help severe premature ejaculation problems that have not responded as well as you might have hoped to the relaxation and awareness techniques. Before you take the time to learn the PC squeeze, though, try an easier option first. Have your partner stimulate you to ejaculation at the beginning of a peaking session. If you ejaculate at the beginning of a session, you won't be worried about ejaculating during the peaking process. This will reduce your anxiety so that you will be able to learn how to peak. Once you have learned the peaking skills with your partner, you will no longer need to ejaculate at the beginning of a session.

If the above strategy does not work, you can learn the PC squeeze. Begin the session with focusing caresses. Then do a nondemand genital caress or oral sex with your partner.

Lie on your back, remembering to focus on the sensations, breathe, and relax all of your muscles. Have your partner begin to caress your genitals as she would during a peaking exercise. When you feel yourself reach a low level of arousal (for example, a 4), squeeze your PC muscle several times until you feel your arousal go down. Repeat this process, squeezing at levels 5, 6, 7, 8, and 9 if possible. It goes without saying that before you can do this exercise, your PC muscle needs to be in good shape, which should have happened naturally already because of the daily exercises you have been doing.

There are several ways you can squeeze your PC muscle. You could do one long, hard squeeze. You could do several quick squeezes in a row. Or you could do three or four medium-strength, rhythmic squeezes that mimic the action of your PC muscle when you ejaculate.

Squeezing your PC muscle in this way during this exercise will probably cause your erection to go down a little. If you squeeze too hard at a high level of arousal before you have done the low levels, you may actually trigger an ejaculation. This is nothing to worry about. It will only happen once. Just wait a few minutes and start the exercise over.

It is possible to overdo the squeezing, and if you do this exercise for more than about half an hour, you may temporarily find yourself unable to ejaculate at all. This is also nothing to worry about as long as you are learning to recognize your arousal levels and to decrease your arousal by squeezing your PC muscle.

For the PC squeeze to control your ejaculation, you must be sure to squeeze only the PC muscle. You must make sure that you are not tensing your abdomen, thigh, or buttocks muscles at the same time.

You may need to repeat this exercise a number of times until you become aware of how hard you need to squeeze to feel your arousal go down but have your erection stay up. When I taught the PC squeeze to clients, I told them they needed to learn to "tap on their brakes" rather than "slam on their brakes."

After you have learned to do the squeeze while receiving manual and oral stimulation, you can also practice it during intercourse. It is possible to squeeze your PC muscle at the moment of ejaculation, which I am told creates some unusually pleasurable sensations. A strong PC squeeze at the moment of orgasm can sometimes cause you to have an orgasm without ejaculating. A few seconds later you could have another orgasm and ejaculate.

This exercise will show you that your ejaculations are under your control, which will help you relax. After you have mastered the PC squeeze so that you can allow yourself to relax, go on to the peaking exercises without the squeeze. Use the PC squeeze only as a tool to enable yourself to become comfortable enough so that you start learning to stay aroused through awareness and relaxation. Squeezing tends to reinforce the idea that you are "working" on your problem rather than relaxing and enjoying the stimulation. Squeezing should be used for only a few sessions, and then you should return to the awareness and relaxation techniques, unless you want to experiment with the squeeze to see if you can have multiple orgasms.

◯ *Exercise 30.* THE PARTNER-SQUEEZE TECHNIQUE

This exercise is different from the PC muscle squeeze, although the exercises have similar names. The squeeze technique involves your partner squeezing your penis. You may be familiar with the squeeze technique, which was invented by Masters and Johnson and is recommended by most sex therapists. I usually teach the peaking process instead, but the squeeze technique is effective for some clients with very severe premature ejaculation problems. Use the squeeze technique only if you have gone all the way through this program and are still not confident that you can control your ejaculations.

Begin as you would any other exercise session, with focusing caresses. Your partner will then caress your penis while you are passive. When you reach the level of arousal right before the point of ejaculatory inevitability, signal your partner and she will squeeze the head of your penis tightly between the thumbs and first two fingers of both hands. After your partner squeezes your penis, you will feel your arousal level decrease. Your erection level is also likely to go down somewhat.

You can repeat the squeeze technique several times in one session, after which you should allow yourself to ejaculate. You can also do the squeeze technique during intercourse, withdrawing your penis at high levels of arousal so that your partner can squeeze it.

Breathe, relax, and focus on the sensations as you would during any other exercise. Again, use the squeeze technique only as a tool to bring yourself to the point where you are comfortable enough to begin the peaking exercises without the squeeze technique.

You can combine the squeeze technique with the peaking process. Do a peaking exercise while your partner stimulates you with her hands. As you reach each arousal level, tell your partner your level and she will squeeze the head of your penis so that your arousal goes down. Then continue peaking up through all of the levels to ejaculation, having her stop the stimulation and squeeze at each level.

෬ *Exercise 31.* EJACULATING ON PURPOSE

Some men have a different issue with premature ejaculation: They literally don't enjoy ejaculation. Because of many bad experiences, they don't feel good about ejaculating, and they don't even really experience orgasm when they ejaculate. The uncontrollable ejaculation is really just the localized genital reflex when the PC muscle spasms and forces semen out of the penis.

Ejaculating on purpose is not exactly a specific exercise. Rather, it is giving yourself permission to learn to enjoy your ejaculations again. In this technique, you have intercourse and try to ejaculate as quickly as you can. It doesn't matter if you come right away, as long as you allow yourself to enjoy your ejaculation as much as possible. Learning to enjoy your ejaculation and to give yourself permission to have one whenever you feel like it is just as important as peaking and plateauing and all the other ejaculation control "skills." Do this exercise if you are starting to feel a bit bogged down by working on your problem. Repeating this experience a few times will give you permission to ejaculate whenever you want to.

෬ *Exercise 32.* MAKING NOISE DURING EJACULATION

Some men have a related issue, which is that they have been embarrassed by their premature ejaculation problem for so long that they try to pretend they're not ejaculating. I guess this is a form of denial. They try to control an ejaculation by not moving or not making noise or not doing anything to indicate that they're aroused. This doesn't work, of course.

If this is the case for you, start making noise as you have intercourse. Role-play someone who is extremely aroused. Grunt or pant as you get close to ejaculation. Really go overboard—loudly say "I'm coming!" Imitate the orgasm scene from the movie *When Harry Met Sally,* but in reverse. This works best if you have already gained some degree of ejaculatory control, so that you can have intercourse without ejaculating immediately.

෬ *Exercise 33.* KEEPING YOUR EMOTIONAL AND
                  PHYSICAL AROUSAL LEVELS TOGETHER

This is an exercise that is especially helpful for flaccid ejaculation. Remember that flaccid ejaculation is a problem in which a man ejaculates before he has a full erection. It is a combination of premature ejaculation and erection problems.

There are two different arousal scales for men. There is the 1-to-10 scale of your internal feeling of closeness to ejaculation. That's the scale you've used in the peaking exercises in this chapter. We can call this emotional, psychological, or subjective arousal.

There's also the 1-to-10 scale describing how hard your erection is. We can call this physical arousal.

So far, you have only used the first scale. I now want you to be aware of the second scale. Normally a man's physical and emotional arousal levels run parallel, with his erection becoming harder as he becomes more emotionally aroused. It is not unusual, though, for the two responses to be a little bit out of sync; for example, your erection could be at level 8 and you could be ejaculating, or your feeling of emotional arousal could be at level 5 but you could have a really hard erection. In flaccid ejaculation, these two responses have gotten completely out of sync. For example, your emotional arousal might be at level 10 (ejaculation), while your erection is a 3 or 4 (not really erect enough for easy penetration).

If you experience flaccid ejaculations, you should do an exercise in which you peak during intercourse in the side-to-side position, gently folding or stuffing your penis into your partner's vagina using plenty of lubrication (the flaccid-insertion technique described in Exercise 26). After you have learned to control your ejaculation by focusing, breathing, relaxing, and peaking, try the following exercise, in which you attempt to keep your emotional and physical arousal levels together.

Begin the session with focusing caresses, and then do a nondemand genital caress or oral sex with your partner. Next, lie on your back while your partner caresses your genitals and does oral sex. Switch your focus back and forth between your erection level and your emotional arousal level. When you feel your emotional arousal level go higher than your erection by one or two levels, ask your partner to stop the stimulation. When your emotional arousal has gone down two levels, ask your partner to restart the stimulation.

You cannot will your erection to become harder so that it matches your emotional arousal, but you can manipulate your emotional arousal level to match your erection level by stopping the stimulation, slowing down the stimulation, breathing, focusing on the sensations, and relaxing. Do four or five peaks this way. You will find that each time your emotional arousal decreases to become more in line with your erection level, your erection level will increase with the next peak. Spend about fifteen minutes on this part of the exercise.

Ejaculate at the end of the exercise if you feel like it. You may need to repeat the exercise several times or alternate it with peaking exercises until you begin to notice a definite improvement in the hardness of your erections.

You can also do this exercise during intercourse in the butterfly position. Your partner lies on her back with her knees bent and her legs up in the air and spread apart. Using plenty of lubrication, kneel between her legs and stroke her vaginal lips with your penis. As you caress the outside of your partner's vagina with your penis, you will be aware that you are reaching a certain level of emotional arousal. If you feel that your erection level is lower than your emotional arousal level, slow down. Use your penis to caress some other part of your partner's body until your emotional arousal level has dropped back down to the same level as your erection.

If your penis is erect enough, insert it into your partner's vagina for the next peak, and repeat the process. Your penis doesn't have to be super-hard to penetrate in this position as long as you use plenty of lubrication. Every time you feel your emotional arousal go noticeably beyond your physical arousal, stop your movement or withdraw your penis until your two arousal levels are more in line with each other.

ᕙ *Exercise 34.* LISTENING TO MUSIC DURING INTERCOURSE

This is an advanced exercise to fine-tune your ability to last longer during intercourse. It can be used in any position. It will remind you to slow down during intercourse.

Choose a piece of music with a very slow beat and put it into the CD player. It should be instrumental; listening to the words of a song will distract you. When you start intercourse, just hold your penis still inside of your partner's vagina, and pay attention to the beat of the music. Slowly start to stroke, switching your focus back and forth from the feelings in your penis to the music. See if you can keep up with the music by matching one stroke per beat or one stroke per two beats. If you are able to do this, for the next exercise you should choose a different piece of music that has a slightly faster beat.

chapter 24

Healing Erection Problems

This is the longest treatment chapter in *Sexual Healing*. In part that's because we know much more than we used to about erection problems. Another reason why this chapter is so long is because in addition to sensate-focus exercises, it outlines medical solutions for erection problems that have a physical basis.

Could Your Erection Problems Be Physical?

If you have decided that you have an erection problem and you wish to heal it, the first thing to do is recognize that your problem might be physical. Before consulting a physician and undergoing a lot of expensive medical tests, ask yourself the following questions:

* Do I have erections during the night, or when I wake up in the morning?

* Do I have morning or nighttime erections, but have trouble when I'm with my partner?

* Do I have erections when masturbating but not when I'm with my partner?

As described in Chapter 7, a healthy man has several erections during the night, and he also has erections with masturbation. If you answered yes to any of the above questions, your erection problems may have a psychological basis, which means you will benefit from the exercises in this chapter.

If you never have morning or nighttime erections and haven't for several years, try the exercises anyway. There is a good chance you have a physical problem, but the exercises won't hurt you, and I've seen them work wonders for men with organic (physical) erection problems because of the powerful effect the mind has on the body. If you go through this program and experience no improvement, I recommend that you consult a urologist who specializes in erection problems. If you do not get erections when you masturbate (that is, when the psychological pressure is off), you might very well have a medical problem, and seeking medical advice is in order.

Now for the exercises. A couple of the early ones were adapted from the second edition of my book *Sexual Pleasure*. Remember to end all of the partner exercises with five or ten minutes of spoon breathing, and then with each partner giving feedback based on the questions outlined in Chapter 15.

❧ *Exercise 35.* DAILY GENITAL MASSAGE

Every day, for ten minutes, gently massage your penis, especially around the base. This is a way to get more blood flowing to the genital area. Put simply, this will help to "prime the pump."

Don't massage to create an erection. Massage to become aware of your penis and its sensations. This will create or reinforce your mind-body connection, which is crucial to experiencing deep arousal. Gentle massage will also help you develop your sensate-focus awareness. Do this massage whether you have an erection or not. I promise that you will see the results in future exercises.

❧ *Exercise 36.* CARESSING YOUR MORNING ERECTION

For many men, the hardest erections they have are the ones they have during their sleep cycles at night or the ones they have when they wake up in the morning. Here is an exercise you can do to use this to your advantage.

Figure out roughly how much sleep you need in order to have your best chance of waking up with a morning erection. Allow a little extra time in the morning, and when you wake up, do a self-peaking exercise (like you learned in Chapter 18). Do the peaking while paying attention to your arousal levels, not your erection levels. Peak for about fifteen minutes, going up to levels 5, 6, 7, 8, and 9, and then ejaculating if you want to. This exercise is good for improving erections because your arousal level will go up and down, but your penis will probably stay relatively hard during the entire exercise.

Many men unconsciously tighten their PC muscle when they feel themselves starting to become erect. Men develop this habit because, at first, squeezing the PC muscle seems to pump up their erection. However, if a man makes a habit of doing this, he may start to notice after a while that it takes longer and longer to get an erection, or that he gets an erection and then has trouble maintaining it. If he reacts to a loss of erection by squeezing harder, he will actually make matters worse. Here's why. If you squeeze your PC muscle when you start to get an erection, your penis will momentarily fill a little bit, because the blood that was already in the shaft past the PC muscle will flow into the penis. After that, however, the temporary squeezing of the PC muscle prevents more blood from flowing into the penis, and the end result is a net loss. You're literally taking one step forward and two steps back. If, on the other hand, you squeeze your PC muscle when your erection has already reached the state of rigidity, your erection will not be affected, because no more blood can flow in anyway.

Squeezing your PC muscle as you are getting an erection also works against your erection in two other ways. First, the sensation of tension travels along a feedback loop between your genitals and your brain. When your brain registers this "tension" message, it reacts in ways that interfere with your ability to feel the first stages of erection. Your body reacts to the tension by beginning the stress response, including the release of adrenalin, which can inhibit erection. Second, the fact that you are "doing something" to get an erection shifts you into a performance mode. Psychologically, this decreases your ability to relax and just allow your erection to happen.

Are you squeezing your PC muscle at an inopportune time? Try the exercise below to see if this is the case. Often, one session is all you need to break any bad habits. That may sound too good to be true, but I've seen it work with clients.

◠ﮩ *Exercise 37.* RELAXING THE PC MUSCLE FOR STRONGER ERECTIONS

This is an exercise that you do with your partner. Start the session with relaxation and focusing caresses. Then pleasure your partner with a nondemand genital caress. Lie comfortably on your side or back in the passive role. Have your partner spend fifteen to twenty minutes slowly caressing your genitals with her hand and mouth. As you become aroused, if she feels you tighten your PC muscle, she will tell you and then wait for you to relax it before she begins the caress again. After your partner has pointed out your unconscious tensing three or four times, you will begin to recognize it yourself, and then you'll be able to keep your PC muscle relaxed without feedback or prompting from your partner.

○ *Exercise 38.* ERECTION AWARENESS

Believe it or not, some men are so out of touch with their bodies that they do not know whether they have an erection. This may sound hard to believe, but it can happen if you have ignored the sensations in your body for a long time. If you have a problem with erection awareness, you may experience pleasant feelings in your genitals even while being unaware that your penis is hard enough for intercourse. I have worked with clients who had this problem. I would do a genital caress for twenty minutes or so, and the client would have an erection for almost the whole time without realizing it. Eventually the erection would go away simply because so much time had elapsed. The client would think that he had never gotten an erection during the session.

Another reason for lack of erection awareness is that sometimes a man specifically learns to ignore his erections because he thinks that is the best way to get an erection. Actually, he is partially on the right track. What he needs to do is stop worrying about his genitals and start feeling them. The feelings of arousal in your genitals are something you definitely want to concentrate on, not ignore!

To practice erection awareness with your partner, think of the hardness of your erection on a scale from 1 to 10 (review Chapter 7 for descriptions of the various erection levels). Level 1 would be a completely flaccid penis, and level 10 would be an extremely hard, almost painful, erection. If you get erections in the morning or when you masturbate, practice describing them using this scale.

Begin your first erection-awareness exercise with focusing caresses. Then you may do a genital caress or nondemand oral sex with your partner, after which you should lie back and relax with your eyes closed.

Women, you will monitor this exercise. Begin a nondemand front caress, and continue to a genital caress or oral sex for about twenty minutes. Ask your partner at various points during the caress how hard he thinks his erection is. If his estimate differs significantly from your estimate, have him open his eyes and look at his penis. No matter what his erection level is, ask him to estimate it five or six times during the course of the exercise. It's just as important for your partner to learn to recognize the lower levels of erection as it is for him to learn to recognize the higher levels of erection.

If your partner describes his erection as a level 2 when in fact it is hard enough for intercourse (a level 5 or 6), he needs to believe this. After he has seen his erection, have him close his eyes again and concentrate on the feelings in his penis so he can learn to recognize those feelings without having to look.

It is important to make sure that your partner breathes evenly and remains relaxed during this exercise. If he holds his breath, remind him to breathe. If he tenses his leg muscles, lightly pinch or tap them as a signal to relax. If he squeezes his PC muscle, remind him to relax it. As always, if he starts to become anxious, caress another body part to take the focus off the genitals. If your partner finds it impossible to relax, back up to an exercise with which he felt comfortable, like a back caress or an upper-body front caress.

Men, do the erection awareness exercise as many times as you need to until you are confident you can recognize, through feeling alone, when your erection is sufficiently hard for penetration.

Maintaining Erections

"What goes up must come down." We all accept this law of gravity in the abstract. However, when it comes to erections, many men believe—or hope—that what goes up should stay up forever. In fact, it is perfectly normal for erections to get harder and softer several times during the course of a sexual encounter, especially as you get older. When men feel their erections start to go down, whether during intercourse or before, they often panic and start frenzied activities to try to regain the erection or to "use it before they lose it." Working at it or trying to keep it hard is the worst thing you can do, as it virtually guarantees that you will lose the erection.

If you are one of those men who panics when your erection starts to go down, you need to learn a new response to this situation. Your previous response has been, "Oh, no! I'm losing it! I need to hurry up and do something with it before it goes down completely!" Guess what? What you really need to do is exactly the opposite. You have learned to believe that once you lose an erection, it will never come back. It is obvious how you learned this. In previous situations, when you lost an erection, you worried about it, which guaranteed that it didn't come back. Now is your opportunity to train yourself to think differently about this natural physiological phenomenon. Whenever you get that panicked feeling because you are losing an erection, use the feeling as a signal to tell yourself the opposite of what you usually tell yourself. Instead of, "Oh, no! I'm losing it," say to yourself, "I now am able to relax and enjoy the sensations in my penis. I won't try to work at anything sexual when I am feeling anxious. Instead, I take a deep breath, I relax my leg muscles, and I focus on how my partner is touching me."

Some men experience a more extreme reaction called *pelvic-steal syndrome.* In this case, the man can get an erection but loses it as soon as he starts to move or tighten his large muscles. The larger muscles, especially the leg muscles, literally steal blood away from the erection. This is a complex phenomenon, and there is some debate over whether it can be cured by anything other than surgery. I believe it can, and I have seen clients improve with this exercise. Whether you experience pelvic-steal syndrome or whether you panic when your erection goes down, the "get-and-lose" exercise will help you practice a new response when you feel your erection going down. You will learn that "what goes *down* must come *up.*"

The physiology of having and maintaining erections is well beyond the scope of this book. In fact, we could write a whole book just about erections. Instead, let's talk about it in simple terms. Think about your partner doing a genital caress or some oral sex with you. When you are breathing deeply and evenly, and not holding your breath, she will be able to feel (or even see) blood flow into your penis. If you hold your breath, she will be able to feel blood flow back out. If you keep your abdomen, thigh, and buttocks muscles completely relaxed, she will be able to feel blood flow into your penis. The instant you tighten up, she will be able to feel the blood flow back out. If you keep your PC muscle relaxed, blood will flow in. If you either consciously or unconsciously tighten your PC muscle, blood will flow back out. This simple in-and-out process, which your partner can easily observe, is the basis of the next erection exercise.

ᜒ *Exercise 39.* GETTING AND LOSING ERECTIONS

Begin the exercise as you would any other session, with focusing caresses. Then you may do a nondemand front or genital or oral caress on your partner. After that, lie on your back with your eyes closed. Your partner will begin a nondemand front caress, genital caress, and oral sex. As always, she will do the caresses for her own pleasure. She should note whether you are breathing evenly and relaxing. If not, she can remind you to do so. Remember to focus on the sensations.

Whenever you get a noticeable erection response, your partner will stop the stimulation and allow your erection to go back down to a level 1 (no erection). Then she will start over with the caress and allow your erection to come back up again. Repeat this pattern as many times as possible during a twenty-minute to half-hour period.

The first time you do this exercise, it may be frustrating. In fact, the first time you do it, you may not have an erection at all because you will be worrying about it. If you do have an erection, you may be tempted to think your old thoughts or go back to your old habits of flexing your PC muscle, tensing your thighs, thrusting your pelvis, or holding your breath when you feel yourself losing the erection. Your partner can give you feedback about whether you are doing these things. She can help you monitor yourself so that you become aware of the simple relationship between tension level and blood flow: Relaxing equals blood flowing in, tensing equals blood flowing out.

Many men develop a habit of tensing their PC muscle group as they are becoming aroused. Tightening your PC muscle may make you feel as if you are pumping up your erection, but in fact, as discussed above, it has the opposite effect: It will cause your erection to go down. An especially negative habit is tensing and holding the area of your PC muscle that includes the anal sphincter. This can cause you to lose your erection quickly. Make sure that you keep your anal sphincter completely relaxed during any sensate-focus exercise, especially the exercises involving genital stimulation. The get-and-lose exercise should demonstrate the relationship between muscle tension and erection quite clearly. You will learn that if you relax, your erection will return, whereas if you become tense or work at getting an erection, your penis will stay soft.

You may also find that you feel frustrated the first few times your partner stops stroking you. You may experience a little reverse psychology, thinking to yourself, "I'll show her! This time I'll get the erection and I won't lose it even though I'm supposed to!"

Finally, the exercise gives you a chance to practice your new responses to the former panic situation. During the first few erection losses you will probably experience frustration and worry. Tell your partner what you are feeling, and have her coach you on relaxing when you feel your erection going down. Repeat this exercise as many times as you need to, until you honestly are completely comfortable with the feeling that your erection is going down.

❧ Exercise 40. PEAKING FOR ERECTIONS

In Chapter 18, on self-touch, you learned how to do the peaking process by yourself. In Chapter 23, on healing premature ejaculation, I described the peaking process with a partner using manual and oral stimulation and intercourse. The peaking process can also be used to help you have firmer erections.

In Chapter 23 I described how to use the subjective or psychological 1-to-10 scale. That scale measures emotional arousal or your sense of closeness to ejaculation and orgasm. If you want to use the peaking process to heal erection problems, you can use either the subjective/psychological arousal scale or the erection-hardness scale. I would suggest that you first use the subjective/psychological scale. Doing so will help your erections, because focusing on arousal instead of erection removes the performance pressure. If you would like to do the peaking process using the subjective/psychological arousal scale, just do the peaking exercises described in Chapter 23 until you are confident that you can have reliable erections at level 6 or 7.

Next, you can start the peaking process based on your erection scale. First, do focusing caresses with your partner. Then have her give you a manual and oral genital caress. This time, instead of you giving her arousal feedback, as you did when you were using the psychological/subjective scale, she will give you feedback about the hardness of your erection. She'll stop at each peak and allow your erection to go down a couple of levels. After you have peaked at levels 4, 5, 6, and 7 (and 8 or 9 if possible), ejaculate if you feel like it or end the exercise however you wish.

You can also do an erection peaking exercise with intercourse. Start with focusing caresses, and then have your partner stimulate you manually and orally until you have about a level-5 erection. Then get into the butterfly position, and, using plenty of lubrication, insert your penis. Thrust and peak up to erection levels 6 and 7 (and 8 and 9 if you can). End the exercise with ejaculation or however you wish.

You can do this exercise using all of the versions described in Chapter 23. You can do several peaks in a row with low-level erections, or several peaks with higher-level erections. Allowing your erections to go up and down will make them not only harder but also more reliable.

In addition, you could do several peaks in a row at the same erection level. This is a really good idea. Do one exercise where you do five peaks at a level-5 erection. Then do a separate exercise in which you do five peaks at level 6. Doing several versions of this exercise at different levels is probably the best way I know of to regain your erection ability. Repeat all of these peaking exercises in all of the intercourse positions, including (in this order) the side-to-side position, the female-superior position, the rear-entry position, and the missionary position.

ᏝᎧ *Exercise 41.* PLATEAUING FOR ERECTIONS

Plateauing using the subjective/psychological arousal scale as described in Chapter 23 will help your erections because keeping your focus on arousal rather than erection takes the performance pressure off of you. You can also plateau using the erection scale, with manual or oral stimulation or intercourse in any position.

You first read a description of the plateauing process in Chapter 18 on exercises you can do by yourself. You know from that chapter that there are four techniques you can use to plateau using the subjective/psychological arousal scale: changing your breathing, squeezing your PC muscle, changing your thrusting, and switching your focus. You also read a description of the plateauing process for premature ejaculation in Chapter 23. We'll modify the exercise somewhat here so you can use it to help with your erections. To plateau using the erection scale, you won't use the PC muscle squeeze, because squeezing the PC muscle can cause your erection to go down too much. Instead, we'll substitute another technique: Your partner will vary the way she touches you. The first version of this plateauing exercise relies on your partner to gauge your erection level and adjust her caresses accordingly.

Start the exercise with focusing caresses, and then give your partner a front caress and a manual or oral genital caress. Next, lie on your back, and your partner will start to caress your penis manually and orally. When she sees that you have reached a level-4 erection (advanced filling), she will tell you that you are at level 4. She will take turns slowing down and speeding up her touch to see if you can stay at erection level 4 for a few seconds to a minute.

She should do the same for levels 5, 6, and 7 (and 8 and 9 if you're really on a roll). You should start the exercise in the passive role, but as you reach the higher levels, you can start moving and thrusting to help you plateau. Finish the exercise any way you both agree on.

Repeat versions of this exercise with your partner doing manual and oral stimulation. You can either change your breathing, change your movement, switch your focus, or have your partner vary the way she touches you in order to plateau at erection levels 4, 5, 6, and 7. Then do a version in which you alternate each of these techniques. In other words, do one erection plateau by changing your breathing, and the next one by switching your focus, and the next one by changing your movements, and the next by having your partner vary how she touches you.

Here's an active version of the plateauing exercise that takes place during intercourse. Do focusing caresses, and then have your partner stimulate you orally up to erection level 5. Next, get into the butterfly position and insert your penis. Slowly thrust until you are at erection level 6, caressing your partner's vagina with your penis. Use whatever combination of techniques (changing your breathing, switching your focus, changing your movements, having your partner vary her touches) that allows you to plateau at erection levels 6 and 7. With intercourse, the best plateauing technique for maintaining your erection at any given level seems to be alternating the speed of your thrusting.

ᕦᕤ *Exercise 42.* KEEPING YOUR PHYSICAL AND EMOTIONAL AROUSAL LEVELS TOGETHER (FOR ERECTIONS)

This is a slightly different version of the exercise described in Chapter 23. This version is amazingly effective for treating erection problems. It is a very advanced exercise because it combines elements of the subjective/psychological arousal scale and the erection-hardness scale, and it also requires a high degree of concentration and awareness of your body.

For most men, erections increase as arousal builds. Although erection and arousal are separate processes, they generally happen simultaneously. Men often have their hardest erections a few seconds before ejaculation. Men with erection problems, however, may notice that their erection tends to lag noticeably behind their arousal level. This partner exercise can help your erection rise with your arousal level. It allows you to alternate an erection peak with an arousal peak.

While you can't will your erection to become harder so that it matches your arousal level, you can manipulate your arousal level to sink until it matches your erection level. Arousal (which is psychological) decreases faster than erection does. As you do this exercise, you will find that each time your arousal level goes down to come into line with your erection level, your erection level will increase with your next peak.

To begin, exchange focusing caresses with your partner so that you are both relaxed. Then pleasure your partner with a sensual caress of her choosing—a front caress, genital caress, or oral sex. Now lie on your back and shift into the mindset of the passive role. Have your partner caress your genitals with her hands or lips or tongue. Focus on the sensations. If you reach arousal level 3 and you don't feel any erection occurring, signal your partner to stop the caress until your arousal level goes down to a 1. Then your partner can start to caress you again.

When you reach a filling-stage erection (level 3 or 4), check your arousal level. If it is higher than your erection level, have your partner stop the caress again until your arousal level is at 3 or 4. Keep peaking at higher and higher levels, alternating an erection peak with an arousal peak. Every time you reach a peak where your arousal level is higher than your erection level, have your partner stop the stimulation until your erection and arousal levels are the same.

If you repeat this exercise a couple of times, you will notice that your erection and arousal levels tend to stay together, especially at the lower levels. You may want to repeat the exercise another couple of times to practice this technique at higher levels of arousal and erection. Finish any of these exercises with orgasm and ejaculation if you feel like it.

You can also do this exercise in any intercourse position. Depending on the position, you or your partner may be responsible for stopping the stimulation to allow your arousal level to decrease. If you use the female-superior position, it will be your responsibility to ask your partner to stop moving. If you do the exercise in a side-to-side position, the butterfly position, or the rear-entry position, you will be responsible for both monitoring your levels and stopping and starting the movement to adjust your arousal and erection levels.

This exercise requires a lot of concentration, but I believe it's worth it. The awareness you will gain of both your arousal and erection levels is invaluable.

ᘓ *Exercise 43.* NONVAGINAL REPETITIVE PENETRATION

A lot of men with erection problems focus totally on being able to get inside their partner's vagina. In this exercise, you will "penetrate" various parts of your partner's body so that you start to think of every part of her body as sexual. Begin with a front caress with your partner. Then caress her genitals with your fingers, lips, and tongue. Put lubrication on your penis (whether it is erect or not) and caress your partner's body with it.

"Insert" your penis into your partner's armpit, elbow, the back of her knee, the space between her thighs, or any other opening you notice. For another version of this exercise, alternate these insertions with insertions into her vagina.

༄ *Exercise 44.* REPETITIVE PENETRATION FOR
           ERECTIONS

Before you begin, exchange focusing caresses with your partner; then do a nondemand front or genital caress or oral sex with her. When you're ready, lie on your back. Have your partner take the active role. She will do a front and genital caress with you and some oral sex if she wishes. When you have an erection of level 5 or 6, switch positions and have your partner lie on her back with her knees bent and her legs in the air (the butterfly position). Kneel between her legs and put a lot of lubrication on your penis and on your partner's vagina. Slowly caress the outside of her vagina with your penis. Caress her outer and inner vaginal lips and her clitoris. Caress your penis with your hand at the same time.

When your erection is at level 7 or so, slowly slide your penis into your partner's vagina. Do a few strokes inside, and then pull out and caress her lips and clitoris with your penis again. Allow your erection to decrease one or two levels by stopping the stimulation to your penis. Then stroke your penis again, and allow your erection to go up to level 8. Slowly penetrate again and do several long strokes, remembering to breathe, relax, and focus on the pleasurable sensations you are feeling in your partner's vagina.

Now withdraw and let your erection go down to a level 4 or 5. Use more lubrication and slowly penetrate when your erection is no higher than a level 5.

Repeat several of these erection peaks with withdrawal until you are confident you can penetrate with any level of erection. Notice that with a lot of lubrication your erection doesn't have to be super-hard to penetrate your partner's vagina. You can do this exercise no matter what your level of erection is.

༄ *Exercise 45.* MAINTAINING ERECTIONS DURING
           INTERCOURSE

Suppose that you successfully have erections and intercourse with the exercises described so far in this book. What should you do if you feel yourself starting to lose your erection after you have been having intercourse for some time? First of all, remember that it is perfectly normal for your erection to get harder and softer during intercourse. For example, you may penetrate with a level-7 erection, feel it go up to level 8, then back to level 6, and so forth. If you feel your erection start to go down, the secret is not to panic. Use the techniques that you practiced in the get-and-lose exercise. Do not immediately start to thrust harder or faster or become more active. Instead, breathe, relax your legs, focus your attention on the feelings in your penis, and start to move more slowly.

The reason you lost your erection in the first place was probably because you were becoming distracted. Ask yourself what is distracting you. Are you thinking about something other than sex, for example, work? Sensate focus is the answer to distracting thoughts of this type. Is your erection going down because you are tired and feel that you have had intercourse for a long-enough time? Remember not to put pressure on yourself. Do not continue intercourse if it no longer feels good, and do not attempt to have an orgasm if you really don't feel like it.

If you still have trouble maintaining erections during intercourse, try this erection-maintenance exercise. You are going to think your erection back up using intense sensate focus. You could call this exercise the "erection elevator."

Be sure that you are having intercourse in a comfortable position rather than a position that is putting stress on your chest and arms. When you feel your erection go down, breathe, relax your legs, stop all movement for a few moments, and focus your attention completely on the feelings in your penis. Slowly begin to caress the inside of your partner's vagina with your penis, making movements that are just barely vigorous enough for you to feel. Feel the warmth surrounding the different areas of your penis. Start with the slowest possible discernible movement and gradually increase your speed as your erection grows. It may also be helpful to think of this in terms of your partner using the inside of her vagina to caress the different parts of your penis.

Instead of relying on your partner to give you some kind of stimulation in order to get an erection, you are mentally providing your own stimulation by a combination of intense sensate focus and barely perceptible movements. For this exercise to be enjoyable, both partners should focus all of their attention on the feelings in the penis and vagina. Take turns moving, or move at the same time.

This exercise can be done in any position. It is easiest to do in a side-to-side position or with the man kneeling in front of the woman (the butterfly position). If you use the butterfly position, start the exercise without an erection. Kneel in front of your partner and begin to caress her vaginal lips with your penis, using lots of lubrication. Breathe, relax your muscles, and focus totally on the feelings in your penis. Use a masturbation motion if it helps you focus. When you have a moderate erection (about a level 6), insert your penis and do a few thrusts. Stop thrusting and allow your erection to go down a level. Then slowly start to move and focus until you are aware that your erection has gone back up. Thrust by tilting or rolling your pelvis rather than by tensing your leg muscles.

This exercise is similar to peaking, except that you use the physical-response (erection) scale instead of the psychological arousal scale. Your partner should remain passive while you practice allowing your erection to go up and down. She should focus intensely on her feelings in order to get the maximum sensual enjoyment from the exercise.

ᑐ *Exercise 46.* ORAL SEX WITH THE MAN ON TOP

Do you have erections fairly reliably but find it difficult to maintain one when you are lying on your back? If so, try this version of oral sex. Have your partner lie on her side. Kneel in front of her mouth. Have her prop herself up on an elbow and hold your penis with her other hand. She can lick your penis and take it into her mouth in this position. She will be going "up" on you rather than going down on you. This position offers a number of benefits for erection maintenance. A lot of men find that gravity gives them a boost of blood flow in this position. Plus, it's very arousing to watch your partner do oral sex from this vantage point.

In another variation on this position, your partner can lie on her back and you can straddle her chest. She can hold your penis and suck on it and lick it. You can be more active in this position and stroke your penis with one hand. You can "feed" it to her and caress her lips and the inside of her mouth with it.

ᑐ *Exercise 47.* FLACCID INSERTION

You may have been getting partial erections but avoided using them for intercourse because you thought they weren't hard enough. The purpose of this exercise (also called *quiet vagina* or *stuffing*) is to dispel the myth that your penis has to be rock-hard in order to have intercourse.

Begin with focusing caresses as usual. Next, you may do a genital caress or oral sex with your partner. Then have your partner do a front caress with you.

For this exercise, it is easiest to use the side-by-side scissors position. You should lie on your right side. Your partner will lie on her back at a right angle to you. She will put her left leg on top of your left leg and her right leg between your legs. Then you should scoot up against each other so your genitals are touching.

Both partners should breathe and relax. Your partner should caress her genitals and your genitals with some lubricant. If you become partially erect, that is fine. No matter what the state of your erection, your partner will gently fold or stuff your partially erect or flaccid penis into her vagina. She should first open her vagina with her fingers and caress the inside of it with lubricant.

It is sometimes helpful to slide the flaccid penis into the vagina by using one or two fingers as a splint of sorts. Rather than trying to insert the head of your penis first, she should place the penis along her vaginal lips with the base of your penis at the vaginal opening. Then she can gently push on the base of your penis to insert it. The head will follow. Your partner can then squeeze her PC muscle to make sure your penis is inside.

The purpose of this exercise is not to become aroused, but rather to experience the feeling of being inside the vagina with no pressure to have an erection or to perform sexually. Once your penis is inside your partner's vagina, it will be tempting to move or thrust. The first time you do this exercise, try to remain as motionless as possible. Breathe and relax your legs. Let your whole body sink into the bed. Focus on the pleasurable sensations of your penis enveloped in your lover's vagina. At most, squeeze your PC muscle a few times to assure yourselves that you are still inserted. Even if you feel yourself start to become erect while you are inside, don't move. Do this for fifteen to thirty minutes, then stop and give each other feedback.

If you repeat this exercise and are comfortable inside your partner's vagina, you may begin to slowly move your penis. You can do this whether you have an erection or not. Think of this as caressing your partner's vagina with your penis. If you become aware that your erection is going down, move more slowly or stop moving completely. Breathe and relax. Both partners should focus completely on the sensations in the penis and vagina. It is easier to focus if you move more slowly.

Practice the flaccid insertion exercise as many times as you need to, with progressively more and more movement, until you are comfortable with the idea that you can be inside your partner's vagina whenever you want to, no matter how hard or soft you are. Repeat the exercise until you can truly allow yourself to relax and leave yourself alone whether or not you have any level of erection.

The flaccid insertion exercise can be done in other positions besides the scissors position. It generally does not work well in the female-superior position, but it works very well in the butterfly position. If you decide to use the butterfly position for this exercise, you rather than your partner will be in charge of inserting your penis. Have your partner lie on her back with her legs up and spread. Kneel between her legs and caress your penis and her vagina with a lot of lubricant. Line your penis up so that it runs along her vaginal opening with the head near her clitoris and the base at the bottom end of her vagina. To insert your penis, gently push on the base. Then hold your partner's hips and move her toward you in order to get inside her vagina as far as you can.

∾ *Exercise 48.* NONDEMAND PENETRATION

There are two forms of nondemand intercourse: the "quick dip" and the longer version.

The Quick Dip

For the quick-dip version of the exercise, you add a quick episode of intercourse (no more than a few strokes) to the end of a manual or oral peaking exercise. Start with focusing caresses. Do a front caress, a genital caress, or oral sex with your partner. Next, she should begin a manual or oral peaking exercise while you remain passive. Peak using arousal levels rather than erection levels. See if you can peak all the way up to level 7 or 8. When you have reached a fairly high arousal level and when your partner thinks you are hard enough for intercourse, instead of doing another manual or oral peak, your partner can climb on top of you, insert your penis into her vagina, and thrust for a few strokes. If you become more aroused and ejaculate during this short bit of intercourse, fine. If not, your partner will climb off and finish the exercise using manual and oral peaking.

The purpose of this version of the exercise is to teach you that intercourse doesn't have to end with ejaculation, and if you feel your erection going down during intercourse, you can always switch to some other activity that you find stimulating and with which you are comfortable.

Longer Version

In the longer version of nondemand penetration, you use the female-superior position. This exercise is very similar to the flaccid insertion exercise. The difference is that you stay totally passive while your partner does all the thrusting. To begin, exchange focusing caresses with your partner. Then give her a front caress, a genital caress, or oral sex. Next, lie on your back and have your partner caress you. She can stimulate you either manually or orally, as long as she is doing it for her own pleasure. During this exercise you are totally passive, meaning that you don't even have to pay attention to your arousal levels or give your partner any feedback about them.

If your partner feels you are erect enough for intercourse, she will climb on top of you and thrust for a few strokes. Then she'll climb off and stimulate you manually or orally again. Your partner will be in charge of this exercise; that is, she will decide when to have intercourse and how many strokes to do at a time. She will have to monitor whether you are erect enough to keep going with intercourse. The first time you do this exercise, you may feel frustrated because you are not in charge of deciding when you will stop and start intercourse. You may feel that your partner is stopping and starting on a whim. Her instructions are to start intercourse if she thinks it would feel good and to stop temporarily if it doesn't feel good any more and go back to a caress that did feel good.

During this exercise, remember to breathe and to keep all of your muscles relaxed, especially your PC muscle. Focus as much of your attention as you can on the feelings in your penis, no matter what kind of stimulation you are receiving from your partner. If you want to, finish the exercise by having an orgasm and ejaculating, with either intercourse, oral sex, or manual stimulation.

This exercise can result in an important change in your thinking about intercourse. It reinforces the idea that you don't have to be rock-hard in order to start intercourse. It also helps you learn to appreciate the unique sensations of intercourse instead of looking forward to intercourse as the "main event" and seeing every other kind of stimulation as second-best. You will learn what you are supposed to from this exercise if you can truly say that you were able to focus so intently on the sensations themselves that you really couldn't tell which type of stimulation your partner was giving you at any particular time.

❧ *Exercise 49.* PHONE IT IN

Do you own a phone with a vibration setting or a beeper? If so, you can use it to train yourself to have erections. Figure out how to set a phone or beeper to go off at random times during the day—say, maybe ten times a day. Whenever the vibrator or beeper goes off, stop what you are doing, find a private place, sit down, relax, and give yourself a short sensate-focus genital caress, whether you get an erection or not. Reset the beeper or phone every day so that it goes off at different times. Do this for about two weeks. From this point on, whenever you feel the vibrator or hear the beeper, you'll start to get an erection.

Physical, Behavioral, and Psychological Issues in Erection Problems

Specific aspects of the mind-body connection may be getting in the way of your ability to have satisfying erections. Let's look at some potential physical, behavioral, and psychological issues that could be at play here.

Health Habits

Take a look at your health habits. Are you overweight? Do you smoke, drink alcohol, or use illegal drugs? As I mentioned in Chapter 17, all of these habits can cause severe erection problems. Quitting these practices will cause dramatic changes in your erections as well as in your sexual fulfillment, your ability to savor sensations, and ultimately your sexual self-esteem.

Medical Conditions

Do you have any chronic medical conditions that might be affecting your erections? Diabetes, prostate problems, and circulatory problems are among the medical conditions that can interfere with erections. In addition, many prescription medications, such as those given for high blood pressure and ulcers, can have a negative effect on erections.

Pelvic-Steal Syndrome

In addition to all of the physical and emotional problems that can affect your erections, it is also possible that you may be doing something during lovemaking that prevents you from having an erection (a behavioral issue). As discussed earlier in the chapter, unconsciously or consciously squeezing your PC muscle during arousal can actually prevent erection. As you become aroused, you may also unconsciously tighten the muscles in your legs, abdomen, or buttocks. Some men do this because they think it helps them get an erection. In fact, it does the opposite, because the blood that could be available for your erection is diverted to the muscles that are tightening up. This phenomenon is called pelvic-steal syndrome because the blood that could be used for your erection is literally being stolen for use by your body's long muscles. To deal with these possible issues, try the exercise for relaxing the PC muscle (Exercise 37) and the "get-and-lose" exercise (Exercise 39).

Attitude

When discussing psychological causes of erection problems, the first place to start is by taking a look at your attitude and sexual awareness. Never pressure yourself to have an erection during any exercise described in this book or during any sexual activity. You can do every exercise in this book, up to and including sexual intercourse, without an erection. While going through the exercises, try to pay more attention to your arousal levels (i.e., how close you feel to ejaculation) than you do to your erections.

Erection problems occur when men expect their bodies to perform like machines. It's unrealistic to expect to get an erection if you're angry, exhausted, stressed out, or have just eaten a huge meal. On the other hand, try to be satisfied with the erection you have. It doesn't do any good to wait for the perfect erection that's somewhere out there on the horizon. Start some sensual contact with your partner and enjoy the level of erection you *do* have.

Attributions

An attribution is an explanation for a behavior. How you explain your erection abilities to yourself can have an impact on those abilities. There are two basic types of attributions: internal and external. In an *internal attribution,* you attribute the cause of your behavior to something inside yourself, for example, your personality or your character. In an *external attribution,* you attribute your behavior to something outside yourself, for example, bad luck or the behavior of another person.

When it comes to erections, you should always attribute your erections to something internal ("I had an erection because I allowed myself to relax," or, "I had an erection because I was horny"). Conversely, you should always attribute situations in which you *did not* have an erection to something external ("I didn't get very hard because I had just eaten" or "I didn't get hard because the noise from the television set was distracting"). Make lists of both internal and external attributions for your erections, and start using them often.

Spectatoring and Performance Anxiety

Finally, are you spectatoring? This is a term coined by Masters and Johnson that refers to watching and worrying about whether you are getting an erection. You can read more about spectatoring in Chapter 3, on the role of anxiety in sexual problems. A watched pot never boils... and a watched penis never hardens.

Medical Solutions for Erection Problems

We live in an age when men are very concerned about erections. A number of medical solutions have been developed over the years to help with erections. They all have downsides. If a perfect erection enhancer existed, everyone would use it.

I list these medical solutions in order from cheapest, easiest, and safest to most expensive, most painful, and most dangerous. When describing drugs, I obtained my information from the product packaging.

Over-the-Counter Erection Enhancers

Go to any health-food store or supplement/vitamin store and you will find a whole wall of products that purport to help erections. Some of these products are herbal remedies, and some are precursors of testosterone or other hormones that help erections. Do they work?

To my knowledge, the only one of these substances that has been clinically tested is yohimbine. Yohimbine is a stimulant made from the bark of the yohimbe tree. It used to be sold by prescription only, but now it is sold over the counter. Yohimbine has been found to enhance erection in some men because it is a stimulant. This means it causes your heart to beat faster and your blood pressure to rise. For some men this translates into a quicker or harder erection. You should not take yohimbine if you have anxiety problems or are on heart medications. Some men report that yohimbine gives them heart palpitations.

Regarding most other herbal products that claim to enhance erections, in general I would steer clear of them. Most of them contain stimulants that are not clearly labeled as such and can make anxiety symptoms worse.

I know many men who have taken supplements like DHEA (a precursor of testosterone) and arginine, because they supposedly enhance erections. Sometimes these supplements appear to work for a couple of sessions. I believe these results are probably due to the placebo effect, which can occur when someone expects a medication to work. (You'll read more about the placebo effect in Chapter 32.)

Vacuum Erection Device

The vacuum erection device (VED or penis pump) is not a drug and is not invasive. It consists of a plastic cylinder that fits over the penis. You put lubrication and a surgical rubber band on one end of the cylinder and fit it over your penis. The cylinder is attached to a pump, which is either battery-powered or operated by hand. The device pumps air out of the cylinder, creating a vacuum, which causes blood to literally be sucked into the penis. When you have pumped your penis up to a full erection, you slide the rubber band down to the base of your penis in order to hold the blood in.

The upside: This device is inexpensive. If you buy it as a medical device, insurance plans will often cover it. You can also buy cheaper versions of it in adult stores or through adult-product catalogs. The device is very good for men whose PC muscle is in bad shape or men who have difficulty maintaining an erection. The downside: Because the rubber band acts as a tourniquet around the penis, you really shouldn't use it for more than twenty minutes. If the rubber band is too tight, in some cases it can rupture a blood vessel in the penis, which can cause bruising and bleeding. Furthermore, it kind of breaks the mood of a sexual encounter if you have to stop and pump up your penis. You need to have erectile tissue to use this device; in other words, men with advanced Peyronie's disease (a buildup of scarring in the erectile tissue) can't use it. The men whom I have seen use this device successfully have been in their seventies and eighties and really had no other options other than a penile implant.

MUSE

MUSE stands for male urethral suppository for erections. It is the brand name for a drug called alprostadil that is administered in a pellet form that is inserted directly into the urethra. This is painless; the pellet is very small. Once the medication is inserted, the user is instructed to walk around for about ten minutes while stroking his penis firmly from head to base to get the medication into his erectile tissue.

MUSE is easy to use and doesn't go through the digestive system, so it doesn't cause stomach problems. In my experience, however, it just doesn't work very well. It is too dependent on the vagaries of individuals' metabolism. Plus, if receiving oral sex is a big part of your sexual repertoire, you definitely don't want to use this drug. A woman can't go down on you right after you insert the pellet because she will suck it right out of your penis. Besides, it tastes terrible and probably doesn't do her any good, either.

Viagra, Levitra, and Cialis

When Viagra was first introduced in 1998, it caused quite a controversy. Most of the hoopla seems to have died down, and many men are using it successfully on a regular basis. In general, Viagra works by relaxing the smooth muscle at the base of the penis (the PC muscle), thereby allowing blood to flow into the penis more easily following direct stimulation.

Viagra comes in doses of 25 milligrams, 50 milligrams, or 100 milligrams. You take it half an hour to an hour before you want to have sex. Viagra cannot be used if you are taking nitroglycerin heart drugs; this combination can be fatal. Since it is taken orally, it has to go through the digestive system and thus can cause indigestion. If you take it with food, it takes longer to work. It can also cause nasal congestion and facial flushing.

I have seen Viagra work really well for many men. It tends to work well for men in their forties, fifties, and sixties who have psychological erection problems, although I have also seen it work for men following prostate cancer and surgery. In my experience, it has not worked well for men in their seventies and eighties. This is probably because the smooth muscle at the base of the penis is in such bad shape.

The newer drugs Levitra and Cialis work on the same principle as Viagra: They relax the smooth muscle, allowing blood to flow into the penis more easily with stimulation. The advantage of Levitra and Cialis over Viagra is that they are purported to work faster and to last for a longer time.

Versions of these drugs are available that can be inserted under the tongue so you don't have to digest them.

Injection Therapy

There are several substances that can be injected directly into the penis to cause erections. Two of them are papaverine and regitine, which are fast-acting vasodilators that literally draw blood into the erectile tissue of the penis. Using a fine-gauge needle, you inject the drug into the corpus cavernosum on one side of your penis. Prostaglandin (or alprostadil), a hormone that also promotes erection, is another substance that can be injected directly into the penis.

Obviously, the downside of injection therapy is the discomfort or pain of injecting something directly into the penis. If you are uncomfortable with the idea of filling a syringe, the manufacturers market a version called Caverject, which comes already filled with a quick-action injection device like the ones used for flu shots. A problem with injection therapy is that if you inject at the same site over and over, you can develop scar tissue that can change the appearance of your penis or further compromise your ability to get an erection. Sometimes the use of penile injections can cause bruising or bleeding. Finally, users have to be careful to make sure they are injecting into the erectile tissue rather than into some other area.

Penile Implants

Penile implants are mechanical devices that are surgically inserted into the penis. They are a last resort for men with serious medical problems who have no other way to obtain an erection. The most likely candidates for penile implants are men who have had their prostate removed and men with diabetes who no longer have nerve supply to the penis.

There are two kinds of penile implants: the semirigid rod and the three-part inflatable implant. The semirigid rod is a silicone-covered rod that is inserted alongside the urethra. It has no moving parts. It makes the penis semihard all the time. When you're not having sex, you just bend it down so it rests against your leg. When you want to have sex, you bend it up. Obviously, having a semirigid rod inserted in the penis will interfere with ejaculation. But a man with advanced diabetes or prostate problems can't ejaculate anyway. He can still have an orgasm.

I believe that the semirigid rod is no longer used very much. The three-part hydraulic implant is now the implant of choice. The three parts of this implant are comprised of a hollow cylinder that is implanted in the penis alongside the urethra, a reservoir of fluid placed in the abdomen, and a valve implanted under the skin of the scrotum. When the user wants to have an erection, he turns the valve, causing fluid to flow from the reservoir into the cylinder located in the penis, making the penis erect. A man with this type of implant can have an orgasm but not an ejaculation. When he's finished having intercourse, he just pumps the implant back down.

As is probably apparent, implants have their problems. There are risks involved with any surgery, and recovery from the surgery takes many weeks. Like any mechanical device, the implants themselves have some percentage of failure. Also, the implants don't go all the way into the head of the penis, so the head may be a little floppy even though the rest of the penis is hard. Implants obviously take some getting used to, but I have seen many men who are happy with them.

Other Surgical Options

Sometimes erection problems occur because blood flow to the groin area is severely compromised. If this is the case, undergoing an arterial bypass may be an option. In other cases, a man can't maintain an erection because some of the valves at the base of the penis that hold blood in the penis are faulty. The valves can sometimes be tied off surgically. Obviously, these two surgical repairs are very serious and should be undertaken only if no other options are available.

chapter 25

Healing Male Orgasm Disorder

In the chapter on healing premature ejaculation, I discussed three things a man needs to do in order to get ejaculatory control. Similarly, if you are experiencing inhibited ejaculation, there are a number of things you will need to do.

Behavioral Changes: A Summary

Like the man with premature ejaculation, you will need to get control of your PC muscle by exercising it (see exercises in Chapter 17). The man with premature ejaculation needs to get control of his PC muscle so he can squeeze it to delay ejaculation. You will need to do the opposite: You will get control of your PC muscle so you can learn to consciously relax it as you near ejaculation. One of the biggest problems in men with inhibited ejaculation is that they unconsciously tense their PC muscle as they approach ejaculation, and we know from the findings of Masters and Johnson that this only leads to more of a problem with ejaculation.

Also, like the man with premature ejaculation, you will need to learn to become more aware of your sensations of arousal. The man with premature ejaculation needs to get experience with the lower levels of his arousal scale. You will need to get experience with the higher levels of your arousal scale— 7, 8, and especially 9. One of the biggest problems with men with inhibited ejaculation is that they start anticipating ejaculation too soon. They start anticipating it at arousal level 7 or even 6, instead of at level 9. They lose their sense of what it feels like to be at level 8 or 9, and they start tensing up and working at ejaculation at low levels. Because of this lack of awareness of arousal levels, the peaking process works very well for both premature ejaculation and inhibited ejaculation. I know it seems ironic that the same process would work well for completely opposite problems, but it's the case.

You will probably also have to change your masturbation habits, at least temporarily, if your habits are contributing to a problem of being unable to ejaculate with intercourse. I've included several suggestions and exercises to help you do this.

Last, but by no means least, in order for you to learn to ejaculate more easily, you will probably have to work on promoting the intimacy in your relationship. Your sense of emotional closeness with your partner will have a huge impact on your ability to ejaculate more easily during intercourse with her.

Before you begin to deal with your inhibited ejaculation problem, there are a couple of things you should stop doing. First, you should limit the amount of time you spend having intercourse. For example, if you find that you are having intercourse for half an hour and are unable to ejaculate even though you want to and are trying to, then limit yourself to a certain time frame. Tell your partner that from now on you will stop at ten minutes or fifteen minutes or some other mutually agreed on comfortable limit, whether you have ejaculated or not. Contrary to what you may believe, it will not hurt you to become aroused and then naturally allow your arousal to go down without ejaculating.

Limiting the time you spend in intercourse will allow you to stop thinking, "If only I had another few seconds (or few minutes, or half an hour), I know I could ejaculate." Women, if you are the partner of a man who is having problems with inhibited ejaculation, there is no need to feel guilty about ending intercourse before he ejaculates. Prolonging intercourse will not help inhibited ejaculation. In fact, it will make it worse. Doing more of what you are already doing will not help. Learning some alternative activities will.

Limiting the time you spend in intercourse will also force you to focus on the sensations of intercourse that are happening in the here and now, rather than on sensations that may happen in the future (orgasm and ejaculation). It will also force you to admit that you have a problem ejaculating, which is something you may not have truly accepted.

Also, resolve that from now on, when you have intercourse, you will do it as slowly as possible, and in a sensate-focus, nondemand fashion. You have probably become used to a hard-driving mode of intercourse that is actually making your problem worse. When you catch yourself going too fast, consciously make an effort to slow down.

The Role of Intimacy

Take another look at Chapter 10 for a discussion of the role of repressed anger in inhibited ejaculation. The anger you are holding inside may be overcome to some degree by fostering intimacy in your relationship, and you can accomplish this by doing the exercises described in this chapter (provided your anger is at a woman from your past, not at your current partner). In order for this to work, you will have to want it to work. That is, you can't do these exercises halfway, as they will definitely produce a certain amount of intimacy. If you know that you do not want that level of intimacy, then do not attempt these exercises.

Although all of the partner exercises in this book will promote intimacy between you and your lover, the two exercises that follow are specifically aimed at building intimacy.

∾ *Exercise 50.* SENSUOUS KISSING

In this exercise to foster intimacy, you and your partner will take turns kissing each other on the mouth. The active person should kiss as if it were a caress. Caress the outside and inside of your partner's mouth with your tongue. Focus, breathe, and relax, just as you would with any sensate-focus caress. The best position in which to do this is lying on your sides facing each other.

Each partner should do the kissing caress for at least five to ten minutes. Stop occasionally and gaze into each other's eyes. Finish the kissing caress with five or ten minutes of mutual kissing.

The goal of this exercise is not to leave each others' lips and tongues sore. The idea is to kiss as slowly, sensuously, and intimately as possible. If you find that you are going too fast, kissing too hard, or unable to maintain concentration, stop for a moment, refocus your attention, and start over more slowly.

It is important that you do this exercise separately from any other exercise at least once. Talk about your feelings about the exercise after you do it. Then, use this kissing exercise as a prelude to the other exercises in this chapter.

If you feel anxious during this exercise, that's because it promotes tremendous intimacy between partners, whether you want it to or not. Many people find kissing on the mouth to be a more intimate act than oral sex or even sexual intercourse. Remember, if you feel anxious or uncomfortable during this exercise, do what you would do if you feel anxious during any exercise: Tell your partner you are anxious, and back up to something you are comfortable with. For example, if you are uncomfortable looking into your partner's eyes while kissing, practice the exercise with your eyes closed until you can relax. Then move on to the more intimate version of the exercise and repeat it as many times as you need to until you are completely comfortable with it.

∿ *Exercise 51.* EYE GAZE

This is a very simple but powerful exercise. Lie together on your bed and face each other. Wrap your arms comfortably around each other and gaze into each other's eyes for a few minutes without talking. Consciously relax your whole body so that none of your muscles are tense.

The Role of Masturbation

In my experience, the most common cause of inhibited ejaculation is probably masturbation habits. If you have learned over the years to masturbate with a harder and harder and faster and faster stroke, pretty soon you will have difficulty ejaculating with intercourse because your partner's vagina cannot provide the same level of physical stimulation that your hand can. Here are some activities that can help you change your masturbation habits.

There are three ways to change your masturbation habits: decreasing masturbation time, decreasing masturbation frequency, and softening your stroke.

∿ *Exercise 52.* DECREASING MASTURBATION TIME

Some men experience inhibited ejaculation with intercourse simply because they masturbate for excessive amounts of time but don't have the stamina to continue intercourse for the same amount of time. Their partner probably doesn't have the stamina either. Research indicates that some men masturbate to ejaculation in a few seconds, while others may spend several hours stimulating themselves before they allow themselves to ejaculate. Chances are, if you have difficulty ejaculating with intercourse, you tend to masturbate for a long period of time. Our goal here is to shorten the amount of time it takes you to masturbate to orgasm and ejaculation.

Don't worry. I'm pretty sure you like your masturbation habits. I am not asking you to change them permanently. Once you have learned to comfortably and predictably ejaculate with intercourse, you can go back to masturbating in whatever way makes you comfortable.

The easiest way to decrease your masturbation time is to simply keep track of your masturbation habits. Don't try to change anything at first. Just masturbate the way you normally like to, but jot down what you do in a notebook. If you like to masturbate while using things like videos or magazines, continue to do so.

Look at a clock before you start masturbating, and then look at it again right after you ejaculate. You may be surprised to discover that you've gone much longer than you thought. For two weeks, keep a chart of your masturbation time. Record how many times a week you masturbate and how long it takes you each time. During week three, try to take five minutes off your time. Each successive week, try to take two minutes off your time until you can easily masturbate to orgasm and ejaculation within ten minutes at the most. At this point you will be ready to begin peaking exercises with your partner.

ᘙ Exercise 53. DECREASING MASTURBATION FREQUENCY

Again, try keeping a two-week record to see how often you masturbate. Then cut down the frequency by about 10 percent each subsequent week until you feel a noticeable increase in your penile sensitivity and a greater ease in ejaculating.

ᘙ Exercise 54. SOFTENING YOUR STROKE

Here is an exercise that will help sensitize your penis. It will help you become more aware of the delicate sensations of being inside your partner's vagina.

Do a genital caress on yourself. Close your eyes and concentrate on the sensations of your touch. As you caress your genitals, slow your stroke down so that it is half as fast as when you began. Enjoy the sensations of this new stroke. What sensations do you feel in your penis, your fingers?

Now slow down a second time, until your fingers and palm are barely moving over your penis. Continue this caress for fifteen minutes whether you ejaculate or not.

Do this exercise on a regular basis to decrease the roughness of your masturbation stroke. To help slow yourself down, try using your left hand if you are right-handed (and vice versa), or try using an open palm or your fingertips alone instead of a closed fist.

Some men find that they can make changes in their masturbation time, their masturbation frequency, and their masturbation stroke during the same week or weeks. Other men find it easier to concentrate on one area at a time; for example, they may concentrate on decreasing masturbation time for a couple of weeks, and then on decreasing masturbation frequency for a couple of weeks, and then on changing their stroke for a couple of weeks. You know yourself, and you will have to decide which of these approaches will work best for you. I believe that working on one thing at a time is best from a behavioral standpoint, but some men get bored with this approach.

Also, try not to get discouraged if this process seems to take a long time. It may take you a good six or eight weeks to change your masturbation habits enough to start doing peaking exercises with your partner. Remember that you can still have sexual intercourse with your partner during this time frame, as long as you set a time limit on the intercourse and never work at ejaculating.

Here are a couple more exercises that use self-touch to help you learn to ejaculate more easily.

∾ *Exercise 55.* SIMULATE THE VAGINA

Another reason why men develop an inability to ejaculate with intercourse is because they are so used to masturbation that the sensations of being inside a vagina are not stimulating enough for them. A solution for this is to introduce something into your masturbation habits that makes masturbation feel more like intercourse.

There are several things you can use to masturbate with that feel more like a vagina than your hand does. Adult stores and catalogs sell many varieties of artificial vaginas. One that is quite popular is shaped like a flashlight and has a removable liner. Other men have used a banana peel filled with lubricant, or an old sock warmed in the dryer or microwave and filled with lubricant. Or you could use a large-size condom filled with lubricant. The point is to thrust into something that is warm and isn't as tight as your closed fist. (Although, as I'm writing this, I'm thinking, when you have intercourse with your partner, don't say to her, "Honey, being inside you feels great. You feel almost as good as an old sock filled with K-Y Jelly.")

To make the most of your vagina substitute, use it during a self-touch exercise. Start by stroking your penis with your hand and doing a peaking exercise as you learned in Chapter 18. Do several high-level peaks while thrusting into your vagina substitute. See if you can ejaculate into it.

꙰ *Exercise 56.* PROLONGING ORGASM

This exercise can help you ejaculate more easily by helping you learn the difference between the sensations of ejaculation and those of orgasm. Remember that orgasm and ejaculation are not exactly the same thing. Orgasm is systemic and includes full-body responses like rapid heart rate, muscle tension, and a feeling of extreme pleasure, whereas ejaculation is the localized genital response in which the PC muscle spasms and forces semen out of the penis.

Start with a slow, sensual genital caress, using plenty of lubrication. Remember to breathe, focus on your sensations, and keep all of your muscles, including your PC muscle, relaxed. Using the psychological/subjective arousal scale, peak up to lower levels like 4, 5, and 6. Let your arousal decrease two levels between peaks. Let each complete peak last three to five minutes. Now peak up to levels 7 and 8.

Next, peak up to level 9. When you reach your point of inevitability, stop thrusting, stop your hand movement, hold perfectly still, close your eyes, and take a deep breath. Focus all of your attention on your pelvic sensations. Feel the semen start to move from your testicle area into your urethra. This is the "emission" phase of ejaculation. Feel the contractions of organs such as your prostate, and then notice how a few seconds later your PC muscle starts to pulse rhythmically. This is the "expulsion" phase of ejaculation. Now breathe deeply again, open your eyes wide, and focus all of your attention on the sensations in the base of your penis. You will feel each spurt of semen distinctly as you ejaculate, and you will experience a sense that your orgasm lasts longer than usual. Experiencing these sensations and the difference between ejaculation and orgasm can help you ejaculate more easily because it will help you look forward to ejaculating without pressuring yourself.

More Behavioral Strategies for Changing Masturbation Habits

Here's a final thought on changing your masturbation habits. Let's say you have learned to decrease your masturbation time, decrease your masturbation frequency, change your masturbation stroke, simulate a vagina, and prolong your orgasm. Do you have any "weird" habits that you think might be contributing to your ejaculation difficulties?

I'm not trying to suggest that your masturbation habits are bad, wrong, or kinky. Rather, I'm pointing out that men who have no difficulty ejaculating tend to masturbate in particular ways that involve no "weirdness." Here's what I mean by "weirdness." Do you masturbate in an unusual position—for example, do you always kneel to masturbate? Do you always use sexually explicit materials when you masturbate? Do you have to have certain objects around you when you masturbate? Do you consistently use an unusual stroke, such as rubbing your penis between your hands like someone trying to light a fire in the wilderness? Do you have to fantasize about unusual scenarios (coercive scenarios or anything else) in order to come? Do you require anal stimulation in order to have an ejaculation when you masturbate?

I'm not saying that any of these things are wrong. I'm saying that they can stand in the way of your learning to ejaculate easily with intercourse. If you have any of these habits, now's the time to taper off the behaviors. You will have the best chance of learning to ejaculate easily with intercourse if you masturbate while lying on your back or sitting up leaning against a wall or headboard. You have the best chance of learning to ejaculate with intercourse if you masturbate by gripping your penis with one hand and moving your hand up and down.

You can taper off any behaviors that you think might interfere with your ability to ejaculate during intercourse using the following strategy:

1. Chart your behavior. For example, let's say you are trying to taper off anal stimulation, because you know your partner won't do it during intercourse. For two weeks, record how frequently and how long you masturbate, and also record what percentage of time you stimulated your anus during masturbation. Chances are it will be for a large percentage of your total masturbation time.

2. For the next two weeks, set a goal of decreasing the amount of anal stimulation by a certain percentage during each masturbation session. For example, if you usually stimulate your anus 80 percent of the time while you masturbate, try to stimulate it only half the time, then a fourth of the time. Get to the point where you only touch your anus right before the point of orgasm. The next step is that you will be able to have an orgasm while merely thinking about touching your anus as you are close to ejaculation.

You can use this behavioral strategy to change any of the habits I've listed above. All of these changes will prepare you to have orgasms more easily during intercourse.

In addition, you will need to "overlearn" the genital self-caress and self-peaking exercises described in Chapter 18. Set aside separate times for having time-limited intercourse with your partner and for doing the genital self-caress. You may do a genital self-caress as often as every day, but allow yourself to go all the way to ejaculation only if you can do so without working at it. During the exercises you do by yourself, train yourself to become aroused with a gentle touch to your penis, rather than the fast or vigorous motions you may have used for masturbation in the past.

A Choice of Approaches for Healing Inhibited Ejaculation

Now we move to what might be called the advanced stage of the program for healing inhibited ejaculation. As a man who has difficulty ejaculating, you have several options for approaching your problem. Read through the three different strategies that follow and use the one that most appeals to you, based on your sense of the problem and your issues. The three strategies are the peaking process, intercourse and masturbation together, and shaping. I would use shaping for a very severe problem with inhibited ejaculation, masturbation and intercourse together if you can ejaculate easily with masturbation and can regularly go up to arousal level 8 with intercourse, and peaking if you have only recently developed the problem with ejaculation. Another strategy would be to try the peaking process first because it's the easiest, and if it doesn't really work for you, then try one of the others. All three programs involve a progression of exercises that should be done as fully structured sensate-focus exercises, with focusing caresses, active and passive roles, and feedback.

The Importance of Peaking

Peaking is just as important for inhibited ejaculation as it is for premature ejaculation. If you would like to use the peaking process, do it as described in Chapter 23, on healing premature ejaculation. You can do the exercises exactly as described there, with one major exception. If you are dealing with inhibited ejaculation, never squeeze your PC muscle during an exercise.

If you opt for the peaking process, do all the exercises in the following order: arousal awareness, peaking with manual stimulation, peaking with oral sex, and peaking with intercourse. When you do the exercise for peaking with intercourse, use the different positions in the following order: side-to-side, butterfly, woman on top, rear entry, and man on top. Remember, you can do one exercise in which you only peak at lower levels, one in which you only peak at higher levels, or one in which you do all the peaks at the same level. In the case of inhibited ejaculation, you will need to focus mostly on the higher arousal levels, because these are the levels with which you have a problem. Do each session of peaking as a full sensate-focus exercise, with spoon breathing, focusing caresses, active and passive roles, and feedback.

The plateauing process will also benefit you. Again, you can plateau with manual stimulation, oral sex, or intercourse in any position. Plateauing strategies include changing your breathing, changing your movement, and changing your focus. If you have inhibited ejaculation, *do not* use the plateauing strategy of tightening your PC muscle.

Important: If you do any peaking or plateauing exercise for inhibited ejaculation, never pressure yourself to ejaculate, and never do anything to try to ejaculate. The goal here is for you to learn the sensations of high arousal levels. If you don't ejaculate during an exercise, that's okay. You've still done the exercise correctly if you remembered to breathe, relax, focus on the sensations, and keep your PC muscle from tightening. Ejaculation will happen when it happens. It will happen when you are so focused on the sensations that you allow it to happen rather than try to make it happen.

In addition to the peaking process as described in Chapter 23, there are a couple of variations you can use for inhibited ejaculation.

❧ Exercise 57. ALTERNATING PEAKS

In this version of the peaking exercise, you alternate peaks with manual stimulation and peaks with oral stimulation. This is really simple. Start with a low-level peak, like a 4, with your partner caressing you with her hand. Then do the next peak (a 5 or 6) as she caresses you with her mouth. Keep alternating manual and oral peaks until you either reach a very high level of arousal or ejaculate.

In another version of the exercise, alternate masturbation peaks with oral sex peaks. This generally works really well for men who have difficulty ejaculating inside their partner's vagina. Have your partner stimulate you to a level 5 with oral sex. Next, allow your arousal level to decrease, and then stimulate yourself up to level 6 with masturbation. Try to use a sensate-focus masturbation stroke rather than a hard and fast stroke. Continue alternating these peaks, and allow yourself to ejaculate with the final masturbation peak. Another way to do this is to masturbate to the final peak of ejaculation and hold your penis up against your partner's mouth as you ejaculate.

If you usually go into another room to masturbate, before you do these exercises you may need to practice masturbating in the same room with your partner. Have her shut her eyes at first if you are uncomfortable with her watching you. If you are able to masturbate with your partner watching, there is an excellent chance that you will be able to relearn how to ejaculate with intercourse.

Intercourse and Masturbation Together

The second strategy for dealing with inhibited ejaculation involves combining masturbation with intercourse. As you'll see, this isn't just one exercise, but rather a progression of exercises.

ᑫᖫ *Exercise 58.* INTERCOURSE WITH MASTURBATION

Begin the session with focusing caresses. Remember the basic sensate-focus principles: Focus on the sensations, breathe, and relax. Move on to a few minutes of mutual sensual kissing. Then lie on your back and take the passive role. Your partner can do a genital caress and oral sex with you. Peak up to levels 7 and 8 if you can. Next, your partner can climb on top of you and insert your penis into her vagina. Again, peak up to levels 7 and 8. At level 8, she should withdraw your penis from her vagina and let you masturbate to ejaculation.

Masturbate without tensing your legs. If you want to move, use pelvic rolls instead. Remember to breathe as you feel yourself getting more aroused. If you tend to masturbate with fast strokes, try to slow down and touch yourself in as sensuous a manner as possible. Either have your partner put her hand on the base of your penis or your scrotum as you masturbate, or have her caress herself.

The next time you have intercourse, alternate the intercourse with masturbation at high arousal levels. Peak up to level 8 during intercourse, withdraw and masturbate, then do another peak. Do three or four combination intercourse and masturbation peaks, and then ejaculate with masturbation.

The next time you and your partner do an exercise, alternate intercourse and masturbation at high arousal levels. This time, see if you can arrange your peaks so that you ejaculate in your partner's vagina.

It doesn't matter which intercourse position or positions you use for this progression of exercises. Part of it depends on which position you are most comfortable masturbating in. The easiest position to use for this progression of exercises is the woman-on-top position, because it's physically easiest to alternate peaks in that position. The butterfly position will also work well, because it's visually and physically stimulating, as well as fairly comfortable. However, if you have trouble ejaculating while kneeling, that might pose a problem. One solution would be to have your partner do the following maneuver. In the butterfly position, when you are doing a really high peak (an 8 or a 9), have your partner grab the arches of her own feet with both hands as you thrust into her. This creates more leverage, which allows her vagina to tighten around your penis, and makes it more likely that you will ejaculate.

Do not pressure your partner to go faster during intercourse. Allow your partner to caress you or have intercourse at her own speed. Breathe and keep your leg muscles relaxed. Focus on your feelings as your partner caresses your genitals with her hand or mouth or moves up and down on top of you. Don't work at ejaculating even if you feel yourself getting close.

You have probably gotten into a habit of anticipating ejaculation before you are close, and then working at it. Use the arousal awareness, peaking, and plateauing exercises to relearn what high levels of arousal feel like. Nothing bad will happen to you if you passively become aroused and then allow your arousal to decrease without ejaculating. What results in negative feelings is working at ejaculating and then being unable to ejaculate because you are working at it.

Women, if you are the partner of a man with inhibited ejaculation, go as slowly as you can during the manual and oral genital caresses. Don't allow yourself to be pressured into moving faster than is comfortable for you. If your partner pressures you, stop having intercourse and back up to a previous exercise for a few minutes.

Shaping for Inhibited Ejaculation

If you can ejaculate with masturbation but never with intercourse, try this strategy. It uses a behavioral psychology technique called *shaping* or *successive approximation of behavior*. You could also think of it as "baby steps," or constant movement toward a goal.

The main idea behind shaping is that if you are trying to reach a particular goal, it doesn't matter how many steps you have to take to get there or how long or short each step is. The only thing that matters is that you always move in the direction of the goal, never away from it. Our goal here is for you to be able to ejaculate with intercourse. Our starting point is that you already know how to ejaculate with masturbation.

If the intercourse with masturbation strategy does not result in ejaculation, there is another way you can approach the problem. Think of these exercises as pleasure, not work. Your problem has been that you feel that ejaculating is something you have to *try* to do. You need to relax so that your body can produce its ejaculation response naturally.

Shaping, or successive approximation of behavior, means you do exercises that take you closer and closer (both physically and emotionally) to ejaculating inside your partner's vagina. Try to determine the exact point at which your sexual response shuts down—the exact point at which you lose your focus on sensations and start trying to ejaculate. Your partner may be able to help you recognize this point, because she may be able to tell when you switch from enjoying yourself to working at ejaculating.

After you are able to recognize this point, you need to overpractice the response you have right before this point. For example, if the point when you start trying or working at it is when you feel yourself reach arousal level 8 inside your partner's vagina, you need to do several exercises (complete with focusing caresses, active and passive roles, and feedback) in which you bring yourself up to level 8 and maintain level 8 by plateauing.

Below, I describe a typical progression of exercises, all of which can be done separately, with focusing caresses beforehand and mutual feedback afterwards. These are the "baby steps" I talked about earlier. The reason why inhibited ejaculation can take so long to deal with is because the best approach for you may be to do each of these steps as a separate hour-long exercise. This sequence of exercises has worked for a number of my past clients with inhibited ejaculation. Remember to focus, breathe, and relax

throughout each exercise. Also, as part of the exercises, give your partner a front caress, genital caress, or oral sex before you begin your part of the exercise.

1. Masturbate to ejaculation with your partner in the room. Close your eyes if you need to.

2. Masturbate to ejaculation while your partner is on the bed next to you and is watching.

3. Masturbate to ejaculation and ejaculate on your partner's stomach while lying on your side facing her.

4. Masturbate to ejaculation and ejaculate on your partner's stomach while she lies on her back.

5. Masturbate to ejaculation and ejaculate at the entrance to your partner's vagina.

6. Masturbate to ejaculation while lying on your back, and signal your partner to climb on top as you are ejaculating (not before). By now you are probably able to know that you are going to ejaculate a few seconds before it happens. Part of your problem before was that you anticipated it too soon. Signal your partner to climb on top only after you have reached the point of inevitability and semen has started to leave your penis.

7. Masturbate to ejaculation while kneeling in front of your partner, and thrust into her vagina as you ejaculate. Continue to have intercourse in a slow, focused manner until your erection goes down.

8. Masturbate and penetrate your partner's vagina when you reach an arousal level of 9. Keep your hand on your penis as you thrust in and out, and ejaculate into your partner's vagina.

9. Kneel in front of your partner, and stroke your penis with your hand as it goes in and out of your partner's vagina. Take your hand off your penis as you ejaculate. Practice this several times, removing your hand from your penis at lower and lower arousal levels.

10. Have intercourse with your partner as you close your eyes, imagining that you are stroking your penis with your hand.

Some Final Suggestions

If you can reliably go up to arousal level 8 or 9 with intercourse, there are a few small behavioral changes you can do at this point to make it more likely that you will ejaculate. These techniques have worked for some of my clients.

If you are uncircumcised, when you are having intercourse in the butterfly position, as you get to level 9, reach behind yourself and gently tug on the foreskin near your scrotum so that your foreskin tightens around your penis. This can often give you the burst of stimulation on the head of your penis that you need in order to ejaculate. Just make sure you tug only on the skin. You don't want to pull your scrotum so that it moves too low.

If you are having intercourse in the butterfly position and you get to level 9, have your partner reach underneath you and gently rub the area behind your scrotum and around your anus. She should do this so gently that you really have to concentrate to feel it.

Some men have used vibrators to sensitize their penis. I recommend this as long as you don't use a vibrator too often. In other words, don't use it every time you masturbate. Use it only during intercourse or masturbation when you are already at level 9 to give you the extra boost that helps you ejaculate.

Learning to ejaculate during intercourse if you have had difficulty doing so is really a matter of identifying your strengths. Until now, I have advised you to try to make your sex life more like that of someone who ejaculates easily. For example, I've advised you to masturbate for shorter periods of time, and to learn to recognize high arousal levels such as 8 and 9. If you can do this, now would be a good time to reconnect with your strengths. For example, is there a particular fantasy that always turns you on? If you can peak up to arousal level 9, use the fantasy at that point. Is there a particular form of pornography that turns you on? Peak up to level 9, and use the pornography at that point. The strategy here is to allow yourself to become as aroused as you can with sensate focus, and then and only then use something that has turned you on in the past.

If you have been troubled by inhibited ejaculation, there are a couple of other things you need to remember. Any time you have intercourse, either during a sensate-focus exercise or after you have completed this program, remember to keep your thigh muscles as relaxed as possible, and thrust by using pelvic rolls rather than keeping your pelvis stiff. During intercourse, any time you feel your emotional arousal level drop below your physical arousal level (your erection), stop thrusting for a moment and allow the two sensations to merge, even if your erection goes down a level or two.

Whenever you do a sensate-focus exercise by yourself or with a partner, you need to be aware of your PC muscle. Many men with inhibited ejaculation problems consciously or unconsciously tense their PC muscle as they reach high levels of arousal. Tensing your PC muscle at high arousal levels can cause an inability to ejaculate. To break this habit you may need to do several sensate-focus exercises (either genital caresses or intercourse) during which you stay aware of the condition of your PC muscle and consciously relax it. It is especially important that you relax the area of the PC muscle group associated with the anal sphincter.

⁓

Dealing with inhibited ejaculation can be a time-consuming process and may become frustrating for both partners. This is why it is important to increase intimacy at the same time as you go through the exercises. Sensuous kissing and mutual eye gazing are two ways to do this. Don't be afraid to tell each other if you feel angry or frustrated. It is possible to talk about these issues without blaming the other person. In fact, sharing feelings about the process is a good way for you and your partner to become more intimate.

Another important thing for men with inhibited ejaculation is to learn to accept pleasure. You are not the whole show. Hopefully, the sexual healing program will teach you that you can ask your partner for activities you like and allow yourself to relax and enjoy them without feeling that you have to return the favor immediately.

chapter 26

Healing Female Sexual Arousal Disorder

Now we turn to the chapters in which we focus on healing women's sexual problems, beginning with arousal problems. Remember from Chapter 8 that the current DSM definition of female sexual arousal disorder focuses solely on a woman's physical signs of arousal. As I said in that chapter, in my opinion the definition should also include recognition of a woman's psychological arousal level because in women the two arousal levels don't always go together. The exercises in this chapter ask you to pay attention to both your physical and your psychological, or subjective, arousal levels.

First, some preliminary questions: Do you have difficulty becoming aroused? Are you aware of your sensations of arousal—both physical and psychological/emotional? Some women get concerned because they don't lubricate adequately or often. However, I have found that lubrication is not always a reliable sign of a woman's psychological or emotional arousal. Furthermore, the amount of lubrication a woman produces can vary with her hormonal levels and her age; it is a physical reflex that is connected to the touching of a particular vaginal area. A woman might lubricate without feeling emotionally turned on at all; conversely, she may be very turned on and still not lubricate.

Try the following three exercises. If you have difficulty lubricating even after doing them, be sure to always use an artificial lubricant during both self-stimulation and stimulation from your partner. Adequate lubrication is important for your comfort and enjoyment during any sensual activity.

Physical Arousal

There are two physical signs that a woman is aroused: lubrication, and increased blood flow to the genitals. The following three exercises will increase lubrication. Remember from Chapter 2 that a woman's body has three sources of genital lubrication: the A-spot, the Bartholin's glands, and the G-spot. Each of these exercises targets one of those areas. After you have done all of the exercises separately, you could do a single exercise in which you combine stimulation of all three areas.

ᕀ *Exercise 59.* STIMULATING THE A-SPOT

The anterior fornix erogenous zone, or A-spot, is the whole front wall of the vagina between the G-spot and the cervix. It appears to be the area that is responsible for most of a woman's vaginal lubrication.

To stimulate the A-spot, sit with your back against a wall or headboard with your knees bent and your legs slightly spread. Caress your vulva using plenty of lubrication. When you are ready to stimulate your A-spot, insert your middle finger straight into your vagina. Keep your finger straight and gently rub the front wall of your vagina between the G-spot and the cervix (see below for information about how to locate the G-spot). Use a slow, sensuous caressing technique. Alternate between stroking the A-spot and stroking the vaginal sponge (the area in front of the G-spot that surrounds your urethra and swells up when you get really aroused). Use long, repeated in-and-out strokes of your finger along the whole length of the front wall of your vagina. Gently rubbing this area for ten to fifteen minutes may cause you to lubricate.

ᕀ *Exercise 60.* STIMULATING THE BARTHOLIN'S GLANDS

The Bartholin's glands secrete a drop or two of very slippery lubrication when a woman is aroused. You can stimulate them during a genital caress. Remember that the Bartholin's glands are located under the skin of your inner vaginal lips, about halfway between the top and bottom of your vagina. In other words, if you were looking at your vagina at the same angle from which your gynecologist sees it during your pelvic exam, the glands would be located at about the middle.

Caress yourself as you normally would, focusing on your sensations and remembering to breathe and relax. At some point during the caress, take the index and middle finger of one hand and lightly press on your inner vaginal lips about halfway between the top and bottom of the vagina. You don't have to rub very hard to stimulate the glands; just lightly pressing or tapping is enough. You won't see the lubrication because it is excreted inside the opening of the vagina. But you can feel it if you gently place your finger about half an inch into your vagina.

∽ Exercise 61. STIMULATING THE G-SPOT

Remember that the Gräfenberg spot, or G-spot, is a very sensitive area located on the front wall of the vagina behind the pubic bone. It's a little difficult to stimulate it yourself with your hand, but some women can do so. Here's how.

Give yourself a sensate-focus genital caress with plenty of lubrication. Caress all the parts of your vulva—your clitoris, inner and outer lips, and vaginal opening. Use a position in which you are sitting up with your back against a headboard or wall. Bend your knees and spread your legs slightly.

Bend all of the fingers of your right hand except your middle finger. Stick your middle finger out like you're giving someone the finger. Bend your wrist and insert your middle finger into your vagina with your palm up. Curl your middle finger back toward the front wall of your vagina and hook it behind your pubic bone, as if you were trying to touch your clitoris from the inside. That's your G-spot. Gently rub the pad of your middle finger on your G-spot and feel it swell and start to pulse. If you're lucky, you'll also feel the area start to lubricate, and if you're really lucky, you may actually feel a gush of fluid. If you have trouble touching your G-spot with your own hand because your arm isn't long enough, either use a dildo to reach it (special curved ones are available for just this purpose) or show your partner how to stimulate it.

The previous exercises stimulated lubrication. The next few exercises stimulate genital swelling—blood flow to the genitals, or what Masters and Johnson called *vasocongestion.*

∽ Exercise 62. STIMULATING THE CLITORIS

There are many enjoyable ways to touch your clitoris. Do this in the context of a sensate-focus exercise so you don't pressure yourself to respond in a particular way.

Use some baby oil or other lubricant and gently start to rub the tip of your clitoris. Feel it start to swell underneath the pressure from your fingertips. Hold your clitoris between two of your fingers and squeeze it as if it were a small penis. Or, if direct stimulation is too intense for you, take two fingers and rub them along the sides of your clitoris. Note your response. Do other areas of your genitals swell up at the same time your clitoris starts to harden? As your level of arousal increases, notice how you can rub your clitoris harder because you can handle more stimulation.

One of the best ways to stimulate the clitoris is to use hot water. (I first read about this technique in *The Sensuous Woman* when I was a teenager.) Buy a shower massage device and install it. Lie in the bathtub and turn the water on your clitoris as hot as you can stand it without hurting yourself. (It's possible to do the same thing using the jets in a Jacuzzi.) Alternatively, I've seen a type of round vibrator that's encased in a sponge for use underwater. Enjoy the intense sensations.

When you caress your clitoris, to further stimulate vasocongestion, cup one hand over your pubic mound and rub. Doing so will stimulate the whole vaginal sponge area.

❧ *Exercise 63.* MASTURBATING WITH A DILDO

Before you begin this exercise, purchase a dildo that is close to the size of your partner's penis. If you're too embarrassed to go into an adult store and buy one in person, you could order one from an adult-products retailer, either through a mail-order catalog or online (see the Sources for Sex Toys section, located in the back of the book).

Lie on your back and, using your hand, give yourself a sensate-focus front caress and genital caress. Next, put some lubrication on your vulva and inside your vagina. Give yourself a slow genital caress with the dildo. Keep your touch sensual, and remember to breathe, relax, and focus on the sensations. Use the dildo to slowly caress the different parts of your vulva, including your clitoris, your inner and outer lips, and your vaginal opening. Slowly run the dildo in a circular motion around your PC muscle. Then insert the dildo and use it to feel your A-spot, your G-spot, your cervix, and your cul de sac if you can.

There is no pressure on you during this exercise to reach any particular level of arousal or to peak up to certain levels. These parts of the program will come later. In this exercise, just relax and notice whether the stimulation of some areas causes you to become more aroused than the stimulation of other areas.

∾ Exercise 64. MASTURBATING WITH YOUR PARTNER'S PENIS

Share a sensate-focus genital caress or oral sex with your partner until he has an erection. Put a lot of lubrication on your vagina and on your partner's penis. Then climb on top of your partner and use his penis to stimulate yourself. Pretending that your partner's penis is a dildo, use it to rub your clitoris and your PC muscle. Continue for about ten to fifteen minutes. Finish the exercise by having intercourse if you both want to.

∾ Exercise 65. GETTING ACTIVE FOR AROUSAL

One of the best things you can do to help yourself experience increased sexual arousal is to take the active role in a sexual encounter. For this exercise, have your partner lie on his back and remain passive. Ask him to close his eyes and try not to move. Pretend that his body is a playground or a toy for you to play with. Or pretend he's asleep. Play with him. Stroke, caress, lick, or suck different parts of his body. Whatever you decide to do, do it slowly, sensuously, and without any pressure on either of you. If you want to climb on top of your partner and have intercourse, do so. Chances are that at some point in the exercise he won't be able to hold still any longer, and you two can revel in your sexual play together.

Peaking

The cornerstone of arousal with a partner is the peaking process. In Chapter 18, you learned what peaking is and you practiced it by yourself. Chances are, doing so helped you reach at least the lower levels on the 1-to-10 arousal scale. If you have difficulty becoming aroused, you especially need to practice the lower levels of the arousal scale with a partner. In this chapter, I'll describe different versions of the peaking process with your partner, as well as other options, so you can take advantage of the many ways that this process can help you learn to become aroused.

Before you begin the peaking process with a partner, review Chapter 8, on female arousal. As I mentioned at the beginning of this chapter, it's important to remember that there are two possible arousal scales for women: psychological arousal and physical arousal. Psychological arousal is your subjective sense of feeling aroused emotionally or mentally. Physical arousal is genital swelling and lubrication. You can do any peaking exercise using either scale or both scales. I'll make specific suggestions at appropriate points during descriptions of the next few exercises.

For all of the partner exercises, remember to begin with spoon breathing and focusing caresses, and to end with spoon breathing and partner feedback. You may want to review the guidelines for partner exercises given in Chapter 19.

◞ *Exercise 66.* AROUSAL AWARENESS WITH MANUAL STIMULATION

This is the same exercise you did by yourself in Chapter 18, but this time you will do it with your partner stimulating you. Begin with focusing caresses, followed by a nondemand front or genital caress with your partner, if you wish. Then lie comfortably on your back with your arms at your sides and your legs spread. Place a pillow under your buttocks if doing so makes you more comfortable. Your partner will then begin a slow sensate-focus front and genital caress. He should remember to do the caress for his own pleasure and to caress as slowly as possible. Men, the way to make sure that your partner enjoys herself and receives the maximum amount of stimulation is for you to focus totally on what you are doing and to enjoy yourself.

Women, every few minutes your partner will ask you what your arousal level is on the 1-to-10 scale. You will be familiar with these levels from doing the self-caressing exercises. If you need to review what the different arousal levels feel like, refer back to Chapter 18. Focus on exactly what your partner is doing. If you are uncomfortable or feel anxious in any way, ask him to caress more slowly. If you feel he is "working at" caressing you, ask him to caress more slowly. When you feel your arousal increase, take a deep breath and relax your leg muscles. Your partner will lightly tap your leg if you hold your breath or tense up.

It doesn't matter how aroused you become during this exercise. During the course of a twenty-minute exercise, your partner can ask you about your arousal level every two to three minutes. Tell your partner where you are; it doesn't matter whether your arousal level is higher or lower than the last time he asked. Keep your focus on the point of contact between your skin and your partner's skin, and relax your body completely.

It also doesn't matter whether or not you lubricate during this exercise. Your partner should use plenty of baby oil or other lubricant so you stay comfortable. Just let your partner know what you feel. Try not to move around, because tensing and moving at this stage won't increase your arousal level; in fact, it will only make it go down. Taking a few deep breaths and relaxing your muscles will allow your body to experience more sexual arousal.

ᕙ *Exercise 67.* AROUSAL AWARENESS WITH ORAL SEX

Repeat Exercise 66, but this time your partner can stimulate you orally in addition to manually. The following instructions are for the male partner.

Begin a nondemand front caress. Caress your partner's genital area with some baby oil. Gently spread your partner's legs so that you can see her inner vaginal lips. Slowly begin to use your tongue. With the tip of your tongue, slowly lick from the bottom of your partner's vaginal opening up the center of her lips. You will feel your tongue go over her clitoris, as if it were a speed bump. Repeat this motion several times, each time more slowly. Use the other oral techniques you learned in Chapter 22. Stimulate your partner with your fingers at the same time you are doing oral sex. During the course of a twenty-minute exercise, ask your partner her arousal level every two to three minutes.

ᕙ *Exercise 68.* PEAKING FOR AROUSAL

Remember that a peak is a wavelike increase in arousal. You learned how to do the peaking exercise by yourself in Chapter 18. Now you'll do it with your partner's help. I'll describe three different versions of peaking exercises with the woman as the focus. They're very similar to the exercises with the man as the focus described in Chapter 23, on premature ejaculation.

Manual Stimulation

The first peaking exercise is peaking with manual stimulation. Begin by exchanging focusing caresses with your partner. Pleasure your partner with a front caress or genital caress or oral sex. Take note as to whether pleasuring your partner causes your arousal level to rise, in either the physical sense, the psychological sense, or both.

To start the peaking exercise, lie on your back in the passive role. Your partner will begin a slow front caress and then will move to your genitals. He should use plenty of lubrication. He can gently caress all of the parts of your external genitals first, including your inner and outer lips, your clitoris, your vaginal opening, and your PC muscle. It's important that he caress really, really slowly, because you need to be able to feel very small changes in sensation. If you feel he's going too fast or rubbing too hard, be sure to let him know so he can slow down. As a part of this caress, your partner can also caress your inner genitals, including your vaginal walls, your A-spot, your G-spot, and the area around your cervix if he is able to reach it easily.

No matter what area of your genitals your partner is caressing, if and when you reach a level 3, let your partner know by saying, "Three," or, "Stop." Your partner will then move his hand to your belly, thighs, or some other part of your body until your arousal has dropped one or two levels. Let him know that your arousal level has dropped, and he will begin to caress your genitals again until you report a level 4.

Remember to stay relaxed and to breathe and focus. As you reach each peak, say the number level out loud, take a deep breath, and relax your PC muscles and other pelvic muscles. Make a mental note to yourself about which body parts tend to trigger the most arousal for you when they're stimulated.

Do the peaking exercise for about twenty-five minutes. It doesn't matter how many peaks you are able to do or how high you are able to go. If you don't go beyond a level 3 or so, don't worry about it. Learning to identify your arousal levels may take some time, and that's okay. The key to learning to become really aroused is first to learn to recognize and become comfortable with the lower levels. If you can, however, continue peaking up through levels, 5, 6, 7, 8, and 9. Who knows? You may even surprise yourself and have an orgasm. If you reach only the lower levels, practice peaking repeatedly at those levels.

Here's what you want to pay attention to: When your partner touches your genitals, do your inner and outer lips respond by feeling bigger or fuller? When your partner touches your clitoris and then moves his hand away, does your clitoris feel harder against his hand the next time he touches it? Do you lubricate when your partner touches your vaginal opening? It may be difficult to tell if you're lubricating because your partner should be using some kind of external lubrication, but sometimes you can tell. These are all signs of physical arousal.

Psychological arousal will feel a little different. Signs of psychological arousal might include drifting into a fantasy or starting to anticipate later sexual activities.

Because this is such a powerful exercise, you will want to repeat it several times, with variations. The first time you do it, keep it as simple as possible. Use the subjective or psychological scale. While your partner is caressing you, in addition to focusing on the exact point of contact between his hand and your genitals, also see if you can open your eyes and focus on a part of him, such as his face or shoulders or anything you find attractive. Then try a version of the exercise using the physical arousal scale. You could also do a version of the exercise in which you alternate between doing one peak with the physical arousal scale and the next one with the psychological arousal scale. When you have enough experience with the peaking process, you may not need to differentiate between the two scales. They'll probably start to blend together in your mind. This is good, because it means that your sense of physical arousal (which is usually easier to recognize) is causing you to become more psychologically aroused. When this happens, your desire level generally increases as well.

For other variations of the exercise, you could do one exercise with only low-level peaks and another with only higher-level peaks. Or you could do an exercise in which your partner caresses only your internal genitals or only your external genitals. Peaking is very versatile—you can make up your own version of an exercise based on your intuition about what you think will help you.

Oral Sex

For peaking using oral sex, begin with focusing caresses. Next, give your partner a sensate-focus front or genital caress, or do oral sex with him. Then lie on your back and relax. Your partner will begin a front and genital caress with his hand. Then he'll start to caress your clitoris, inner and outer lips, and vaginal opening with his tongue. Take about twenty-five minutes and peak up to levels 3, 4, 5, 6, 7, 8, and 9 if you can. You may need to repeat this exercise several times in order to reach some of the higher levels, and that's okay. Take your time and don't pressure yourself.

The first time you do this version of the peaking exercise, stay relaxed. Then, when you are more confident with the exercise, add some pelvic rolls or thrusts, which can help increase your arousal. Remember to keep breathing regularly during the stimulation. Breathe at each peak, and keep your PC muscle relaxed.

When peaking with oral sex, you could do one exercise in which you focus only on physical arousal, and then another exercise in which you focus only on psychological arousal. Or you could alternate one physical arousal peak and one psychological arousal peak. After you have a lot of experience with peaking, your sense of physical and psychological arousal will probably start to blend together.

ᴄᴠ *Exercise 69.* PEAKING WITH INTERCOURSE

Peaking can also be used with intercourse. The position that eventually will be most arousing to you will probably be the female-superior position, but for now I recommend that you start with the butterfly position. This position is also really arousing because it allows contact with so many of your genital erogenous zones. In addition, you'll probably find it easier to focus if you're in a more comfortable physical position (lying on your back versus kneeling).

Begin with focusing caresses. Then give your partner a front caress, a genital caress, or oral sex. When your partner has an erection, lie on your back, spread your legs, and bend your knees. Remember to stay comfortable. If that means your legs are straight up in the air rather than bent, that's fine. Your partner will kneel in front of you and put a lot of lubrication on both his penis and your genitals. He should then slowly begin to rub his penis against your clitoris. Breathe, relax, and stay focused. If you reach arousal level 3, tell him. He'll stop the stimulation so your arousal level can go back down. See if you can do two or three peaks with stimulation from your partner's penis on the outside of your genitals.

When your partner is ready, he can insert his penis. He should slowly caress the inside of your vagina with his penis. Have him caress your A-spot, your G-spot, and the area around your cervix if he can reach it. Peak at levels 3, 4, 5, 6, 7, 8, and 9 if you can. Spend about twenty to twenty-five minutes doing several peaks at whatever levels you can reach.

Like the other peaking exercises, peaking with intercourse in the butterfly position is very versatile. You could do one exercise with only low-level peaks, and one with only higher-level peaks. Or you could do one exercise in which you do several peaks at the same level. You could do an entire peaking exercise using only stimulation of the outer genitals and another using only stimulation of the inner genitals. You could do one exercise using only stimulation of the A-spot and another using only stimulation of the G-spot. You could alternate physical and psychological arousal peaks. I'm sure you'll think of other variations.

A variation on the male-superior position that is specifically recommended for clitoral stimulation is the coital alignment technique (the CAT position). Lie on your back and have your partner lie on top of you. He will then pull himself up toward your shoulders so that when he thrusts, his penis goes in and out of you more vertically than horizontally.

Here's another variation that can give you more stimulation: While you and your partner are in the missionary position, twist your legs together. This will squeeze your partner's penis between your thighs. Or you can press one of your feet on top of the other, which also tightens your grip on your partner's penis.

After you have a lot of experience peaking in the butterfly position, you will want to try all of the peaking variations in the other positions. The side-to-side position is good because it's really comfortable, but it doesn't provide much stimulation of the female genitals. If you want to do a peaking exercise in the side-to-side scissors position, it's very easy for your partner to reach down and stimulate your clitoris with his fingers. In addition to all of the peaking variations I described above, in the scissors position you could alternate peaks with stimulation from your partner's hand and peaks with stimulation from your partner's penis.

Although the rear-entry position can also be highly stimulating, I don't generally recommend it for peaking. Due to the lack of eye contact, it's sometimes difficult to communicate with your partner about when to stop and start the stimulation. Plus, the position itself makes it difficult to focus on the sensations in your genitals. There's just too much going on.

If you are practicing peaking exercises in order to learn to become more aroused, you will definitely want to use the female-superior position at some point. Sex therapists agree that it tends to be the position in which women become the most aroused. If you have practiced peaking in the butterfly position, you have learned to peak while remaining fairly passive. Once you decide to use the female-superior position, your partner will be passive and you will be active. This way, you will be able to control the timing, depth, and angle of thrusting during all of your peaks.

∾ *Exercise 70.* PLATEAUING FOR AROUSAL

Remember from Chapter 18, on self-touch, that plateauing is very similar to peaking. The difference is that in a peaking exercise, you allow your arousal to go up to a certain level, recognize the level, and stop the stimulation so your arousal goes down. In plateauing, you reach a certain arousal level, recognize it, and then try to maintain your arousal at that level for anywhere from a few seconds to a couple of minutes.

You can use any of four techniques to plateau: changing your movement, changing your breathing, changing your focus, and squeezing your PC muscle. In this chapter, you'll use only the first three methods. Squeezing your PC muscle changes your arousal level by lowering it, and for the purposes of increasing a woman's arousal, we don't want that. (In the chapter on female orgasm, you'll learn that squeezing your PC muscle at the moment just before orgasm can often trigger or enhance your orgasm, but we don't want to use the PC muscle at the lower arousal levels because doing so can decrease arousal.)

The exercise I describe below is a theoretical plateauing sequence; that is, I describe how it *could* happen. It doesn't have to happen exactly this way or in exactly this order. If you can do the exercise exactly the way I describe it, that's great. Remember that you are never under any pressure to reach certain arousal levels during any exercise. Focus on and approve of whatever levels you reach, even if they're low levels.

Begin your first plateauing session with focusing caresses. Then give your partner a front caress, a genital caress, or oral sex. Lie on your back and relax. Your partner will start a front caress with you, moving to a genital caress with his hand. When you reach arousal level 4, instead of telling your partner, speed up your breathing. This should cause your arousal to increase about half a level. When you feel you are slightly above level 4, slow your breathing down. This will cause your arousal to drop back to level 4. See if you can stay at level 4 by alternating between slower and faster breathing. Then just relax. Your partner will continue to caress you.

Allow yourself to reach level 5. When you feel you are at level 5, thrust your pelvis against your partner's hand. This will cause your arousal to go up about a half level. Remember to stay relaxed when you do pelvic rolls and thrusts, as you learned in Chapter 17, so you don't tense up. Now stop your thrusting. See if you can maintain your arousal at level 5 by starting and stopping your movement. Then relax again.

For the next plateau, try a level 6. When you reach a level slightly above 6, switch your focus to a part of your body that your partner isn't caressing. For example, if your partner is caressing the inside of your vagina, mentally switch your focus to your clitoris. Can you still feel your clitoris even if your partner isn't touching it? See if you can stay at level 6 by switching your focus back and forth between the area your partner is caressing and an area he's not currently caressing.

At this point, you can keep going. See if you can plateau at levels 7, 8, and 9, using either a change in your breathing, a change in your movements, or a change in your focus. Once you have practiced all of these techniques, you'll be able to use two of them or all three of them at the same time. Try to do a plateauing exercise for twenty or twenty-five minutes, no matter what levels you reach.

From here, you can go in many different directions. You could do an entire plateauing exercise, practicing just one technique. You could have your partner add oral stimulation. You could do an entire plateauing exercise repeating several plateaus at the same level. Plateauing can also be used during intercourse. The best positions for doing so are the butterfly position, the side-to-side position, and the female-superior position.

Using Erotica

Until now, I have advised you to keep things simple—to do your sensate-focus exercises in a room with no distractions and to use only a bare minimum of supplies, like baby oil and towels. When people have sexual problems, I generally don't recommend accessories like lingerie and X-rated videos. These additions usually complicate an already confusing situation. I believe that in order to solve most sexual problems, it's best to make the sexual situation as basic as possible. But there's an exception to this rule, and it has to do with women's arousal problems.

In the case of women's arousal problems, I often recommend the use of sexually explicit materials. From an evolutionary standpoint, both men and women have evolved to become physically aroused at the sight of a naked person of the other sex. Most of us probably still have this ability. However, when many women view erotic material, they often have mixed feelings about it. Research shows that most women lubricate fairly rapidly at the first sight of a sexually explicit image. But then they start to pay attention to their psychological arousal, and many women are very turned off by the content of a lot of pornography, because it's mostly designed for male tastes. So although a lot of women have the ability to become physically aroused by viewing pornography, many shut down because they focus on the idea that a lot of sexually explicit material can be disgusting. Women's taste in erotica tends to be material that appeals to psychological arousal rather than physical arousal. For example, romance novels rather than still pictures of genitals tend to appeal to women.

Women can sometimes learn to become more aroused by retraining themselves in the ability to feel physical arousal at the sight of sexually explicit images. There is no specific sensate-focus exercise using sexually explicit materials, but you could buy some magazines that contain images of naked men or of couples making love and look at the pictures while you relax, paying attention to your physical arousal rather than your psychological arousal. See if any of the images cause you to lubricate. Or you could caress yourself while looking at pictures. The trick is to find images that aren't a psychological turn on but are physically arousing. With everything that's available on the Internet, you should be able to find something to fit the bill.

Vibrators

Earlier in this chapter I described the use of a dildo to stimulate various areas of your genitals. A dildo is a penis-shaped sex toy. Some dildos vibrate and some do not. Up to now I have described exercises with dildos that don't vibrate. Now let's talk about vibrators. Vibrators come in many shapes and sizes. They aren't necessarily shaped like penises. Some are meant to be inserted into the vagina, but many aren't. If you have never used a vibrator, getting one (or a whole collection of them) could be a valuable aid in healing your arousal and orgasm problems.

The most common types of vibrators are penis-shaped ones, small ones about the size of a car cigarette lighter, and large ones (about the size of your forearm) that have a round, vibrating head. If you have arousal or orgasm problems, I think you owe it to yourself to peruse a sex toys catalog or website or to visit an adult store to see the seemingly countless different kinds of vibrators that are available. Once you have selected one (or more), you can use it as an addition to many of the exercises in this book. You can do any caress on your external genitals using a vibrator in addition to your hand, or you can use a vibrator as an adjunct during oral sex or intercourse if it helps you get more aroused. For all sorts of additional creative ideas about how to use your new toys, get a copy of the book _The Many Joys of Sex Toys_, by Anne Semans (see Recommended Reading). Just remember to follow the sensate-focus principles: focus on the sensations, breathe, and relax.

Lubricants

Some women experience psychological arousal and vasocongestion (swelling) in their genitals, but they don't lubricate. They need to use some form of externally applied lubricant to stay comfortable, especially during intercourse. Even women who lubricate naturally when they are aroused sometimes experience a little vaginal dryness and need to have a commercial lubricant handy. Here's my point: It's a good idea for all women (and men, too) to keep a sexual lubricant on hand for either self-pleasuring or sensual encounters with a partner. No one should feel embarrassed about using artificial lubrication.

Many different commercial lubricants are available. There's no single lubricant that's perfect for every woman. The two main types of lubricant are oil-based and water-based. Oil-based lubricants include mineral oil, baby oil, and petroleum jelly (Vaseline). Some people use food oils such as vegetable oil or olive oil as sexual lubricants. Water-based lubricants include K-Y jelly and some of the products that claim to mimic natural vaginal lubrication, such as Astro-Glide. Water-based lubricants such as K-Y jelly have medical uses in addition to sexual ones. Adult stores offer large selections of flavored lubricants that are designed specifically for use on the genitals. Personally, I prefer oil-based lubricants, but a lot of people think they are too greasy. Water-based lubricants tend to stay cold on the body and to impart a clammy feeling. Plus, after being exposed to the air for a while, they can become sticky or tacky.

As part of the sexual healing process for your arousal problems, you will probably want to purchase several types of lubricants and use them during genital caresses on yourself to see which ones you like best. Be aware that if your partner uses condoms for intercourse, you need to use a water-based lubricant with the condom. Oil-based products cause condoms to fall apart. (As a side note, also be aware that if you use condoms for contraception—and not just for protection from sexually transmitted diseases—you need to use a spermicide to give the condom maximum effectiveness. Spermicidal jellies lubricate the vagina; other types of spermicides, such as suppositories and foams, do not.)

Medical Solutions

A number of herbal products that are sold over the counter in health-food stores claim to increase a woman's sexual arousal. To my knowledge, none of them have been tested to see whether they work better than a placebo. In addition, a number of testosterone-based creams are available through compounding pharmacies. These are applied topically, usually to the thighs, for several weeks. Apparently they can increase desire and the ability to become aroused. See Chapter 28 for a more thorough discussion of testosterone therapy in treating low sexual desire.

Men can take Viagra, which works by promoting blood flow into the penis, to improve their erections. If the drug increases genital blood flow in men, there's no reason why it shouldn't do so in women, but to my knowledge it has not been shown to be effective for women in clinical trials. However, some physicians prescribe it anyway, and some women have found that it increases their physical arousal.

Another over-the-counter product, Zestra, is a botanical massage oil that's applied directly to the vulva. It has been shown to increase desire, arousal, and genital sensations. Finally, the Eros clitoral stimulator is similar to the vacuum erection device for men, but as the name implies it's designed for women. It looks like a small oxygen mask and fits over the pubic mound. An attached pump is used to pump the air out of the device, which creates a vacuum that draws blood into the clitoris and surrounding area. This action can definitely increase a woman's sense of physical sexual arousal.

❧

Research on female sexuality has historically lagged behind research on male sexuality. The good news is that we are finally starting to catch up. I predict that in the very near future you'll see a lot of new medical and behavioral options for women with sexual concerns.

chapter 27

Healing Female Orgasm Disorder

Remember from Chapter 11 that there are many kinds of orgasm problems. Some women don't have orgasms at all, some only have them unreliably, and some only have them following very specific types of stimulation. But no matter how a woman's problems with orgasm manifest themselves, there are some prerequisites to healing them that are common to all women. If you have a problem reaching orgasm, no matter what type of issue it is, before you do the exercises in this chapter you'll need to set the stage for your healing process by doing the relaxation exercises in Chapter 16, the sexual fitness exercises in Chapter 17, and the self-touch exercises in Chapter 18. It is essential that your PC muscle be in good shape, that you are comfortable touching your genitals, and that you are able to peak and plateau.

What If You've Been Faking It?

A lot of women pretend they are having an orgasm when they're not, especially during intercourse. The most common reason for faking an orgasm is to show your partner that you're enjoying sex. Women don't really fake orgasm to be intentionally deceitful. Usually the first time a woman fakes orgasm it's because intercourse is going on for a long time and she wants it to be over, since many men don't want to ejaculate until they think their partner has had an orgasm. Then faking becomes a habit.

There's nothing wrong with making a lot of noise during intercourse. If your doing so makes your partner believe you're having an orgasm when you're not, in a sense that's his problem, not yours. It's different if he asks you if you've had an orgasm and you say yes even though you haven't. Now we're into the realm of lying, and that's a problem.

If you've been faking orgasm and/or lying about it, you don't necessarily have to come clean in order to learn how to really have orgasms. If you would like to use the techniques in this chapter to learn to have orgasms, all you have to say to your partner is something like, "I've been reading this book about sex and I want to practice some new ways to have orgasms. So for a while I'm going to stay quiet during intercourse and learn some new ways to focus on what I'm feeling." You don't necessarily have to say that sex hasn't been satisfying for you up to now. You can just frame your explanation in terms of learning *new* techniques.

Discovering Your Orgasm Triggers

A goal for many women is to learn to have orgasms with intercourse. The first step in being able to do so is learning to have orgasms by yourself (which is also an end in itself, obviously). Furthermore, learning to have orgasms by yourself can help you discover several different ways to have orgasms with a partner that don't necessarily include intercourse (such as orgasms with oral stimulation or from having your partner caress you with his hand). Remember from Chapter 2 that your body has many sites in the genital area that can trigger orgasm. The external sites are the clitoris (which I've nicknamed Old Faithful, because for many women it is the most reliable orgasm trigger), the inner and outer vaginal lips, the opening of the vagina, and the PC muscle. The internal sites are the G-spot, the area around the cervix, and the cul de sac. Any of these locations can be stimulated by either yourself or a partner in such a way that may cause you to have an orgasm.

Talking about the various orgasm triggers on a woman's body raises the topic of clitoral orgasms versus vaginal orgasms, a potential source of worry and performance anxiety for some people. I'd like to lay to rest the controversy surrounding this issue. One type of orgasm isn't "better than" the other. They're different—that's all. Our knowledge of female anatomy tells us that the two stimulate the nervous system differently, and thus produce different kinds of sensations. But whether a woman prefers one type of orgasm over the other is strictly a matter of personal preference.

You will begin by going through the entire female arousal process described in Chapter 26. As a prelude to becoming orgasmic, you need to do all of the arousal exercises, including peaking and plateauing by yourself (Chapter 18), basic partner exercises (Chapter 22), and peaking and plateauing with your partner (Chapter 26). Those exercises are powerful and can often cause you to become aroused enough to have an orgasm. Start with the exercises that focus on using two different arousal and orgasm triggers: the clitoris (Exercise 62) and the G-spot (Exercise 61). Then try the following exercises to get in touch with your cul de sac before you try to have orgasms with intercourse.

For all of the partner exercises, as outlined in Chapter 19, remember to start with spoon breathing and focusing caresses, and to end with spoon breathing and partner feedback.

ᨑ *Exercise 71.* TIGHTENING YOUR PC MUSCLE AROUND A DILDO

For this exercise you will need a dildo that fits comfortably inside your vagina. One of the main reasons why women have difficulty reaching orgasm during intercourse is because their PC muscle is out of shape. Remember that the PC muscle spasms when you have an orgasm. The better shape your PC muscle is in, the easier it will be to have an orgasm.

It's easier to have an orgasm with manual stimulation or oral sex than it is to have one with intercourse, because your PC muscle has to be in really good shape to spasm when there's something inside your vagina. The basic PC muscle exercises described in Chapter 17 will get your PC muscle in good enough shape to spasm with manual or oral stimulation. But you may need to get it in even better shape in order to have orgasms with intercourse. That's where this exercise fits in.

Lie on your back and caress your genitals using plenty of lubrication. Insert your dildo into your vagina and use it to do a few low-level peaks. Now just hold the dildo in your vagina and alternate tightening and relaxing your PC muscle around it. Do twenty-five repetitions. Use either the dildo or your hand to continue peaking, going as high as you can.

ᨑ *Exercise 72.* VAGINAL BREATHING

This exercise will help you identify the cul de sac and the muscles that support your uterus. The contraction of these muscles can greatly enhance your experience of orgasm. The way to learn voluntary control of these muscles is to practice sucking air into your vagina and blowing it back out.

Start the exercise by lying on your back and relaxing. Raise your knees, and experiment with tightening various muscles in your lower abdominal area. If tightening any of these muscles causes air to be sucked into your vagina, then you are using the correct muscles. If you can't locate the right muscles while lying flat on your back with your knees bent, try an old calis-thenics position—the upside-down bicycling position. Lie flat on your back and lift your lower body up by bracing yourself on your elbows. You don't actually need to move your legs. The position alone will cause your uterus to settle on top of your vagina. When you return to a lying position, air will blow out of your vagina. Practice alternating the bicycling position with tightening your muscles while lying down until you get a sense of which muscles are at work. Then start to tighten them while lying on your back. Once you've identified the correct muscles, practice sucking air into your vagina and blowing it back out.

ᐸᐳ *Exercise 73.* USING A DILDO IN YOUR CUL DE SAC

For this exercise you will need a dildo that fits comfortably into your vagina. Lie on your back and caress your genitals. Put plenty of lubrication on your dildo and stroke your clitoris with it. Peak at low levels, for example 4, 5, and 6, using the stimulation of the dildo on your clitoris.

Now insert the dildo into your vagina. Bend your legs and slowly thrust with the dildo as if you were having intercourse. At the same time, tighten your muscles as you learned to do in the vaginal breathing exercise. Your cul de sac will open up and you will be able to insert the dildo into it. This should cause some particularly pleasurable sensations. Practice moving the dildo in and out of your cul de sac. Finish peaking with this stimulation if you can.

Orgasms with Intercourse

Difficulty reaching orgasm during intercourse is one of the most common sexual complaints women have. Some women strive for orgasm during inter-course not so much because it feels better than orgasm triggered by other types of sexual activities but because they wish to share this loving expres-sion of intense arousal, vulnerability, and abandon with their partner. You will find that in addition to making it more likely that you will have an orgasm during intercourse, the following exercises will heighten your senses and deepen your intimacy.

ᐸᐳ *Exercise 74.* ORGASM AT THE POINT OF PENETRATION

This exercise helps you get rid of the myth that it takes a long time for a woman to have an orgasm with intercourse. It's possible to learn how to have an orgasm immediately upon penetration. This exercise uses the peaking process to help you learn to do just that.

Begin the exercise with focusing caresses (such as back caresses) by each partner. Then have your partner lie on his back. Do a front caress, genital caress, or nondemand oral sex with your partner for your own pleasure—whatever you like and whatever is easiest for you to focus on. Your partner will remain passive during this exercise. When your partner becomes erect, kneel over him and use his penis to pleasure yourself. Masturbate with his penis. Remember to breathe and to keep your leg muscles as relaxed as you can in this position. Use your partner's penis to slowly peak yourself up to high levels of arousal, including 6, 7, 8, and 9 if possible.

If you start to feel anxious, you know what to do: Refocus on the pleasurable sensations, and/or back up to a previous part of the exercise with which you were more comfortable (for example, doing a genital caress with your partner). When you are more comfortable and focused, start peaking again.

Peak up to level 9 by slowly rubbing your partner's penis on your clitoris and the outside of your vagina. Masturbate with your partner's penis rather than touching your clitoris with your fingers. When you are on the brink of orgasm (a level 9-plus), open your eyes wide, take a deep breath, and thrust yourself all the way down on your partner's penis. You will probably have an orgasm within the first few thrusts.

The secret to being able to do this is the peaking process, not the penetration itself. Before intercourse, you may need to spend fifteen or twenty minutes using your partner's penis to peak yourself up. Don't forget to allow your arousal to decrease somewhat between peaks. While caressing your partner and masturbating with his penis, it is important to focus on exactly what you are doing and to stay in the here and now. If you anticipate an orgasm or worry about it, it won't happen. Your ability to concentrate, peak yourself up to level 9, and totally focus on the level-9 state of arousal is what will produce an orgasm upon penetration or shortly thereafter.

A variation on this exercise is to peak yourself up to level 9 several times in a row (rather than just once) and then thrust down on your partner's penis. Whichever way you decide is best for you (of course, you could always do both), it is likely that this exercise will show you and your partner that you don't need long sessions of intercourse in order to reach orgasm.

Remember that the primary sign of orgasm is a rhythmic spasming in the PC muscle that lasts for a few seconds. The following three exercises focus on the PC muscle. They will help you learn to make it spasm.

ᐸᐧ *Exercise 75.* SHALLOW PENETRATION

Begin the exercise with focusing caresses. Then give your partner a manual and oral genital caress until he has an erection. Get into the butterfly position. Using lots of lubrication, have your partner insert his penis.

With your partner doing deep thrusts into your vagina, peak up to arousal levels 6, 7, and 8. When you reach a level of arousal beyond 8, tell your partner. At that point, he will adjust his position so that he is thrusting only an inch or so into your vagina at most. He should slow down his thrusting so that he is barely moving, and he should use the head of his penis to tease your PC muscle by moving both in and out and in a circular motion. You will probably feel your PC muscle start to twitch with some preorgasmic spasms. When you are on the brink of orgasm, tell your partner. He can then resume deep thrusting, which should send you over into orgasm.

ᐸᐧ *Exercise 76.* STIMULATING THE PC MUSCLE FOR ORGASM

This is similar to the previous exercise but focuses exclusively on the PC muscle. Give your partner a manual and oral genital caress. When he has an erection, get into the butterfly position. Put a lot of lubrication on both your vaginal opening and your partner's penis.

Have your partner rub his penis over your clitoris and along your vaginal lips. Peak up to levels 6, 7, and 8 with this stimulation. Then have your partner insert his penis no more than half an inch into your vagina. His penis should stay within the area of your PC muscle and not enter the vaginal canal itself. You'll be able to tell that his penis is in the correct position because you'll feel your PC muscle gripping it. Have your partner very slowly move his penis in and out of your vagina to tease your PC muscle. This can often trigger orgasm.

ᐸᐧ *Exercise 77.* USING THE PC MUSCLE TO TRIGGER ORGASM

Use this exercise if you are able to peak all the way up to arousal level 9 but can't seem to go over the edge to orgasm. Begin a peaking exercise with your partner. Give him focusing caresses and then manual or oral stimulation. When your partner has an erection, climb on top of him and use his penis to peak yourself up to levels 4, 5, 6, 7, 8, and 9 if you can. Take your time doing these peaks.

When you reach level 9, squeeze your PC muscle as hard as you can two or three times in a row. Often, this is all that is necessary to trigger orgasmic spasms.

◠◡ Exercise 78. IMITATING ORGASM

Imitating orgasm in the way that I describe here is very different from faking an orgasm to please your partner or because you think your partner expects you to have one. What you will learn here is how to fake yourself into thinking you are having an orgasm. This in turn can actually trigger an orgasm.

If you have experienced the peaking process with intercourse both actively and passively and have tried the female arousal techniques in Chapter 26, chances are good that you have had an orgasm (or several). However, if you have not yet experienced orgasm, try this exercise. It is most likely to help you if you can successfully peak up to level 9 with different kinds of stimulation but cannot seem to go over the edge.

Remember that the orgasmic response is a full-body response, not something that occurs only in the genitals. At the moment of orgasm, your face contorts, your arms, legs, and neck spasm, and your PC muscle begins to contract. Your breathing and heart rate reach peaks. The key to faking yourself into orgasm in this exercise is realizing which of those orgasmic body responses are under your potential control and which aren't. Spasms of your arms, legs, neck, and PC muscle can be under your voluntary control. So can your breathing. Your heart rate is not under your voluntary control. If, when you are at arousal level 9, you enact the bodily responses that are under your control, there is a good chance that you will trigger an orgasm. The secret is to do these things because they feel good, not just in order to have an orgasm.

Begin this exercise however you would like—with focusing caresses or by giving your passive partner a genital caress or oral sex. When your partner has at least a partial erection, get into the butterfly position. I find that position to be the best for the orgasm-imitating technique. Using lots of lubrication, have your partner peak you up to low levels of arousal by stroking his penis on your clitoris and vaginal lips. Then he can penetrate and you can peak up to levels 6, 7, and 8. Don't forget to allow your arousal to decrease between peaks.

When you are at level 9 or slightly above, take a deep breath, suck in your lower abdomen, hunch your shoulders into the bed, open your eyes wide, and relax your PC muscle. This may trigger an orgasm, which you will experience as a fluttering or spasming of the PC muscle.

Another way to imitate orgasm is to pretend you are having an orgasm and act the way you think highly orgasmic women act. Moan, flail your limbs, or imitate an orgasm vocally like Meg Ryan did in the movie *When Harry Met Sally*. Research shows that the more we express an emotion or sensation, the more deeply we experience it, and this is true of orgasm. Sometimes women can't reach orgasm because they are embarrassed to let loose and make a lot of noise.

You can do this version of imitating orgasm with any activity and in any intercourse position. Do it when you are at a very high level of arousal. This is a more mental version of the exercise that may involve moaning, contorting your face, or pretending that you are with a particular fantasy object. It can work best if what is holding you back is your image of yourself as someone who "doesn't do that sort of thing." Pretending that you are a highly arousable and orgasmic woman may allow you to practice orgasm techniques in a nonthreatening way until you feel more comfortable with them.

Both of these ways of triggering orgasm have several things in common. First, you have to be able to focus, breathe, and relax well enough to allow yourself to get up to arousal level 9. If you're unable to do that, you need to focus on treating your arousal issues using the exercises in Chapter 26. You also have to be able to focus well enough so that you avoid having any distracting thoughts when you are at level 9.

As with any skill that involves learning complex patterns of behavior and combining them, the first few tries may feel artificial. But after you have practiced the techniques for a while, they will become habits and your ability to focus at level 9 will trigger an orgasm.

○✎ *Exercise 79.* BRIDGE MANEUVER

Although this sounds like something out of civil engineering, it is actually a gratifying way to bring your self-discovery together with your sexual partnership. This technique creates a psychological/behavioral bridge between your ability to have an orgasm when stimulating your clitoris yourself and your ability to have an orgasm during intercourse. This is the exercise that all sex therapists recommend for a woman who can have an orgasm by herself but has difficulty having an orgasm during intercourse. The best intercourse position for this exercise is the female-superior position.

Your partner will lie on his back as you do a front caress and genital caress to arouse him. When he becomes erect, climb on top of him and begin peaking and/or plateauing, using his penis to pleasure yourself. As you reach the higher peaks or plateaus (levels 7 and 8), stimulate your clitoris with your fingers. Masturbate to orgasm by stimulating your clitoris as your partner strokes the inside of your vagina with his penis. Notice the added sensations you feel with simultaneous masturbation and intercourse. With some practice, you will need less and less direct clitoral stimulation with your fingers, and your ability to have an orgasm will transfer to the stimulation of intercourse. Because you receive stimulation both on your clitoris and deep inside your vagina, this exercise may allow you to experience one of those "blended" orgasms I mentioned in Chapter 2.

There are a few variations on this exercise. Both work best if you are on top. Ask your partner to stimulate your clitoris with his fingers instead of doing it yourself. Or either one of you can use a vibrator or dildo to stimulate your clitoris during intercourse. You can also practice alternating peaks with a dildo, your fingers, your partner's fingers, and your partner's penis.

Using Fantasy to Trigger Orgasm

Many women are able to have orgasms through their fantasies alone, or during periods of REM sleep. Here are a few suggestions to make that more likely to happen for you:

　＊ Fantasize while you are doing any exercise that involves self-touch.

　＊ Read or look at erotic visual material while you do any self-touch exercise.

　＊ Fantasize before you go to sleep, but don't finish the fantasy. Go up to the point right before you have an orgasm. Then go to sleep. You may wake up having an orgasm.

✳ Read erotic materials or look at sexually explicit materials right before you go to sleep. You may wake up in the middle of the night having an orgasm.

All of the above activities can help you reconnect with your ability to have an orgasm with very little genital contact. Many of us had that ability when we were children and have simply forgotten how to do it.

chapter 28

Healing
Low Sexual Desire

Unlike most of the previous chapters in Part IV, this chapter does not contain specific exercises to treat the condition listed in the chapter title. Instead, I'll point out how and when some of the exercises from other chapters can be helpful for increasing sexual desire. Much of the material contained in this chapter is more theoretical in nature, although toward the end of the chapter I make many very specific suggestions for increasing sexual desire.

This chapter is largely geared toward women. That's not to imply that men can't experience low desire, too. And, of course, men can follow the suggestions offered here. But in my experience, low sexual desire in men is usually caused by one of about six things: low testosterone, anxiety, depression, use of prescription drugs, work-related stress, or the prior existence of other sexual problems such as premature ejaculation or erection problems. Women's desire problems tend to be more complicated.

Understanding and Dealing with Low Sexual Desire

If you are experiencing low sexual desire, you should begin your healing process by doing the relaxation and breathing exercises in Chapter 16. Try doing them on a daily basis. You should also do the sexual fitness exercises in Chapter 17. It's especially important to make sure your PC muscle is in good shape. In addition, do the self-touch exercises in Chapter 18. The exercises in those three chapters can often jump-start a person's sexual desire. Other than that, no specific progression of sensual and sexual exercises exists to help heal low sexual desire, as it does for erection problems, female arousal problems, and most of the other sexual dysfunctions. Low sexual desire is not a dysfunction as such. By this I mean it's not that the genitals aren't working right. Low sexual desire is more of a psychological issue.

Having said that, absolutely the first thing you should do if you are experiencing low sexual desire is to have your testosterone level checked. This applies whether you are a man or a woman, and it applies no matter how old you are. It is especially true if you have experienced desire in the past and are not experiencing it now, and it is also especially true if you noticed that your level of sexual desire seemed to decrease abruptly for no reason that was obvious to you.

If you are a man and you are found to have low testosterone, the hormone can be administered to you in various ways. It used to be given in the form of a shot, but that method made it difficult to regulate the level of hormone in the person's system throughout the day. The goal is to have a steady level of testosterone throughout a twenty-four-hour period. Now testosterone is mostly administered in the form of a skin patch that is attached to the scrotum and that continually releases the hormone.

If you are a woman with low testosterone, the situation is a little more complicated. Women don't need as much testosterone as men, but they need some. I know that some forms of hormone replacement therapy combine estrogen and testosterone, but hormone therapy is usually used only for women during or after menopause. Unfortunately, we now know that administering estrogen after menopause may have some serious side effects. A new herbal preparation called Avlimil is available that supposedly enhances sexual desire in postmenopausal women. I don't have any experience with it, but it might be worth asking your health-care practitioner about it.

Another solution may be to use the testosterone skin patch that men use, applying it on an area of the lower body such as the buttocks. For many women, however, the patch may prove to be too strong and may cause masculinizing side effects such as hair growth and acne. A number of testosterone-based creams have recently come on the market. Designed to be rubbed onto the thigh area, they are formulated by compounding pharmacies based on the needs of the individual woman. Effects will kick in after about two weeks of use. If I were a woman experiencing low sexual desire due to a testosterone deficiency, I would definitely consult an endocrinologist about the possibility of having a custom-made hormone mixture designed for me.

If you are a woman, it will help to recognize a few really important things about low sexual desire so that your expectations are in line with reality. First of all, women regularly undergo many hormonal events throughout their lives that can have profound effects on their sexual desire. One is pregnancy, which the majority of women in the world go through at least once. Pregnancy and its aftermath (childbirth and breastfeeding) can affect a woman's sex drive in a number of ways. Many women report that they experience increased sexual desire during some phases of pregnancy, but many women report a sharp decrease in sex drive right after childbirth, especially if they breast-feed. There are a number of reasons for this. Pregnancy and childbirth greatly affect the body's hormone levels. And if you breast-feed, you secrete more than the usual amount of oxytocin, the so-called bonding hormone. Oxytocin can temporarily suppress testosterone. Many new mothers experience a sharp decline in sex drive due to a combination of lack of sleep, feeling out of shape physically, and the change in self-image from "hot babe" to "mother." Many women become extremely upset after childbirth when their sex drive fails to return right away. The reality is that it can take as long as two years for it to return to normal. The good news is that, like postpartum depression, hormone-based loss of sex drive is temporary. It will come back; it just takes time.

Another hormonal event that women undergo that can affect their sex drive is menopause. Unlike men, women do not maintain their fertility throughout their lifetime. Somewhere in her forties, a woman's estrogen levels start to drop, and by her early fifties she has usually stopped ovulating and stopped having menstrual periods. Some women report a decrease in sex drive during this process, which is not a one-time event but lasts for several years. Again, this decrease in sex drive is usually temporary.

Men also appear to undergo hormonal changes starting in their late forties. The major differences between the so-called change of life for men and for women is that women can no longer conceive, but men are more likely to experience behavioral sexual changes such as erection difficulties, less urgency to ejaculate, or decreased desire. Surprisingly, most research shows that menopause does not usually affect a woman's ability to become aroused or have orgasms.

Women who take birth control pills (oral contraceptives) may also notice a decline in sex drive after several years of use. This is unfortunate because oral contraceptives are so effective at preventing pregnancy. The drop in sex drive related to oral contraceptives can be a serious problem, and many women have opted for a different form of contraceptive in order to restore their sexual desire to its former level.

If you are a woman, there is another important thing you need to recognize about low sexual desire. This one has to do with societal expectations about women's sexual behavior. Our definition and diagnosis of low sexual desire is highly influenced by a woman's relationship status. We tend to think that women are only likely to consider low sexual desire a problem if they are in a relationship. In this case, of course, the symptom would be that a woman lacks interest in having sex with her partner. Our stereotypical view of the woman with low sexual desire is usually a woman in her fifties who has gone through menopause and has been with the same partner for over twenty years. But single women can also experience low sexual desire. If you are a single woman, it's really important for you to recognize the difference between sex drive (the physiological component) and sexual desire (the psychological component). If you don't have a current sexual partner or love interest, you could still feel "horny" due to your testosterone level. You might experience this feeling as an urge to fantasize, masturbate, or look at erotic materials. It's also normal when you're single to feel a high level of sex drive but at the same time to have a low level of sexual desire, and that's not a clinically significant problem. In fact, if you don't currently have a partner, a strong libido can be a curse, because it's really frustrating to be horny and have no one to have sex with. So you need to ask yourself, "Do I really want to increase my sexual desire?" It might be better to just put it on hold for a while. I believe that women who are between partners should maintain a basic level of sexual functioning by using self-touch and some combination of daily sensual activities like massage and PC muscle exercises. You want to be ready when the right man comes along. But there is nothing wrong with you if you experience a drop in sexual desire when you are between men. That's completely normal.

Are there drugs that have been shown to increase sexual desire? Not really, in any reliable sense. Health food stores sell herbal preparations that purport to increase desire. If they have any effect at all it's probably due to the placebo effect: expectations. None of these substances have been scientifically tested and found superior to a placebo.

In terms of the effects of drugs on sexual desire, what you're *not* taking is more important than what you are taking. We have already seen that oral contraceptives can lower sexual desire. Commonly prescribed antianxiety agents, such as Prozac, Paxil, Zoloft, and other, similar drugs, are also notorious for decreasing sexual desire. This class of drugs is called the selective serotonin reuptake inhibitors (SSRIs). If you have problems with sexual desire, you should never take any of the SSRIs.

There are no specific sensate-focus exercises that are designed to treat low sexual desire. However, you can still use this book, because many of the exercises that work well for other sexual problems also work especially well for low sexual desire. If you are having a problem with low sexual desire, after you have started practicing the relaxation, sexual fitness, and self-touch exercises, begin to work with your partner on the basic partner exercises (the face caress, the back caress, the front caress, the genital caress, and oral sex).

A funny thing sometimes happens in sex therapy with couples who are experiencing low sexual desire. I might ask them to do the basic partner exercises, and after either the genital caress or oral sex, the couple comes into my office looking kind of sheepish. I ask them what is wrong and they say, "Well, after the genital caress, we were feeling so good that we went ahead and had intercourse, and it was great!" Often, if your sexual desire problems are due to overwork and poor time management, the basic sensate-focus exercises are essentially your "cure." It's not so much that these exercises increase desire as such. It's more that making time to spend with each other in a place free of distractions increases desire.

That's why, for couples who are having problems with low desire due to stress, overwork, and any of the lower-level causes I described in Chapter 5, the standard advice from sex therapists is to schedule a weekend together free of distractions and plan to have sex all weekend. This will actually work if your problems aren't too serious, especially if you start slowly, using the basic sensate-focus exercises and massage as foreplay before you proceed to intercourse.

If you and your partner have gone through the five basic sensate-focus partner exercises and still feel that your desire level could use a little more of a boost, the peaking and plateauing processes are dynamite for low sexual desire, because they boost your production of endorphins, the pain-killing and pleasure-causing brain chemicals. Endorphin production is extremely reinforcing, in that it leads you to desire sex more the next time.

Detailed descriptions of the peaking and plateauing processes appear in this book in Chapter 23 (from the male point of view) and Chapter 26 (from the female point of view). If you want to use peaking and plateauing to heal low sexual desire, do the following:

1. Do a peaking exercise with manual stimulation with the man as the focus, then do the same with the woman as the focus.

2. Do a peaking exercise with oral sex with the man as the focus, and then do the same with the woman as the focus.

3. Do peaking exercises in the different intercourse positions with each partner as the focus.

4. Do intercourse peaking exercises in which the man and the woman alternate peaks.

5. After completing these exercises, follow the same progression with plateauing exercises: Use all of the different forms of stimulation, all of the different intercourse positions, and all of the different plateauing techniques.

If you do two exercises a week, this progression of exercises will keep you busy for quite a while. I guarantee you that at some point in this process you're going to look at each other and say, "I can't believe this. I'm feeling sexual again."

The guided activities and exercises in Chapters 34 through 37 will also help you. They don't progress in a particular order, so read through them and choose whichever ones appeal to you.

More Suggestions to Jump-Start Your Sexual Desire

This section describes other factors that have been reliably shown to increase sexual desire. Many of them don't sound overtly sexual. We could probably call this section "Things that don't seem like they would increase your sexual desire but do." I put the list together from many different sources. Especially helpful was the book *Why We Love,* by Helen Fisher (see Recommended Reading), but I've arranged the material according to my own take on sexual desire.

Actually having sex is probably the most important thing you can do to increase your level of desire. The problem is, most people don't want to have sex if they don't feel like it. But it's okay to have sex even if you don't feel like it, and it can boost your desire for the following reason, which has to do with attitude-behavior relations. An attitude is a positive or negative

evaluation of something. Most people believe that the attitude-behavior relationship is a one-way street. We have a positive attitude about a certain
behavior and then we do the behavior. And, of course, for most of us it does
work that way a lot of the time. The seeds of behavior are often attitudes or
intentions. But it can also work the other way around. Behavior can precede
attitude. If you actually do a behavior even though you don't feel like it, it
can cause you to have a more positive attitude about the behavior in the
future and to want to do it again.

An example that's relevant to sex is physical exercise. How many of us
have vowed to start an exercise program on the morning of a certain date,
and then when that morning came along, we didn't feel like getting out of
bed and going to the gym? If you actually start exercising even though you
don't feel like it, after a few sessions you will start to like it. That's why personal training is so popular. Once you've been motivated to start that first
behavior change, you'll like it so much you'll want to stick with it. And the
same thing is true of sex.

This next suggestion may be a little harder to implement. Being in love
usually causes an increase in sexual desire. Besides heart-pounding excitement, some of the other factors that are involved in being in love include
uncertainty about the nature of the relationship and artificial barriers to
being together. This one is a little tricky, because obviously you love your
partner, or you wouldn't care about jump-starting your sexual desire. But
your relationship may have reached a stage where the love you feel for each
other is more a companionate or friendship love than wild, sexual passion.
You can help bring some of that passion back into your life by injecting a
small element of uncertainty into your relationship—a bit of playing hard to
get, for example. You could also create minor artificial barriers to being
together and then overcome them.

Here's one way to create a small artificial barrier to being together: If
your partner asks whether you would like to go out for dinner on the weekend, instead of readily agreeing, you could hesitate a moment and then say,
"Can I let you know tomorrow? There's a possibility I have something else
to do that day." Then just agree to the date tomorrow. This creates enough
uncertainty to pique your partner's interest.

You can play hard to get sometimes when your partner asks you to have
sex. You can say, "Talk me into it. Tell me everything you want us to do
together and how it's going to feel." You fully intend to go to bed with your

partner, but you put him or her off for a few minutes, during which he or she has to plan some sexy activities and talk you into them.

Another way to use romantic love to boost your sexual desire is to utilize your memory. Think back to when you did have that head-over-heels romantic feeling for your partner and fantasize about it. Or maybe there's a person for whom you feel passionate love or even just plain lust, but you haven't acted on it. Fantasize about that person. It's okay—you're not going to act on it with that person; you're going to act on it with your partner. Your partner will be the beneficiary of your fantasy about a past or current lust object. The lust object doesn't have to be anyone you know. It could be someone unattainable to you, like a celebrity or authority figure.

Which brings me to my next suggestion—fantasy. Research shows that sexual fantasy is highly related to sexual desire. People who report that they fantasize more also report that they feel more sexual desire, and vice versa. You are free to fantasize about anything you like. It doesn't have to be about sex with your current partner. If you've had problems with low sexual desire for so long that you literally can't even think of anything to fantasize about, then visit a bookstore and browse through the shelves of erotica and the collections of typical fantasy scenarios to help you get started.

And, of course, related to fantasy is the use of sexually explicit materials. These could include written erotica or visual materials such as still pictures or videos, or even recordings of sexual words. I call this stuff sexually explicit material rather than pornography. A lot of people are turned off by the concept of pornography, because much of it is either sleazy or totally male-oriented (or both). A lot of pornographic material contains images that are either demeaning or insulting to women. But it's possible to find sexually explicit materials that are milder but that still have the potential to be arousing. Research has long shown that viewing sexually explicit materials leads to temporary increases in both sexual desire and sexual behavior. In fact, this was one of the major findings of the Meese Commission on pornography back in the 1980s. I'm not trying to talk you into becoming a porn connoisseur. However, the correlation is so strong that I think if you are having problems with low sexual desire you should at least try to find some kind of sexually explicit material that is both acceptable and arousing to you.

Another factor that has been shown to be highly and reliably related to sexual desire is novelty. We usually think of novelty in terms of having sex with different partners. Most people's relationships probably aren't set up to allow for that sort of thing. But you can introduce novelty into your relationship by having sex in different settings, in different positions, or introducing new elements into your sexual situations.

Situational factors that can be especially potent in terms of heightening desire are a couple of glasses of wine, special foods, a situation with few distractions, music, or making love with some or all of your clothes on. If you want to use music to set the sexual scene, it's probably best to use instrumental music, especially at first. Song lyrics can be distracting in a sexual situation. Also, don't have the television on if you want to increase the desire potential in a sexual situation. Women in particular have reported that a television playing the background is a huge turn-off. Many people find that receiving compliments during sex is a turn-on. So is intellectually stimulating or challenging conversation.

Your body image has a very big effect on your level of sexual desire. Gaining weight can cause you to experience a decrease in sexual desire. Exercising, changing one's diet, and losing weight have all been shown to increase desire. Exercise is especially important. Any form of physical exercise (whether it's walking, running, swimming, having sex, or whatever) will increase the dopamine levels in your brain. Dopamine is a brain chemical that's related to enjoyment of life. It's especially active when you're in love. Even mild forms of exercise increase it. Diet is important, too. Eating a lot of heavy carbohydrates can make you feel sluggish, and eating too many fats can actually interfere with arousal, especially with erections in men. As I said in Chapter 17, on sexual fitness, just about any kind of physical exercise will ultimately benefit your sex life. The exception is cycling. While it's really good for you from an aerobic standpoint, it can put pressure on the blood vessels in the groin area and can potentially interfere with arousal and erection, although just like any other form of exercise, cycling should increase desire. Some companies make special bicycle seats that have openings where the pubic bone and surrounding areas generally come into contact with the seat. This type of seat could potentially help with arousal problems that stem from pressure on the blood vessels in the groin area.

A few other miscellaneous things have been shown to increase sexual desire, especially in women. Believe it or not, many women report that sunbathing causes them to feel sexual. Meditation and relaxation exercises also increase desire, even though they seem as though they would relax you rather than cause you to feel desire. Yoga is especially good.

Women often experience ebb and flow in their levels of sexual desire depending on their monthly cycle. It would make sense from an evolutionary standpoint that a woman should feel the highest levels of sexual desire during ovulation, when she has the best chance of becoming pregnant. But that's not always the case. Every woman is different, and some women report their highest levels of sexual desire right before their period or even during their period.

The potential influence of pheromones on sexual desire is controversial. Pheromones are chemicals excreted by the body that may have an effect on the sex drive of potential mates. Pheromones regulate sexual behavior in the animal kingdom. They exert their action through the sense of smell. For example, neither rats nor dogs mate unless the females produce certain pheromones that attract the males. The complete influence of pheromones on human behavior remains unknown, although it has been found that exposure to certain animal pheromone compounds can cause reactions in human females. Women who wear clothing that has had male scent applied to it often experience changes in their levels of desire or in their menstrual cycles. Many women like to wear their partner's clothes and take in his scent. It's even been shown that there are components in semen that can increase a woman's level of sexual desire. That's still another reason why actually having sex can increase your desire: Exposure to your partner's semen in your vagina can boost libido.

Many of the above suggestions are pretty basic, I admit. Now we come to some of the heavy stuff—or I guess we could call them *the intangibles*. Women especially are turned on when they feel an emotional connection to a partner. That's not something you can fake, and it's not something you can create by using some gimmick. Generally, women feel intimate when they feel safe and feel that they can trust their partner. They also feel intimate when they are looking at a partner face to face. Many women report that an evening of watching a romantic movie together (no television with advertising, please) and then lying together and talking about the movie leads to a sense of intimacy.

To me, the biggest factor in sexual desire is what I would call involvement in life. This is really more of a philosophical issue than a sexual one. Would you expect to feel interested in sex if you weren't interested in anything else in your life? Of course not, and yet some people have no passion for anything but still expect themselves to be sexual dynamos in bed. It's just not going to happen. Passion outside the bedroom transfers to passion inside the bedroom. I'll tell you an anecdote that illustrates this point. Many years ago a couple I knew was in marriage counseling. When the counselor met with each person separately, he asked the wife, "What's your main complaint about your sex life?" She replied, "It's boring." The counselor said, "Boring people have boring sex." I couldn't agree with him more. Remember back in the 1970s when Henry Kissinger was quoted as saying something like, "Power is the ultimate aphrodisiac?" Why do you think powerful people are so sexually attractive? I suspect one of the main reasons is because they're passionate about their cause (even though the cause may be misguided). Involvement in life is sexy, whether it's on the global level or the one-on-one interpersonal level. To help your partner increase his or her sexual desire, you must convey to your partner that you are involved and completely focused.

Another huge psychological factor in sexual desire is the power of memory. Research shows that most of us don't have an especially good memory for specific sexual episodes, but most of us have a very good memory for the first time we fell in love. Being able to reconnect with those memories can help us jump-start our libido in adulthood. Most people report that their first crush, or their first inkling of what sexual love might be like, took place when they were between the ages of eight and twelve. Being able to reconnect with the memories of a first teenage or preadolescent crush might help your current level of libido, even if the person you first fell in love with is not your current partner. This can be true whether or not you had any sexual contact with your first love.

There are so many potential ways that you can boost your libido. I'm sure you'll come up with some of your own in addition to my list. A temporary bout of low sexual desire provides unlimited opportunities for sexual healing.

chapter 29

Healing Sexual
Aversion Disorder

A nxiety is a subject that's very close to me. I've suffered from anxiety all my life, ranging from mild anxiety to panic attacks, although my anxiety has been unrelated to sexual concerns. Basically, I seem to have anxiety about nearly everything *but* sex. Yet, when I was a surrogate partner, I was very successful at helping people who suffered from intense sexual anxiety. I have no idea why this was true, considering that I'm the anxiety disorder poster child myself. Maybe my clients looked at me and figured their anxiety level wasn't so bad.

Here are a couple of hints to help you reduce anxiety in general, not just sexual anxiety. If you do any stimulants, give them up now. I'm not only talking about illegal stimulants like cocaine or amphetamine, but it goes without saying that if you have anxiety and you use those substances, they are causing your anxiety to be much worse. I'm talking about legal, over-the-counter stimulants like nicotine and caffeine. If you use these substances and have anxiety, you need to stop using them now. You may not believe it, but they are making your anxiety much worse. Too much caffeine (the amount contained in a few cups of coffee or soft drinks) on a daily basis can send you from moderate but manageable anxiety to full-blown panic attacks. No one told me this, so I had to learn it the hard way. A couple of panic attacks on the freeway was all it took for me to give up caffeine completely. Even a piece of chocolate sends me into an episode of rapid heart rate.

Besides giving up stimulants, if you have a tendency toward anxiety you must practice some kind of relaxation training in addition to the sexual exercises you will learn in this book. Possibilities include meditation, listening to music, and yoga. You must set aside half an hour each day just to relax, with no outside mental stimulation.

Another suggestion is worry beads. They are unfamiliar to many Americans, but they are used in Europe, especially in the Mediterranean countries. (They probably need them over there, because they smoke a lot and drink a lot of coffee.) People carry a string of beads in their pockets and play with them when they are under stress. Any string of beads will do. Alternatively, you could wear a watch or a bracelet that can function in the same way. When you become aware that you are stressed out, slowly stroke the beads. Doing so will calm you down.

The most common symptoms of anxiety are rapid heart rate, dizziness, and shortness of breath. Although these symptoms may not sound all that bad, they can have very serious consequences. They can be debilitating and interfere with your life. One example of an incapacitating form of anxiety is agoraphobia, which is a fear of leaving one's house. It literally makes a prisoner out of the person who has it.

The good news is that anxiety is highly treatable. The reason why sexual problems respond so well to treatment is because the treatment is based on anxiety-reduction strategies. Anxiety problems probably have the highest cure rate of any of the psychological problems. Even if you suffer from severe sexual anxiety, there is hope.

I'll include one caveat here. If you suffer from very severe anxiety, you may need the help of a qualified therapist and/or medication to get you to a place where you can deal with sexual stimulation. However, keep in mind that if you take one of the most commonly prescribed antianxiety agents like Prozac, Paxil, Zoloft, or other chemically similar drugs (the SSRIs), they *will* reduce your anxiety, but they've also been shown to depress sexual desire and to delay or interfere with orgasm. In the case of severe, life-altering anxiety, the trade-off may be worth it, at least temporarily. Even if you think you may need a therapist or medication, you can still try the exercises in this book. They can't hurt you, and you might reap some benefit from them before you decide to see a therapist.

Unlike many of the other chapters on healing specific sex problems, such as premature ejaculation and orgasm difficulties, this chapter doesn't contain specific exercises for sexual aversion disorder. Instead, I offer four typical treatment programs: one for mild sexual anxiety, one for moderate general sexual anxiety, one for specific sexual fears, and one for severe sexual anxiety, including fears of touching or being touched.

To help you with any of the programs outlined here, you will want to obtain a medical device that can display and record your pulse rate, such as a home blood pressure monitor. A device is available that fits over one finger and displays both pulse rate and blood pressure.

Mild Sexual Anxiety

Do you experience rapid heart rate when you think about having sexual contact? Does even this mild level of anxiety cause you to avoid sexual situations? Do you tense up when your partner touches you?

On the other hand, were you able to read through all of the exercises in this book without being scared? Could you picture yourself doing the exercises? If so, your anxiety level is probably low enough that you can use the program in this book without any modifications. Go through the chapters in the following order:

1. Do the relaxation exercises in Chapter 16 on a daily basis. Use your pulse monitor to check your pulse before you start the relaxation exercises and then again when you finish. When you see that you can control your anxiety level and cause it to go down, you will feel a sense of mastery.

2. Put yourself on a program of relaxation training for twenty to thirty minutes a day. Use meditation, yoga, listening to music, or commercial relaxation tapes. You can learn both meditation and yoga from books or videos if you would rather not take a class.

3. Do the sexual fitness exercises in Chapter 17.

4. Do the self-touch exercises in Chapter 18. If you feel anxious during any of the exercises, back up to a previous exercise with which you felt comfortable, and then try the new exercise at a later date.

5. Do the basic partner exercises in Chapters 19 through 22. Again, if you feel anxious during any exercise, back up to a previous exercise or to a body part you felt more comfortable with. Then, try the new exercise again next time. Or stop in the middle of the exercise you are uncomfortable with, do some deep breathing or muscle relaxation, and then resume the exercise. The basic sensate-focus partner exercises will help you relax while touching your partner's genitals and having your partner touch yours.

6. For more advanced training and sexual enjoyment, do the peaking and plateauing processes with your partner. If you are a woman, do the peaking and plateauing as described in Chapter 26, on female sexual arousal disorder. If you are a man, do the peaking and plateauing processes as described in Chapter 23, on premature ejaculation.

Congratulations! Now you're ready for anything. With this background you should be able to do any of the other exercises in this book. If you find that once the anxiety is gone you have issues with arousal or orgasm, do the exercises in the appropriate chapters.

Moderate Generalized Sexual Anxiety

Does the thought of sexual contact literally make you queasy but not to the level of actual panic? Do you avoid not only actual sexual contact but also reading about sex or looking at sexually explicit materials? If so, your personality has probably acquired an element of erotophobia, a generalized fear of all things sexual.

If you seek drug therapy for moderate levels of anxiety, in addition to drugs like Prozac, Paxil, and Zoloft, watch out for high blood pressure medications and alpha and beta blockers. Some of these are often prescribed for anxiety, but in some people they do the opposite: They increase an already rapid heart rate and its accompanying anxiety sensations.

Of course, you might be scared of sexual contact for a very good reason. Perhaps in the past you suffered child molestation or some other sexual trauma, or you caught a sexually transmitted disease. These are all good explanations for your fear of sex, and again, you may need some individual therapy to help you deal with past issues.

There's also the possibility that your anxiety might be telling you something. Two of the biggest sources of anxiety are living with someone you don't want to live with and doing things you don't want to do. If at some level you are uncomfortable around your partner because you don't trust him or her, that's a bit more complicated than just a fear of sex.

If you've ruled out all of the above causes for your anxiety, you are ready to proceed with this program. You will get over your moderate level of sexual anxiety using the same program I described above for mild anxiety, with a couple of additions: desensitization and shaping.

Desensitization means the gradual presentation of sexual material that is more and more explicit. To help you get over the anxiety you experience in an actual sexual situation, it will help if you can desensitize yourself to sexually explicit materials in general. I'm not going to try to turn you into a porn addict, but you need to be able to look at adult materials without being embarrassed or anxious. Sexually explicit materials range from four-letter words, written descriptions of sexual activity, and sex scenes in mainstream movies all the way up through very graphic X-rated or hard-core materials like still pictures, videos, or live streaming content on the Internet.

Before you try to desensitize yourself to adult materials, start doing the breathing and relaxation exercises in Chapter 16 on a daily basis. Use your pulse monitor to check your heart rate both before and after the exercises. Give yourself a pat on the back when you notice progress in learning to control your anxiety symptoms.

Once you feel like you've had some success using relaxation techniques to control your anxiety symptoms, and once you've made these practices a part of your daily life, you're ready to move to the next step in the program. Here are some suggestions for desensitizing yourself to general sexual concepts and adult materials:

* Read informational books about sexual techniques.

* Take a human sexuality course at a local college.

* Make a list of four-letter words or sexual words that you are uncomfortable with. Write each word several times in a row. Repeat each word out loud while looking in a mirror until you can say all of the words without becoming anxious.

* Read passages of a sexy novel out loud while looking at yourself in a mirror.

Next, put together a collection of sexually explicit materials that ranges from mild to very graphic. These could be still pictures or video clips or whatever. Arrange the materials in order from least graphic to most graphic. Starting with the least graphic material, look at each picture or clip for a few seconds. If you start to get anxious or experience rapid heart rate, back up to some of the material you were more comfortable with, or do some deep breathing and relaxation exercises. Your goal here is to be able to listen to or view the whole range of sexually explicit material without experiencing rapid heart rate. Keep a record of what you looked at, how much time you spent looking, and your anxiety level during each session, so you can see your progress.

After you have successfully desensitized yourself to a variety of sexually explicit materials, do the sexual fitness exercises in Chapter 17 and the self-touch exercises in Chapter 18. Before you start the basic partner exercises in

Chapters 19 through 22, I will explain again what shaping is (also see the discussion on page 240). Shaping is successive approximation of behavior. You may know shaping as the "baby steps" approach. This means that you identify a goal and are always moving toward it, no matter how small the steps you take or how little progress you make in every session, or whether you have to repeat behaviors or exercises a number of times.

I'll give you an example of shaping from animal psychology. Have you ever seen a movie or TV program that portrayed experiments that reward a rat with food pellets for pressing a lever in a certain corner of its cage? Does the rat press the lever correctly on the first try? Of course not. How do you think the scientists get the rat to figure out that pressing the bar causes food to appear? Through shaping. If you're trying to teach the rat to press a lever for food, first you reward the rat with food whenever it goes to the side of the cage where the lever is. Then you reward the rat with food if it sniffs around the lever. Then you reward the rat if it touches the lever with its paw. Finally you must reward the rat with food every time it presses the lever. (This keeps the researcher busy—it kind of makes you wonder who's really in charge.)

To use this technique in treating anxiety problems, first you identify the particular behavioral goal you would like to reach. This will be different for each specific exercise. Let's say the first exercise that causes you anxiety is a sensate-focus caress on your own genitals for twenty minutes. (This self-touch exercise is described in Chapter 18.) Let's say you experience anxiety with this exercise after only one minute of doing it. Make yourself a chart labeled "1 minute," "2 minutes," etc., all the way up to "20 minutes." The first day, do the exercise for one minute, and then follow with a session of deep breathing and muscle relaxation exercises. Check off on your chart that you completed one minute. Next time try for two minutes. Keep on doing these baby steps until you are up to twenty minutes.

Then move on to the next exercise (arousal awareness or peaking), and make a "baby steps" chart for it. Break the exercise into as many small steps as you think you need to. All you need to do is make sure you're always moving in the direction of the goal. This is important. The key to success using shaping is that in the next session you always either repeat a previous exercise or move on to the next step. You always move toward the goal, never away from the goal. Design your baby steps to ensure your success. If this means breaking your baby steps down into half minutes instead of whole minutes, then do it. The size of the steps doesn't matter. What matters is that you proceed toward the goal. This approach may seem like it will take forever, but it doesn't. At the "baby-steps rate" you can do several sessions a day.

Once you have completed the self-touch exercises, you will be ready for the basic partner exercises in Chapters 19 through 22. Again, if you need to, break these exercises down into baby steps. The following are several ways to do this:

1. If your goal is to be in the passive role in an exercise for twenty minutes, break it down into one-minute segments. Progress to the point where you can complete the full twenty-minute passive or active role before beginning the other role.

2. Alternatively, you could alternate a minute in the passive role with a minute in the active role. Don't forget to do deep breathing and relaxation after your successful completion of each baby-step interval. This is your reward for doing the exercise.

3. If you have a problem doing the basic partner exercises at all, start with something even more basic, like a hand caress instead of a face or back caress. If either caressing your partner or being caressed causes you anxiety, start with something less anxiety-provoking like simply resting your hand on your partner's hand or having him or her rest a hand on you for a short period of time.

4. Devise some other system of rewards besides just breathing and relaxing. For each small assignment you complete successfully, reward yourself with something you like to do—watching a favorite television show, reading a magazine, eating a special food, relaxing in a hot tub, whatever.

Remember, one of the principles of shaping is that if a particular activity seems scary to you, you can always think of something that is conceptually close to the activity but is less scary (e.g., a hand caress in place of a face caress).

After completing all of the basic partner exercises, do the peaking and plateauing processes as described in Chapter 23 if you are a man or Chapter 26 if you are a woman.

Specific Sexual Fears

If you have a specific sexual phobia, do all of the preliminary exercises you can without triggering the phobia. Here's an example of a woman who has a specific fear of doing oral sex with her male partner. She could do all of the relaxation exercises in Chapter 16, the sexual fitness exercises in Chapter 17, and the self-touch exercises in Chapter 18. She and her partner could then do all of the basic partner exercises up to the oral genital caress without triggering a phobic reaction.

Next, she should make a chart that breaks oral sex down into baby steps. The steps might include resting her cheek against her partner's penis without his moving, or resting her lips against her partner's penis without moving. Then the steps could include licking her partner's penis for thirty-second or one-minute intervals. She should be able to think up ten or fifteen baby steps that each move her closer to the goal of having her partner's penis inside her mouth.

After she has successfully done oral sex a few times, she and her partner should work through the peaking and plateauing processes with intercourse. The strategy here is to alternate a fun and rewarding exercise like intercourse with the oral sex practice, making progress one baby step at a time.

Remember that when you are learning to do an activity that you previously feared, you can't expect to enjoy it right away. You have to get over your discomfort first. You go from discomfort to comfort before you get to enjoyment.

Basic Desensitization and Shaping Chart for Someone with a Fear of Nudity and a Fear of Being Touched

Here's another example of a more basic and universal phobia. Let's say a man has a fear of being touched anywhere on his body. He can start the sexual healing program with breathing, relaxation, sexual fitness, and self-touch. Then he's going to have to make several charts—one for each basic partner exercise in Chapters 19 through 22. He and his partner may be unable to start with a face caress or even a hand caress. Rather, his first chart may look something like the following:

✳ He and his partner sit together on a couch with clothes on but without touching.

* He and his partner sit together on a couch with clothes on and with their thighs against each other.

* He and his partner lie next to each other on a bed with clothes on but without touching.

* He and his partner lie together on a bed with clothes on and their bodies against each other.

* He and his partner sit together on a couch with clothes on holding hands.

* He and his partner sit together on a couch partially clothed without touching.

And so on, up through being able to touch his partner's face for a few minutes with clothes off. At this point he will be desensitized enough to continue with the partner exercises. Note that you can make any of the above steps into even smaller steps by breaking them down into time periods like thirty seconds or a minute. And remember to always follow each baby step that you accomplish with breathing and relaxation exercises.

Finally, it's important that you set up a reward system for yourself that has nothing to do with sex. Always keep your eventual goal in sight, and reward yourself for each step you successfully complete. The way to set up a reward system is to use the Premack Principle, in which you follow a behavior you don't do often with one you do often. Here's an example: Let's say there are several things you like to do every day, such as read the newspaper, read a book, play the piano—whatever activity you enjoy enough that you try to do it every day. Every time you successfully complete a baby step in your sexual healing program, follow it with one of your enjoyable behaviors: Read a newspaper, read two chapters in a book, play piano for half an hour.

You can see that you can make behavioral charts for any sexual phobia you have, including fear of fantasy or fear of sexually explicit materials. (A note to women: If you have a fear of vaginal penetration, you have vaginismus, for which there is a very specific treatment. See Chapter 30.)

Severe Sexual Anxiety

Let's say that your sexual anxiety is so severe that you freak out and have a panic attack at the very thought of being touched. In this case we're going to have to bring out the big guns: intense systematic desensitization. Remember that systematic desensitization involves gradually exposing yourself to more intense versions of the feared stimulus. You relax and breathe deeply each time a new stimulus is presented.

There are two forms of systematic desensitization: in vivo and in vitro. In vivo (literally, "in life") desensitization means that you learn to do a previously feared behavior in the real-life situation in which it occurs. Examples of in vivo desensitization are outlined in the preceding section, on treating specific sexual phobias, where I instructed you to treat them by gradually actually touching or being touched by your partner. However, some people have such intense sexual anxiety, often involving panic attacks, that they must first be desensitized in an artificial situation (in vitro, literally "in glass") before they can relax enough to deal with their problems with a real partner.

I'll give you an analogy involving fear of flying, a fear with which I have extensive experience, believe me. In most cases of phobias involving flying, the treatment involves actually being in an airplane and doing deep breathing and relaxation exercises. However, there are some people who have such an intense fear of flying that they can't go anywhere near an airplane without completely decompensating (falling apart). They have to be desensitized in an artificial situation before they can be desensitized in the real situation. This is sometimes called in vitro desensitization.

In vitro desensitization is accomplished using what's called an *anxiety hierarchy,* which is a person's individual list of everything he's afraid of, from least scary to most scary, along with point values on a scale of either 1 to 10 or 1 to 100. The list usually contains about fifteen items. A typical anxiety hierarchy for a person with fear of flying might include the following:

1. Buying a plane ticket

2. Packing the suitcase

3. Driving on the freeway to the airport

4. Parking at the airport

5. Checking in at the ticket counter

6. Going through security

7. Hearing the flight called

8. Boarding the plane

9. Starting of the engines

10. Backing away from the gate

11. Taking off

12. Hearing an unusual noise during the flight

13. Turbulence

14. Landing

Let's say you're working with a therapist. Once you have compiled your anxiety hierarchy, you lie in a lounge chair. The therapist reads aloud each item in the hierarchy, starting with the least anxiety-provoking item. When the therapist reads an item, you close your eyes and visualize yourself in the scene. You breathe deeply and relax your muscles as you picture each item. You don't move on to the next item until you have relaxed completely with the previous one.

Obviously, you don't do the whole list in one session. In fact, some people are so anxious that they need several sessions just to relax with one item. After you have completed the whole list, you're ready for the *in vivo* (real life) desensitization process—in this case, actually getting onto an airplane and learning to relax in flight.

Let's translate this approach to a sexual situation. The first step would be to make up your anxiety hierarchy based on your particular sexual fears. Remember to list the items in order from least anxiety-provoking to most anxiety-provoking. For a man with generalized sexual anxiety and fear of nudity, the list might look like this:

1. Being in the same room with a woman with the door closed

2. Sitting on the couch next to a woman

3. Sitting on a couch with a woman with thighs touching

4. Holding a woman's hand

5. Kissing a woman

6. Sitting on a couch with a woman while you're naked from the waist up

7. Sitting on a couch with a woman with both of you naked from the waist up

8. Sitting on a couch with a woman while you're wearing only your underwear

9. Sitting on a couch with a woman with both of you wearing only underwear

10. Sitting on a couch with a woman with both of you naked

After you create your anxiety hierarchy, lie in a reclining chair or on a bed. Relax and take some deep breaths. Starting with the least anxiety-producing item, close your eyes and imagine the scene in detail. Relax and breathe as you visualize the scene. Use your heart rate monitor to see that your anxiety is decreasing. When you are able to breathe and relax with one item, move on to the next one.

It's a little tricky to do this without a therapist to monitor your progress, but it can be done. After you have completed the hierarchy, you will be able to move on to desensitizing yourself in an actual sexual situation.

You can see that you can make up an anxiety hierarchy for any sexual fear or fears. I've just given one example here. If your particular fear is oral sex, make up a ten- to fifteen-item hierarchy that breaks down the oral sex situation into tiny components. If your particular sexual fear is intercourse, break down the situation leading up to and having intercourse into very small steps, all of which lead toward the goal.

Prescribing the Symptom

Some people have anxiety that is very severe and very resistant to treatment. There is another technique you can use if shaping doesn't work for you. It's called *paradoxical intention,* or *prescribing the symptom.*

Prescribing the symptom works because of the way the human nervous system is set up. Remember from Chapter 3 that the two branches of the autonomic nervous system are the sympathetic nervous system (the fight-or-flight response) and the parasympathetic nervous system (the relaxation response). What I didn't say in Chapter 3 is that these two responses run on the same nerves, meaning that they can't both happen at the same time. You can't be anxious and relaxed at the same time. They are called *incompatible responses.*

Prescribing the symptom is typically used in cases of fear of public speaking. Instead of learning relaxation techniques, the person with fear of public speaking is instructed to try to make himself as anxious as he possibly can. In fact, this has the opposite result, because you can't will yourself to become more anxious than you already are. The net result is that you realize that nothing bad happens to you if you are anxious.

This same technique can work for sexual situations. Instead of trying to activate your relaxation response, go into a sexual situation trying to make yourself as anxious as possible. Tell yourself, "I'm really scared. My heart is racing. I'm starting to sweat. Something really bad is going to happen to me." You'll find that the more you try to make yourself anxious, the more the opposite will occur. You'll relax somewhat and realize that nothing bad will happen to you. (I suppose this also works because people are as contrary as they are.)

An intense form of prescribing the symptom is sometimes used for people who have panic attacks. They are instructed to create the symptoms of a panic attack by spinning around and around really fast. Again, what they learn is that nothing bad happens to them. Prescribing the symptom helps a person get used to anxiety symptoms so that he or she is no longer bothered by them.

≫⚘≪

Let me again reassure you that problems with anxiety are among the most readily treatable psychological issues. The sexual healing program will work for your sex-related anxieties. But the cure is behavioral in nature. That means you must change your behavior. To change anything you must be willing to at least try. I encourage you to give the program presented in this book a try. I believe you'll feel pleased and empowered with the results of your efforts.

chapter 30

Healing Vaginismus

lthough vaginismus feels very scary and hopeless to the woman who experiences it, it is the sexual dysfunction with the highest cure rate: over 95 percent, especially in the case of acquired vaginismus. Essentially, once you have experienced one instance of successful penetration with a penis, you are cured. Read Chapter 29, "Healing Sexual Aversion Disorder," very carefully. Since vaginismus is a phobia (the fear of penetration), many of the concepts outlined in that chapter will apply here also.

The traditional treatment for vaginismus involves the use of dilators, which are rods of graduated width starting with one about the size of a Q-tip. The largest dilator is about the size of an average penis. The woman learns to insert the dilators, beginning with the smallest and moving to the largest. She also learns to breathe and relax her PC muscle as she inserts each dilator and allows it to remain in her vagina for a few minutes.

To cure vaginismus, I could just advise you to go out and buy a set of dilators and learn to use them. But I have a few objections to the use of dilators. One is that they are a prescription item and are therefore expensive. Also, inserting something the size of a Q-tip into your vagina is actually more difficult than inserting a small dildo. When inserting a Q-tip, it's easy to miss the vaginal opening and hit a vaginal lip or your urethra by mistake, which could be painful. Plus, using dilators is neither fun nor sensual. Dilators do not help you get comfortable with the five penetrations described in Chapter 12. You already possess an alternative to dilators that is fun, free, and easy to use: your own fingers.

Progression of Exercises for Vaginismus

If you are trying to heal vaginismus, you should do the breathing and relaxation exercises in Chapter 16 on a daily basis. You should also do the sexual fitness exercises in Chapter 17. Pay special attention to the PC muscle exercises, since this is the muscle group you have a problem with. Make sure that you have located the muscle and are exercising it correctly. Focus on the part of the exercise in which you relax your PC muscle after tightening it. None of the exercises in Chapters 16 and 17 should cause you a problem, as none of them involve penetration. You should also be able to do the basic partner sensate-focus exercises in Chapters 19 (face caress), 20 (back caress), and 21 (front caress). When you get to the genital caress (Chapter 22), have your partner caress just the outside of your genitals. Don't attempt finger penetration if you are still afraid of it. At this point, use the exercises in this chapter instead of the genital caress.

In addition, start the self-touch exercises in Chapter 18. When you get to the vaginal self-caress, if you can't do it as described, that's fine. Break it down into two different exercises, an external vaginal caress (the clitoris, inner and outer lips, and pubic mound), and an internal caress (the inside of the vagina). If you can only do the outer vaginal caress because you can't yet insert a finger into your vagina, that's okay. You can break the genital caress down into baby steps. I'll describe how to do this soon. First, there are a couple of other specific exercises I want you to do that involve the PC muscle.

∾ *Exercise 80.* PC MUSCLE FOR VAGINISMUS

Lie on your back. Relax and breathe. Put some baby oil on your hand and do a genital caress on your external genitals. Now rest one hand lightly over your vaginal opening. Do your PC muscle exercises with your hand resting on your vaginal opening. Squeeze your PC muscle, hold it for two or three seconds, then relax it. Do twenty-five repetitions, all with your hand resting lightly over your vaginal opening. If this exercise causes you to be so tense that your hand isn't relaxed, instead of using your whole hand, just lightly rest one or two fingers on your vaginal opening. As you do the exercise, you will be able to feel your vagina slightly opening and closing each time you tense and relax your PC muscle.

∾ *Exercise 81.* ADVANCED PC MUSCLE FOR VAGINISMUS

Do this exercise as described in the exercise above. Rest your hand or a couple of your fingers lightly against your vaginal opening. Instead of squeezing your PC muscle and holding it for only two seconds, slowly squeeze it to a count of five, hold it for a count of five, and then relax it for

a count of five. This is similar to the regular **PC** muscle exercise, but you are drawing it out so that one entire repetition lasts about fifteen seconds. Work your way up to ten of these advanced squeezes per session.

Shaping for Vaginismus

Once you are able to caress the outside of your vagina and do the above PC muscle exercises, you are ready to set up a shaping program similar to those I described in Chapter 29 for sexual aversion disorder. Always remember that your eventual goal is to be able to have sexual intercourse with your partner inserting his penis into your vagina. Accomplishing this will require the following steps:

1. Insert each of your fingers, one by one, into your own vagina and hold each one there for a couple of minutes, starting with your pinky finger and ending with your thumb.

2. Insert each of your partner's fingers into your vagina and hold each one there for a couple of minutes, beginning with his pinky finger and ending with his thumb.

3. Insert a small (three- to four-inch-long) dildo into your vagina and hold it there.

4. Insert your partner's flaccid penis into your vagina in the side-to-side scissors position and leave it there without moving for ten minutes.

5. Insert your partner's erect penis into your vagina in the female-superior position and hold it there for five minutes without moving.

6. Insert your partner's erect penis into your vagina in the butterfly position and hold it there without moving for five minutes.

7. Insert your partner's erect penis into your vagina in the side-to-side position, the female-superior position, and the butterfly position. You thrust, but your partner doesn't.

8. Insert your partner's penis into your vagina in any position and have your partner move.

9. Your partner inserts his erect penis into your vagina in any position and you both thrust.

Do each of the above steps as a full sensate-focus exercise. Start with spoon breathing and shared focusing caresses, and give your partner a genital caress either before or after your part of the exercise. Finish with spoon breathing and partner feedback. Use plenty of lubrication for each of these steps. For these exercises, you really can't use too much lubrication.

If you are able to work through the above progression, do two versions of each step. Do one version in which you keep your vagina relaxed, and do another version in which you do your PC muscle exercises around whatever is inside your vagina—a finger or a penis.

If you are too anxious to be able to work through the above progression of steps, you can break each of the steps into smaller steps. Here is an example showing how you could break Step 1 into a series of smaller steps. You could do all of these baby steps in one session, you could do all of them in one day, or you could do just one baby step per day.

Step 1 is to insert each of your fingers into your vagina and hold each one there for a couple of minutes. First, lightly rest your pinky finger along your vaginal opening for two minutes. Then insert the first joint of your pinky finger into your vaginal opening and hold it there for two minutes (or one minute, or thirty seconds—whatever works for you). Breathe normally and relax all of your muscles, especially your PC muscle. Insert your pinkie finger into your vagina up to the second joint and hold it there for two minutes. Breathe and relax. Insert your pinkie finger all the way into your vagina and hold it there for two minutes. Breathe and relax.

You can see that you can break all nine steps into a series of smaller steps. You could insert each of your fingers one joint at a time, and each of your partner's fingers one joint at a time. When it comes time to use a dildo, buy a soft rubber one, mark divisions on it in ink, and insert it a little farther each time you do an exercise. When it comes time to insert your partner's penis, you don't have to mark divisions on it. Just take your time and insert half an inch or so at a time and hold it there.

Proceed at your own pace. You could do several finger joints a day or only one. It doesn't matter, as long as you are always either reinforcing a previously successful step or trying a new one. That way you are always moving in the direction of your goal.

If you choose to do this shaping approach, you should make a series of charts to review your progress, and you should set up a reward system for yourself. I described how to do that in Chapter 29.

There is another way to structure an experience to heal vaginismus, based on the five penetrations I talked about in Chapter 12. Remember that those five penetrations are a tampon, a medication applicator, a speculum, a finger, and your partner's penis.

To heal vaginismus based on the five penetrations, buy a box of small-size tampons (I think the size is called "Junior") and a package of yeast-infection medication that includes an applicator. Buy the type of tampons that have a plastic applicator. They're much easier to insert than the cardboard kind. Ask your gynecologist to give you a speculum, or call a women's health center and see if the center can provide you with one.

Work through each of these penetrations in the way I describe for finger and penis penetration; that is, break everything down into baby steps. For example, take a small tampon and make ink marks every half inch along it. For the first exercise, just rest the tampon against your vaginal opening. Remember to relax your PC muscle and breathe. Next, using plenty of lubrication, insert the tampon into your vagina up to the first mark, then the second mark, etc. Hold the tampon in place at each mark for two minutes (start with smaller increments of time, if necessary, and work your way up to two minutes). Remember to breathe and relax your PC muscle. Then actually push the applicator in and insert the cotton part of the tampon. Leave it in for a couple hours. When you remove the tampon, be sure to relax your PC muscle. If you have never done it before, removing a tampon is an unusual sensation that takes a few times to get used to. Once you are able to insert a small tampon comfortably, work your way up through the other sizes until you can comfortably insert the size labeled "Super Plus."

Do the same progression for the medication applicator. When it's time to use the speculum, make ink marks on it, insert it sideways, and hold it. Then insert it sideways and turn it so that it's pointing the same way it would during a pelvic exam. Have your gynecologist or someone at a women's health center show you how this works if you're unsure. Then get to the stage where you can open the speculum inside you. You don't have to open it all the way the first time. It has ratchets so that it can be partially opened. Once you are able to open the speculum inside of yourself, it would be a really good idea to take a flashlight and a mirror and look at the inside of your vagina. This will help demystify things for you.

The other two penetrations are finger and penis. Work through them in the way I described above, using the shaping approach.

◯⌣ *Exercise 82.* ALTERNATING INSIDE AND OUTSIDE STIMULATION

You can do this exercise after you have completed a shaping program using either your fingers and your partner's penis or the five penetrations. You can do the exercise either by yourself or with your partner. If you want to do the exercise by yourself, lie down, relax, and give yourself a genital caress using plenty of lubrication. Caress your clitoris for a minute. Remember to breathe and relax. Now relax your PC muscle, slide one of your fingers into your vagina, and caress the inside of your vagina for a minute. Continue the caress for ten to fifteen minutes, alternating a caress on the outside of your vagina with one on the inside.

If you want to do this exercise with your partner, use the side-to-side position. Put plenty of lubrication on your vagina and on your partner's penis. Hold his penis and use it to caress your clitoris for a minute. Then relax your PC muscle and insert all or part of your partner's penis into your vagina. Keep your hand on his penis and use it to caress the inside of your vagina for a minute. Alternate caressing the inside and outside of your vagina with his penis. It doesn't matter whether he has an erection or not for this exercise. You can do it either way. You could also repeat this exercise in different positions.

A Possible Medical Solution?

Many physicians and psychologists have recommended drugs such as tranquilizers to help women relax enough to allow penetration. Alcohol has also been recommended. I don't believe these strategies work, because you can develop a tolerance to tranquilizers and alcohol, meaning that you will gradually need more and more of the drug to achieve the same level of relaxation.

I was talking with my gynecologist recently about vaginismus and sexual pain. He has seen many cases of these conditions and has been frustrated because many of his patients have been very difficult to treat. He believes that both vaginismus and sexual pain are due to lifelong chronic tension in the PC muscle. He told me that he and his colleagues are considering the use of Botox injections to relax the PC muscle, the same way it relaxes the facial muscles that cause frown lines between the eyebrows. As of this writing, I have not read anything about this line of treatment for vaginismus, but it will be interesting to see whether Botox is approved for this use at some point in the future.

Additional Suggestions for Comfort with Penetration

Here are some additional facts about the vagina and tips that may help you get more comfortable with penetration. One of the most common mistakes made by women with vaginismus is trying to insert something (whether it's a penis or a tampon) at the wrong angle. The vagina doesn't point straight up. When inserting a tampon while standing up, aim it toward the small of your back. Even the most experienced tampon users occasionally experience vaginal dryness and miss the opening or don't insert the tampon far enough and have to take it out and use another one.

If you want to practice inserting a dildo, the best position to use is the butterfly position—on your back with your pelvis tilted and your legs spread. Point the dildo toward the small of your back. It's not going to hit anything. Use plenty of lubrication.

The best way to learn how to insert a finger is to smear plenty of lubrication all over your vaginal lips and then just rub a finger all over the whole area. You will discover a place where your finger slides in. That's your vaginal opening.

If you are working through the progression of exercises using your fingers and your partner's penis, you may make an unexpected breakthrough. When you attempt to insert a half inch of your partner's penis, the whole thing might slide in. What should you do? Enjoy it! If you are able to experience penetration and it feels okay, go for it! Women are often spontaneously cured of vaginismus in situations like the one I have just described. Remember, once you successfully experience comfortable penetration, you're cured.

When you are able to experience penetration with your partner's penis in all the different intercourse positions, continue your sexual education by doing advanced sensate-focus exercises like the peaking and plateauing processes. These are described from the woman's point of view in Chapter 26. Or you could go through any of the other exercises in the female arousal and orgasm chapters to learn more about your arousal and orgasm triggers.

The difficulty with inserting a penis is that there's a person attached to it. You don't just aim the head of the penis toward where you think the vaginal opening is and push. There's kind of an art to it. Use plenty of lubrication, and start by gently inserting your fingers into your vagina to open it up and to make sure there's lubrication all along the vaginal canal, not just at the opening. Rub your partner's penis up and down, over your clitoris and vaginal lips, until it feels some give and slides in.

One of the biggest psychological issues with women who have difficulty with penetration is their feeling that penetration is not under their control. They view a man's penis as a kind of weapon that is forced into them. Healing yourself of vaginismus will ultimately require you to realize that you have a choice about whether or not to have sexual intercourse. The exercises presented in this chapter should help you to tap into your sense of empowerment about your sexuality.

chapter 31

Healing
Sexual Pain

This chapter deals exclusively with treating female sexual pain. I know of no treatment options for men who experience psychologically based sexual pain. When men experience pain during sexual intercourse, in the majority of cases a physical cause can be found for the pain.

If you have sexual pain, you should first do the breathing and relaxation exercises in Chapter 16. Then start the sexual fitness exercises in Chapter 17. When you do the self-touch exercises in Chapter 18, leave out any exercises in which you explore the inside of your vagina if they cause you pain. For the basic partner exercises in Chapters 19 through 22, do all of them except the internal genital caress if it causes you pain.

If you have both vaginismus and dyspareunia, or if you have superficial dyspareunia (pain at the vaginal opening), do the progression of exercises in Chapter 30 instead of the exercises in this chapter. I think they will work better for you. The progression of exercises in this chapter is really intended for women who have deep dyspareunia (psychologically based pain *inside* the vagina during intercourse).

The first three exercises for deep sexual pain involve exploring your own vagina. You should do these exercises even if you experience sexual pain only during intercourse.

ᥱ *Exercise 83.* GENITAL CARESS FOR DEEP SEXUAL PAIN

This is a basic genital caress with a few modifications that will help you have something inside your vagina without pain. Lie on your back and caress your body with some lotion. Remember to breathe deeply and relax all of your muscles. Have some lubricant handy.

Put plenty of lubricant on your hand, and also spread some on your vaginal opening and vaginal lips. Lightly and slowly run your fingers over your vaginal lips, clitoris, and vaginal opening. If you have deep sexual pain, this part of the caress will not cause you any problems. Do the caress in the sensate-focus manner. Relax and breathe. Stay focused, and stay in the here and now. You may need to keep reminding yourself to go as slowly as possible. Your hand should barely move.

Now slowly insert the first joint of your index finger into your vagina. Gradually keep inserting your finger, millimeter by millimeter. Slowly and completely caress the following areas inside your vagina: the vaginal sponge, the A-spot, the G-spot (if you can reach it), the walls on both sides, and the cervix (if you can reach it). If you discover an area that causes you pain when you caress it, avoid that area. Your goal here is to obtain psychological awareness of every millimeter of your vagina that you can reach with your finger.

ᔑ *Exercise 84.* VAGINAL CLOCK

Having done the previous exercise, you're ready to explore your vagina with a slightly different perspective. Think of your vaginal opening as a clock, with twelve o'clock at the clitoris and six o'clock at the base of the vaginal opening.

Begin a sensate-focus body caress and genital caress as above. Use plenty of lubrication on both your hand and your vaginal opening. Insert the first joint of your index finger into your vagina, and press it against twelve o'clock. Slowly move your finger around about an inch inside your vagina so you feel all of the clock numbers. Touch twelve, three, six, and nine, holding your finger against each spot for a few seconds. Then make another circle around your vagina, this time touching all twelve numbers and holding your finger on each for a few seconds.

It might sound funny to someone whose vagina feels too sensitive, but the goal of this exercise is actually to make your vagina more sensitive. As you touch each area, notice the sensations. As you hold your finger on some of the vaginal areas, they will develop a pulse. Some of the areas will feel more sensitive than others. This exercise will help you discover which areas of your vagina are most sensitive and which are least sensitive.

After you have gone around the clock with only one finger joint inserted, put your finger in a little bit farther and go around the clock again—slowly. Really take your time with this exercise. Go all the way around your vagina again, pressing and holding at each clock number. Keep pushing your finger in deeper and deeper, following the clock pattern, until your finger is inserted as far as it will comfortably go. Now withdraw your finger a little bit and do the clock again several times in reverse (i.e., counter-clockwise), each time gradually withdrawing your finger.

During this exercise, if you touch an area that is painful, avoid that area. Do not do anything that causes you any pain. However, see exactly how close you can get to the painful area without actually touching it. This exercise should give you an excellent idea of the exact areas inside your vagina that are painful.

However, it's possible that this exercise will not trigger pain for you if your pain only occurs with partner activity or intercourse. It's also possible that your finger isn't long enough to touch the areas inside your vagina that are painful to you. Don't worry; the exercises later in this chapter deal with this issue. If you are able to complete the vaginal clock exercise without pain, good for you.

○ Exercise 85. EXPLORING YOUR VAGINA

During a genital caress, insert a finger into your vagina as far as is comfortable. When you reach a point right before you feel pain, back off and only do the caress up to the point just before you experience pain.

You can also do this exercise using a small dildo instead of your finger. Insert the dildo to the point where you are afraid you might feel pain. Relax your PC muscle and see if you can insert just a tiny bit farther without feeling pain. Remember to breathe normally and to keep your legs and all other muscles relaxed. Make an ink mark on the dildo to show how far you inserted it. Each time you repeat this exercise, see if you can insert the dildo a little farther without pain. Your goal is to become comfortable with penetration, so you can experience it without pain.

Don't be concerned if you don't feel any sexual pleasure or arousal when you do any of these genital caresses. Eventually you will feel pleasure with penetration. Our goal here is just to make you feel comfortable with penetration.

○ Exercise 86. DRAWING YOUR VAGINA

The cornerstone of the sexual healing program for deep sexual pain is a visualization technique. Using the information you learned from doing the vaginal clock exercise, draw a picture of your vagina. Draw it however you picture it mentally—tube-shaped or as a flat surface. Start by just making a simple line drawing. Now take a colored pencil or marker and shade in the area(s) that you perceive as painful. Make the shaded area(s) as small or as large as you perceive it.

Now you're going to do a genital caress, using this drawing as a map to guide you. Lie down on your back and put plenty of lubrication on one hand and on your vagina. Hold your drawing with one hand so you can see it. Insert a finger and caress any parts of the inside of your vagina that don't hurt. Look at the drawing while you do this. As you touch the inside of your vagina, picture what it looks like based on your drawing, and imagine yourself avoiding the shaded area. Make sure you stop just short of experiencing any pain.

Now file that drawing away. A couple of days later, make another drawing without looking at the previous one. Repeat the genital caress exercise using the new drawing. Then repeat this exercise a couple of times a week. After a couple of weeks, take all of your drawings out and look at them. What you will notice after several drawings and caressing exercises is the shaded area growing progressively smaller in each drawing. Keep repeating this exercise until your drawing shows no shaded area.

You can also do the whole progression of exercises using a small dildo instead of your finger. Use a small, rubbery, flesh-colored one. Keep redoing your drawing, and use it as a guide when you insert the dildo into your vagina and caress yourself with it. Make ink marks on the dildo to show how far you are able to insert it.

Once you are able to caress the inside of your vagina with your finger and/or a dildo without experiencing any pain, you can start to work with your partner. You can do a whole progression of partner exercises similar to the ones outlined in Chapter 30. Use the "baby-steps" principles I described in the chapters on treating anxiety and vaginismus. Do each of these activities as a full sensate-focus exercise, with spoon breathing, focusing caresses, and partner feedback.

The following is one example of a possible progression. Remember, each of these larger steps can be broken down into several smaller baby steps.

1. Progressively insert each of your partner's fingers one by one, from smallest to largest, and just let each finger relax in your vagina without moving.

2. Have your partner caress the inside of your vagina with each of his fingers.

3. Have your partner caress the inside of your vagina with a dildo.

4. Using a lot of lubrication, insert your partner's flaccid penis into your vagina in the side-to-side scissors position. This is a good position for you because you can adjust it so penetration isn't very deep. Just relax and let his penis sit inside you without moving.

5. Stimulate your partner so that he has an erection, and insert his penis into your vagina in the side-to-side scissors position.

6. Now try the flaccid insertion or quiet vagina exercise in any other position that is comfortable.

7. Stimulate your partner so that he has an erection. Now climb on top of him and try intercourse in the female-superior position. You control all of the thrusting. He doesn't move.

8. Have your partner enter you in any comfortable position. This time, he does all of the moving.

You can do any or all of the above activities that you are comfortable with, as long as you remember the following caveat: Don't do any activity that causes you pain. If you experience pain, return to an exercise or part of an exercise with which you were comfortable.

Also, if you find that you are having trouble with a certain activity or position (you find that you start to tense up, or you are afraid it will cause you pain), remember that you can do any of the above activities using the drawing technique. You can make a drawing of your vagina and put it where you and your partner can see it while you insert his penis into your vagina.

⁓

Dealing with sexual pain can be frustrating and can take a long time. Be sure to regularly remind yourself that this healing process *will* work, and that you deserve to have intercourse that is not only pain-free but is intimate, enjoyable, and ecstatic.

Part V

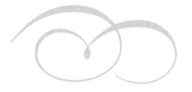

ADVANCED SEXUAL HEALING

In this final section, you'll find chapters on using lovemaking to heal physical and emotional problems and relationship issues. I also provide many exercises for using intercourse for sexual healing and for combining sexuality and spirituality.

chapter 32

Lovemaking to Heal Physical Problems

The area in which I received my doctorate is called health psychology. When I was a graduate student, health psychology was a relatively new area of psychology, but now it is very well established. Health psychologists study the ways in which our bodies (our physical selves) and our minds (our psychological selves) interact and affect each other. This chapter will give you some information about physical and psychological aspects of sexuality that will help you set the stage for using sexuality to heal your physical and emotional problems.

The Unity of Mind and Body

Historically, psychologists have focused their study on the mind rather than the body. However, recent advances in both psychology and medicine have shown the importance of considering the body and the mind as a single unit, a whole. The mind and the body function together, but they interact in ways that make them seem separate. In other words, it is possible for us to be more aware of one or the other at a given time. What is the importance of these concepts for our sexuality? Sexuality and sexual activity are areas in which the mind and the body interact closely. Whether we experience sexual issues as mental or physical, research shows that we need to work with both the body and the mind to enhance our sexual awareness, overcome sexual problems, and possibly heal our bodies.

A basic concept in health psychology is the idea that all physical problems have psychological aspects, and that many (if not all) psychological problems have physical aspects. This idea is the foundation for the program described in this book. At times we have focused more on the body, and at other times we have turned our attention to the mind, but hopefully so far the result has been that you have learned to experience both the mental and physical aspects of sexual arousal and enjoyment. Now, in this final section of the book, we turn our attention to sexual healing of physical problems, emotional problems, relationship problems, and spiritual issues.

In previous chapters, I outlined some of the ways in which breathing, touch, and deep muscle relaxation can have a positive effect on your health, both mental and physical. As we have seen, there is a long tradition in psychology linking mental and physical health. Anxiety is a health destroyer. In the sexual healing program, you learned to recognize anxiety and deal with it. You also learned to slow your body down and to promote the action of your parasympathetic nervous system (the relaxation response), which can also benefit your health. Stress is another health destroyer. The relaxing sexual activity that you have learned to experience with your partner can provide an antidote to any bodily tension that has built up from stress over the day or week.

Perhaps most importantly, sexual expression can provide a "natural high." Sexual activity, beginning from a relaxed state, allows your brain to produce endorphins, the body's natural painkillers. Instead of numbing yourself with alcohol and drugs and getting sex "over with," you can now use relaxing sexual activity to promote your physical health. To my knowledge, no psychologist has studied exactly what kind of sexual activity releases endorphins. But I know from experience that the peaking process seems to train the brain to systematically release these chemicals. Exercises that involve mutual peaking at high levels of arousal seem to be best for simply making you feel good, physically and mentally.

Do you have physical problems that need healing? Or perhaps you suffer from mild anxiety, depression, or other negative emotions. Maybe you are physically and emotionally fit but feel a vague spiritual unease, a yearning for meaning in your life. Better yet, you are happy with yourself and satisfied in your relationship, and you believe that life can be even better. If any of these descriptions fit you, you could benefit from advanced sexual healing.

What do these issues have to do with making love, you may ask. Believe it or not, making love can heal many aspects of your life. Sex is often put down, taken for granted, described as just a physical release or something that animals do, or even regarded as basically sinful. Of course, sex is much more than any of these things. Making love is an expression, an exchange, an involvement that connects you—whether you like it or not—not only sexually and physically, but also mentally, emotionally, and even spiritually with another person. Because lovemaking involves you so completely, it can affect you and your partner in any or all of these areas. In this chapter and the ones that follow, I will explore the vast healing potential that lovemaking holds and how it is powered by your mind, body, and soul.

How can sexual healing help if you're well to begin with? The power of sexuality is generally positive and healthful. When channeled toward a specific ailment, it has curative effects. When embraced by a healthy person, it brings about greater strength, vitality, and well-being.

As you read about the various aspects of sexual healing, consider which will benefit you most and decide how you would like to begin bringing these benefits into your life. The mind and the body affect each other, working together as a system. As a result, you can tap into any aspect of the system—that is, you can work to heal physical, emotional, sexual, or spiritual problems—and *every* part of you will feel the benefits.

The Physical Benefits of Lovemaking

Do you complain about any of the following: ulcers, migraines, asthma, chronic pain, circulation problems, skin problems, general malaise, or a general lack of physical fitness? Complain no longer, for I have seen lovemaking work wonders on these conditions. When I worked as a surrogate partner, many of my clients had physical conditions such as asthma, ulcers, or other gastrointestinal problems. When they realized healing in sexual areas, their physical condition improved as well. Making love generally produces great overall physical benefits.

Lovemaking offers so many healthful perks that it is hard to know where to start describing them. The act of making love is a physical process that involves the interplay of many bodily systems, especially respiration and circulation (blood flow). Since making love stimulates breathing and increases oxygen intake, it can increase lung capacity. When you breathe, oxygen is drawn into your lungs and then is absorbed into your bloodstream. Sex deepens your breathing, increases the oxygen you take in, and helps get your blood pumping, which moves that oxygen through your body. When you make love, a great deal of blood flows to your genitals to cause arousal, erection, and lubrication. When you become highly aroused to the point of orgasm, circulation increases in all areas of your body, especially in your skin and the muscles of your arms and legs.

Lovemaking is also a well-known analgesic: It relieves pain. When we experience significant arousal or engage in strenuous physical activity, our brain releases chemicals called *endorphins*. Endorphins have been likened to opiates such as morphine or heroin and have painkilling properties and are responsible for altered states of consciousness, such as "runner's high."

I have found that the best way to get the body to produce these fabulous endorphins is to allow one's sexual arousal to climb in predictable patterns (like the peaking process, described in several chapters of this book). Then, orgasm triggers a tremendous release of endorphins, which can stop pain for up to several hours. Can you think of a better way to find pain relief? That standard cliché, "Not tonight, dear, I have a headache," should really be the opposite: "Let's make love tonight, honey—I have a headache!" The pain-relieving endorphin effect can work to alleviate both short-term, acute pain, such as that produced by a migraine, and chronic pain, such as the pain of arthritis.

The release of endorphins offers an added benefit aside from pain relief: It boosts the immune system in both the short and long term. The endorphin release produced by arousal and lovemaking encourages relaxation in much the same way as meditation, exercise, and yoga do, and this strengthens your immune response. People who have more reliable releases of endorphins tend to report fewer symptoms and to get sick less often. This means that sexual touch, arousal, and lovemaking can be a delightful way to help dispense with some of the pain that comes with immune-related conditions such as rheumatoid arthritis.

Lovemaking can also be very good for relieving physical problems related to the reproductive system. As many women have discovered, often by accident, making love is especially effective for menstrual difficulties, including painful periods and premenstrual syndrome. Many men with prostate problems experience relief by using the sexual healing techniques for arousal and ejaculation.

Are you worried about your bones? Lovemaking can help ward off osteoporosis because it involves physical exercise. Making love often, whether vigorously or for long periods of time, exercises the long muscles of the arms and legs, and gives the body a more sculpted look. For the same reasons, making love can increase your metabolism and help you lose weight. Lovemaking makes you look and feel better overall: Your hair is shinier, your eyes are brighter, and your skin is fresher and more radiant—all benefits of enhanced circulation.

As wonderful as lovemaking is, there are some things it cannot do for your health. It can't make up for horrible health habits such as eating junk food, smoking, taking drugs, or using alcohol excessively. But with all the good feelings that come from sexually inspired health, you may find yourself drawn to healthier habits anyway.

I believe very strongly in the healing power of lovemaking because I witnessed some incredible physical healing take place when I did surrogate work. I believe that if this type of healing can develop between a client and a surrogate partner, then the intimate bond that exists between long-term lovers—the physical, emotional, mental, and spiritual mutuality you share with your partner—should provide the ideal context for advanced sexual healing. Imagine the power you can create when you make love with the intent to heal yourself and your partner.

Many people believe in the abstract that lovemaking can positively affect physical health, but here, for the first time, I am presenting self-help exercises that show you how to tap into this potential. First, I categorize physical ailments into groups. Then, I discuss the concepts of mind–body healing and how sexual union specifically nourishes the mind–body connection. I offer specific strategies for healing the different types of physical conditions, using exercises from previous chapters as well as some new ones that you will find rewarding if you have physical limitations.

For the purposes of healing, I divide illness into four main categories: psychosomatic illnesses, stress disorders, chronic illnesses, and physical conditions resulting from trauma. See the sections that follow for descriptions of each. As a surrogate partner and therapist, these categories served me well when developing healing approaches and designing programs for clients. By understanding the root cause of an illness, you can emphasize exercises that address that cause as well as the symptoms.

Psychosomatic Illness: How Mind Affects Body

Most people are familiar with the concept of psychosomatic illness: the idea that our mental state, such as attitudes and emotions, can influence whether we get sick, how quickly we get better, or even the development of chronic health problems such as heart disease and cancer. The idea that an illness is psychosomatic does not mean that it is "all in your head" or is not real. On the contrary, psychosomatic illnesses involve observable tissue damage.

Psychosomatic means that our psychology plays some part in an illness, no matter how small a part. In a sense, all medical problems are psychosomatic, because being sick affects us psychologically. The fact that the mind can influence the body has made it possible to design treatments for cancer that include aspects such as relaxation and visualization.

What is the tie-in to sexuality? People experiencing sexual problems often report one or more psychosomatic symptoms, such as migraine headaches, stomach problems, or skin problems. When their sexual problem is successfully treated, their medical problems often become less severe or disappear entirely.

Sigmund Freud was one of the first to recognize psychosomatic illness and its links to sexuality. Freud thought that repressed sexual conflicts could emerge as physical symptoms, and he seems to have been correct. If sexual interactions are a source of conflict or anxiety for you, they could definitely have a negative effect on your physical health. Many people intuitively recognize that their sexual interactions are a source of stress, and thus they attempt to avoid sexual activity. Unfortunately, ignoring the problem will not make it go away, and many people find that even if they give up sexual activity, their psychosomatic complaints remain. The complaints may take on a different physical form, but they remain because the lack of sexual activity is itself a source of unconscious conflict. If you have a fear of sexuality that is reflected in health problems, the exercises in this book provide a way to relearn your sexual expression in a gradual and nonthreatening manner, and to use this positive sexual experience as a way to heal your body and your mind.

Let me caution you that the relationship between sexuality and health has not been proven by psychologists; we only know that these things *seem* to be related to each other in predictable ways. I would like to be able to say unequivocally that improving your sex life will improve your overall physical and mental health. However, there is no absolute scientific proof that positive sexual activity keeps you healthy or that lack of sexual expression causes illness. Believe it or not, no psychologist has ever tried to research these connections! That said, let me repeat what I touched on earlier: Based on my experience with clients, it does appear that many people who are cured of sexual problems find that certain health problems they had been experiencing go away. And it is definitely the case that resolving a sexual problem results in lower levels of anxiety and depression, which can in turn reduce health problems.

While psychology plays a part in creating or maintaining a psychosomatic illness, let me also repeat that both the pain and the tissue damage are real. I believe that most illnesses have a psychosomatic component and can be partially healed psychologically. I have even seen serious medical conditions such as cancer respond to psychological intervention. When medical professionals talk about psychosomatic illnesses, they are usually referring to specific conditions, including cardiovascular problems, ulcers and other gastrointestinal problems like irritable bowel syndrome, asthma, skin problems such as psoriasis, immune disorders such as certain forms of arthritis, chronic pain, migraines, and menstrual problems.

Stress Disorders

Psychologists usually refer to stress disorders as "psychological factors affecting physical conditions." This category includes any medical condition in which stress plays a role. Stress grows out of the necessity to adjust to changes in one's environment. That means stress-related disorders can include psychosomatic illnesses as well as vaguer conditions such as fatigue, and short-term conditions such as heartburn or neck pain.

When you experience long-term stress, your sympathetic nervous system is chronically activated. Your adrenal glands secrete hormones that degrade your organs over time. The difference between psychosomatic illnesses and stress disorders is the cause of the ailment, not the actual physical symptoms. Stress disorders are linked to environmental factors, whereas psychosomatic illnesses are generally caused (or at least worsened) by long-term anxiety, repression, anger, or depression.

Chronic Illnesses

Chronic illnesses are ongoing, incurable, and usually degenerative conditions that a person copes with on a daily basis. For example, lupus, diabetes, multiple sclerosis, Parkinson's disease, cancer, cerebral palsy, Huntington's disease, and amyotrophic lateral sclerosis (ALS) are all considered chronic illnesses. We could also include the sexually transmitted viruses like herpes and HIV in this category because living with them certainly requires adjustment. Sexual healing can help alleviate the discomforts of chronic illness, strengthen the immune system, and feed a person's overall well-being—all keys to living successfully with chronic illness.

Physical Trauma

In this category I include conditions resulting from accidents and surgery, such as spinal cord injury, major burns, paralysis, and limb amputation. I also include severe obesity and genetic defects here, because many of the healing issues are the same. Conditions resulting from physical trauma are likely to be disfiguring, and as such they call on special elements of sexual healing. In our culture, physical attractiveness is a big part of sexual attraction, and conditions that make a person look different require the healing qualities of self-acceptance and self-worth. If you are the partner of someone with a condition resulting from physical trauma, sexual healing can also heal issues or attitudes you may hold about health and physical appearance and how they relate—or don't relate—to making love.

The sexual healing of physical ailments draws on the holistic power of an individual's mental and physical self. However, there are types of illnesses that, because of their causes, cannot benefit from sexual healing, and so I do not address them here. Such problems include schizophrenia, severe depression, dissociative identity disorder (formerly multiple personality disorder), and forms of dementia such as Alzheimer's disease. These illnesses have mental or physical causes and symptoms and require specific, professional psychological or medical intervention.

Sexual Healing of Specific Psychosomatic Illnesses and Stress-Related Conditions

I have used the sexual healing program for all of the following conditions. I have seen it work wonders for many people with psychosomatic and stress-related problems.

Cardiovascular Problems

Cardiovascular problems include angina, chest pain, shortness of breath, high blood pressure, and poor circulation, especially in the lower half of the body. Many men who take high blood pressure medication wish to go off it because it can affect erections. To help treat high blood pressure, make ample use of the breathing and muscle relaxation exercises described in Chapter 16. For angina, do the same; you should try to promote relaxation as much as possible. For poor circulation, when you receive a back caress or front caress, have your partner massage *toward* the affected part of your body, literally forcing blood flow from the center of your body to your arms and legs. Although your partner will need to use a stronger massage technique for this stroke, the caress can still be done in a focused, sensual way.

For all circulatory problems, I also recommend nurturing and trust-based partner exercises that can "open your heart," such as those described in Chapter 34. And be sure to do any exercises in this book in which your partner places his or her hand or face on your heart; this will strengthen your healing connection and intentions.

Breathing Difficulties

These include asthma, allergies, and sinus problems. Many people with asthma are afraid to become aroused or have an orgasm because doing so may trigger an asthma attack. As a result, they become dependent on an inhaler. If you want to use sexual healing for respiratory ailments, pay special attention to the breathing, relaxation, arousal awareness, and peaking exercises, and do them by yourself before you do them with your partner. Doing the exercises alone, at first, will help you learn to become aroused slowly and to breathe more deeply as you become aroused. If during any exercise your breathing becomes ragged, back off to an exercise with which you were comfortable and didn't have breathing difficulties.

Skin Problems

These include conditions such as eczema and psoriasis. If you use a topical medication, apply it by rubbing it on in a sensate-focus way, or have your partner do it. If your condition is contagious, your partner can wear gloves. Your focus in healing skin problems is to bring blood flow to the skin. All of the arousal exercises will accomplish this, including those for arousal awareness, peaking, and plateauing. Any exercises that include intercourse and/or that lead to orgasm will also produce a healthful skin flush.

Immune-System Disorders

These include conditions such as rheumatoid arthritis. If you have painful, swollen joints, you may be unable to caress yourself, so you may need your partner to do it. Find comfortable positions in which your weight is not on your joints; for example, use a side-to-side position for intercourse. Pay special attention to genital caresses. Your goal is to become as aroused as you can without making painful body movements. This will increase endorphin production and relieve some of your pain. You may also find it helpful for your partner to give you mild sensate-focus caresses on the affected joints.

Chronic Pain

Chronic pain can occur anywhere in the body. Sexual healing is especially good for pain in the muscles of the neck, back, and shoulders. Relaxation, breathing, and sensate-focus caresses on the affected area will help relax your body and alleviate pain. I recommend caressing for about fifteen to twenty minutes in a warm, comfortable room. Exercises that encourage prolonged arousal will also stimulate painkilling endorphins. For the special case of pain during intercourse, see Chapter 31.

Migraines

A migraine is a specific, severe form of headache caused by blood-flow problems and muscle tension, usually triggered by stress. To treat migraines, the goal is either to increase blood flow to the head or draw the flow away from it. Both approaches will work. If you are not in the middle of a migraine attack, usher more blood flow into your head by having your partner do a face caress. Have your partner pay special attention to the frontalis muscle, which is located between the eyebrows. If you are in the middle of a migraine attack, have your partner try a front caress and a genital caress to increase blood flow to the genital area. This will also increase endorphin production and relieve pain. Then continue with relaxation exercises, and eventually move to arousal awareness and peaking.

In some rare cases, migraines can occur after orgasm because of changes in the blood-flow patterns. If this is a problem for you, you might prevent it by altering your arousal pattern to include slow, predictable stimulation, or by becoming multiply orgasmic and having a series of small orgasms instead of one strong orgasm that is more likely to cause a migraine.

Gastrointestinal Problems

These include illnesses such as ulcers, colitis, and irritable bowel syndrome. Such conditions are very common in men with premature ejaculation and in women with inhibited orgasm. Again, sensate-focus exercises will bring blood flow to the pelvic and lower abdominal area from the periphery of the body. To bring about healing, try genital caresses, peaking, plateauing, and orgasm—any exercise or series of exercises that relaxes your abdominal muscles and increases blood flow to your pelvis.

Menstrual Problems

These include premenstrual syndrome (PMS), cramps, or irregular periods. Pelvic problems and PMS respond well to sexual healing; in fact, these conditions are among the easiest health problems to treat. Pelvic massage and orgasm are well-known effective treatments for menstrual cramps. In addition, relief can be found with sensate-focus caresses on the abdomen, genital caresses, peaking, and any other sexual healing exercises that lead to orgasm.

Prostate Problems

There is some controversy about the effect of sexual activity on the prostate gland. On the one hand, I have read that men who engage in a lot of sexual activity with several different partners are more susceptible to infections of the prostate gland and eventually to prostate cancer. (They obviously would also be putting themselves at increased risk for contracting a sexually transmitted disease.) However, I've also read that men who engage in more sexual activity tend to have better prostate health.

As far as I know, regular ejaculation can have a beneficial effect on benign prostate hypertrophy (BPH), commonly called an *enlarged prostate*. But how often is "regular," especially if you are an older man? You can usually tell by the color of your semen. Healthy semen is whitish, not yellowish. However, don't force yourself to ejaculate if you don't feel like it; this can contribute to a problem with male orgasm disorder. Regular ejaculation will not help prevent prostate cancer, which usually has a genetic or environmental basis.

It is important for men over age forty to undergo a regular rectal digital examination of their prostate gland, plus a prostate-specific antigen (PSA) test. Some experts on tantra and other Eastern modes of sexuality believe that a man should practice orgasm without ejaculation, because ejaculation depletes the chi or vital essence. All medical research I am familiar with, however, recommends regular ejaculation, especially for men over fifty.

General Lack of Physical Conditioning

You can actually use lovemaking to help yourself get into better overall shape. This is an extension of the line of thinking presented in Chapter 17, "Sexual Fitness." Making love is a great aerobic activity. Furthermore, positions that require you to kneel, stand, squat, or put your legs up will all help develop your flexibility.

Sexual Healing of Chronic Illnesses and Conditions Caused by Physical Trauma

Sick people need love too. In fact, they probably need it more than the rest of us, but for various reasons chronically ill people are less likely to make love. It is heartbreaking to visit a hospital and see chronically ill people shriveling up from lack of human contact because others are afraid to touch them. If you have a chronic illness, one that is not considered "curable," you may be looking for relief on a daily basis. Sexual healing for you focuses on how to cope and make love, rather than on how to specifically heal the illness. This is an area where healing comes from the power of your loving relationship.

One sexual issue that people with chronic illness are often confronted with is the possibility that a form of treatment for their illness may severely compromise their sexual functioning and enjoyment. An example would be treatment for prostate cancer. A man with prostate cancer might be placed in a position of making a decision between the lesser of two evils. A decision to have his prostate removed may mean that he will never again have a natural erection. Yet the decision not to undergo surgery for a cancerous prostate could ultimately kill him.

A similar choice is often faced by women with breast cancer. Research shows that surgery for breast cancer often has a detrimental effect on a woman's body image and therefore a potential effect on her sexual functioning and enjoyment. But delaying surgery or deciding against it could be fatal. Similarly, sometimes women with gynecological cancers have a choice between chemotherapy or radiation. Both of these can affect a woman's sex life. Chemotherapy can leave her feeling weak and unattractive, whereas radiation can destroy her body's natural ability to produce vaginal lubrication. People with chronic illness are sometimes faced with these extremely tough choices, and there are no easy answers. Physicians often fail to recognize that patients take their sex lives into account when they make treatment decisions.

Chronic illnesses such as lupus, Parkinson's disease, and multiple sclerosis (MS) present special healing challenges. Although these illnesses often don't have sexual side effects, they may have psychological ones. This is because our society harbors negative attitudes toward sick people. We sometimes blame a person for the illness and hold it against him or her. We focus on the connection between appearance and sexuality. And we project our own fears onto people who are chronically ill—our fear of disfigurement, fear that all illness is contagious, fear that an ill person will smell bad, fear that making love will hurt the person who is ill. Therefore, touch becomes even more important to a person who is chronically ill, because of the physical and psychological distance from others he or she is forced to endure.

I have had unique experiences with clients living with a variety of chronic illnesses. As a surrogate, I worked with clients who had cancer, heart disease, MS, ALS, Parkinson's—just about every condition you could name. Some people were affected sexually, others were not. Many simply had to make adjustments in the way they made love. My background in health psychology and my familiarity with all of these issues put me in a unique position to work sexually with these clients. I understand the stigma that chronic illness can create, but I also understand that a person's brain and skin are his or her true sex organs. Intimacy and genital sexuality are not the same thing. Everyone appreciates touch, no matter what he or she looks like. If you have a partner with a chronic illness, the best thing you can do to heal your partner is to embrace this attitude.

Many of the same challenges face people who have medical conditions resulting from physical trauma. Some must endure physical or mobility challenges. Others may be disfigured. These conditions can limit a person's sexual potential, from his or her ability to feel sensations to his or her ability to have intercourse. They may also limit the potential for a person to find a sexual partner through the most commonly used channels.

If you or your partner has either a chronic illness or a medical condition resulting from physical trauma, which exercises will help you heal? The answer is any and all of them that you are able to do. I encourage you to do all of the exercises that you are able to. If you have physical limitations, work around them. Be creative. The major adjustment to make is in your attitude, not in the extent of your physical limitations. While I am not naive enough to think that lovemaking will *heal* a chronic degenerative disease or a serious medical condition that results from physical trauma, I have seen truly miraculous changes take place in relationships in which one partner had such a condition. I'd like to share with you other people's experiences of the wonderful power of sexual healing in the hope that their stories might help and inspire you.

As a sex therapist, I once treated a couple in which the husband had prostate cancer. He opted to have his prostate removed. As a result, he was incontinent for a few months. What adjustments did he and his wife make so they could still make love? They had to change a bed sheet once in a while—that's it. Eventually he had a penile implant inserted, which required a bit more adjustment. This was where sensate focus was really important; it helped his wife get over the feeling that she was having sex with a machine rather than a person. His adjustment involved realizing that having an erection whenever a man wants to doesn't mean that he feels like making love. What exercises did they find especially healing? They used the sensate-focus caresses, such as the genital caress.

A colleague of mine treated a woman who developed breast cancer and had a mastectomy. Her cancer was very advanced with a poor prognosis, and there was a strong chance that she wouldn't make it. Her husband spent time physically loving her with massage, caressing, peaking, and plateauing. Through work with the body-image exercises (Chapter 35), she and her husband made such strides in healing their relationship that their lovemaking became better than ever. She survived. And when she was out of the woods, she opted not to have her breast reconstructed.

I knew a woman, Alicia, who was about one week away from dying of an extremely rare form of lung cancer. I believe that her husband, Tom, kept her alive through his sheer force of will. Somehow, even when things looked darkest, he managed to convey to her the expectation that she was going to make it. Even when Alicia gave up, Tom wouldn't let her go. He did this by keeping and sharing his sense of humor throughout her illness. When she was well enough to leave the hospital, she had a port inserted in her clavicle area for delivery of medication. She wanted to go to the water park with her daughter, but her daughter was concerned how people would react to the tube in her mother's neck. Tom told their daughter, "Just tell everyone you have an inflatable mom."

As a surrogate partner, I treated a client, Jerry, who had early-stage multiple sclerosis. Before coming to therapy, Jerry had been very depressed and was drinking a lot. He sought therapy because he wanted to know how much he could still feel and how much he would be able to do if he was actually in a relationship. The sensate-focus techniques helped him realize he could make love, and they gave him the confidence to seek out a loving partner. I credit sexual healing with his turnaround.

The tragic case of actor Christopher Reeve has focused attention on the realities of life for people with spinal cord injuries. From what I understand, he and his wife had the potential for a sexual healing relationship. What can a person experience after a spinal cord injury? Some men can have erections, which is what everybody focuses on; others cannot. It depends on the extent of the injury. Research shows that many women with spinal cord injuries not only enjoy sexual contact, but in many cases are able to have orgasms.

People's range of feeling and their awareness of arousal vary. I worked with a client with quadriplegia, who had movement only in his face. Fortunately, this included his tongue. We were creative and worked with touch he could feel, such as massage. With position adjustments, he found he was able to kiss and have oral sex. Although his physical sensations were limited, his senses of arousal and physiological response were acute. He described what he experienced as "brain orgasms."

Another client of mine, Mark, had cerebral palsy, which limited his voluntary movement to the use of one arm. His speech was slow and barely understandable and he used a wheelchair. However, because the penis has no voluntary muscles, he discovered that his erections were unaffected, and so his sexual response was completely normal. Through sexual healing, Mark realized his sexual potential. He left therapy feeling that there was another aspect of life that was open to him, in addition to being a lecturer, writer, and advocate for independent living.

If your partner has a chronic illness or a physical condition caused by trauma, you will need to make some adjustments, too. Ultimately, the lesson here is not to focus on what a person with a disability can or cannot do, but to share fully in healing touch.

Additional Healing Exercises

The following are some sexual healing exercises that I have used with clients with various physical problems.

↬ Exercise 87. NONTOUCHING CARESS

Begin by doing a slow, focused front caress with your partner. Then concentrate caresses on one area of your partner's body that needs healing. After focusing your healing energies, raise your hand just off your partner's skin and hold it there.

Let's say your partner has menstrual cramps, and you wish to help heal her. Caress her abdomen, then lift your hand a tiny bit away from her skin's surface so your hand is not touching her skin but is still so close that you can feel the energy flow between you. Alternate actual light touching and not touching so that you almost can't tell whether you are touching unless you look. You can use this caress on any part of the body.

ᑬ *Exercise 88.* FROM THE HEART

Caress your partner's body, giving time to the area that needs healing. With healing intention, place your other hand lightly over your partner's heart. Do a nontouching caress over your partner's heart as you simultaneously caress the part of his or her body that needs healing. You may also want to try lightly placing your ear over your partner's heart during the caress.

If Intercourse Is Not in the Cards

If you are a person whose partner needs healing from trauma or is otherwise differently abled, you may need to explore and redefine your understanding of sex, sexiness, and sexual consummation. You may be unable to make love with your partner in a conventional way. If this is the case, remind yourself that the point of lovemaking is much bigger than "conventional" sex. Sexual relating is a unique, individual union between every couple. If intercourse is not an option for you, there are other ways of making love that are. You might consider joining a support group in which people who have made similar adjustments share their experiences.

If you are a person who needs physical healing and you don't have a partner, I hope this book encourages you to seek healing help. I only wish there were more surrogate partners out there to help you.

The following exercises are sensual activities that don't involve intercourse.

ᑬ *Exercise 89.* MUTUAL MASTURBATION

Masturbation is one of the most personal, intimate things we experience. Many of us feel that it is so private that we are hesitant to share it with a partner. However, if illness prevents you from having intercourse or otherwise caressing each other, try sharing masturbation. There are two ways to do this. One way is for both of you to masturbate at the same time. Lie together on the bed, and stimulate yourself the way you would if you were alone. Pay attention to your own arousal, and send that energy out to your partner. If you wish, look deeply into each other's eyes as you become more and more aroused.

Another way to do this is to take turns masturbating while the other person watches. This is a very intimate act, as it involves sharing your most private activity with another person. Try not to be self-conscious about your partner watching you; instead, concentrate on sexual energy. Relax, close your eyes, and pleasure yourself the way you most like to.

Mutual masturbation will cause sexual energy to flow between the two of you, even if you can't caress or make love in more conventional ways. As a result, healing can still take place.

ᕳ *Exercise 90.* SHARING FANTASIES

Here is another exercise you can do if illness or physical limitations prevent caressing. It is commonly used by people who have spinal cord injuries. If you can talk, you can share a fantasy.

Share a fantasy, caressing each other with words. As you talk, the person who is able to can caress the person who is ill or disabled. Or the person who is able to can masturbate. Again, focus on the flow and exchange of sexual healing energy. This technique can also be used to share erotic readings with each other.

※

With some creativity and a bit of can-do attitude, seemingly endless options exist for lovemaking to heal physical problems. Many illnesses and physical conditions now have Internet chat rooms and users' groups devoted to them. It may be worth joining one of these online groups. Not only can you get emotional support for living with your condition (or your loved one's, if you're the partner of someone who is ill). You can also ask other group members to share how they've modified their sensual relationship to both enhance it and to tap into the possibilities for sexual healing.

chapter 33

Using Lovemaking to Heal Your Emotions

A re you already in good physical shape? Then you can enjoy the physical well-being that sexual healing inspires and focus on bringing healing to other areas of your life. Our emotions color the fabric of our sexual life. They provide the context in which we make love—or abstain from it. What most people don't realize is that the way in which we make love can nourish our emotional state. Depression and anxiety are the two most common emotional issues that affect our sex life and that, in turn, can be positively affected by lovemaking. I'll address them specifically, because they are the roots of many sexual problems and much deep lack of fulfillment.

Depression refers to a general feeling of misery or sadness that usually includes loss of appetite, loss of sex drive, excessive sleep, and general feelings of worthlessness. Depression can also result in complete loss of interest in life and lack of motivation. In extreme cases, a person may contemplate or attempt suicide. Reactive depression is caused by a sad life event, such as the death of someone to whom you are close. Biochemical depression is caused by an imbalance in brain chemistry that is probably genetic. As severe as depression can be, in the majority of cases it's temporary. If you are severely depressed for a long period of time, you may need professional help—a psychiatrist or other medical doctor who can prescribe medication.

Depression is a huge enemy of satisfying lovemaking. In fact, one of the most common symptoms of depression is temporary loss of sex drive. (To potentially complicate matters, as I've mentioned several times elsewhere in the book, one of the unfortunate side effects of the class of antidepressant medication known as the SSRIs is a loss of sex drive. For this reason I don't recommend this class of medication for people wanting to tap into the healing power of lovemaking.) The solution for depression is to take action. The best treatment for depression is to do something physical—and making love is one of the best physical things you can do. Sexual arousal is a powerful antidote to depression.

Anxiety is a more complicated issue, as you read in Chapter 3. It is also strongly related to sexuality. It is the root cause of all of the sexual dysfunctions, but it can also exist in relation to any other fears. The physical symptoms of anxiety include sweating, muscle tension, shortness of breath, cold hands and feet, and rapid heart rate. Mental symptoms of anxiety include worry, obsessing, and an inability to relax. These symptoms, both physical and mental, directly affect your ability to experience arousal, feel sexual pleasure, and enter an intimate, loving sphere.

Somatopsychology

In the previous chapter you read about psychosomatics: the study of how the mind affects the body. Somatopsychics is the study of how the *body* affects the *mind*. Let me give you a few examples.

When we move our facial muscles into expressions of emotions, to some degree we experience those emotions. Studies in psychology laboratories have shown that people who are instructed to turn up the corners of their mouths and hold them that way but are not told why they are doing so report more feelings of happiness than people who are not asked to change their expressions. Another example is one way in which many women have learned to have orgasms. By imitating the facial expressions and bodily movements of orgasm when they are highly sexually aroused, they actually have orgasms. Furthermore, studies consistently show that physical exercise, such as jogging, aerobics, or cycling, decreases depression and anxiety and increases positive emotional states. On a simple biochemical level, physical exercise stimulates the production of endorphins, brain chemicals that kill pain and promote euphoria. During states of sexual arousal, we also produce these natural euphorics.

The field of bioenergetic psychotherapy also supports the idea that the body influences the mind. Bioenergetics, as described by Alexander Lowen (who founded the field based on the theories of Wilhelm Reich), is a type of therapy that uses the idea that psychological conflicts are expressed in the ways in which we hold our bodies. By helping clients change their body positions, bioenergetic therapists hope to help them understand and resolve their conflicts.

So if you suffer from mild to moderate depression and would like to use lovemaking to help, the first step is this: Don't wait until you feel sexual to make love—you could be waiting a long time. Start scheduling time for yourself and your partner to do the exercises in this book. Forget spontaneity. Until you jump-start your sex drive you will have to schedule time for lovemaking. Believe it or not, one of the best ways of coping with depression and anxiety is through the use of routine, something you can plan for at the same time every day—and what better thing to count on than a comforting touching exercise, either for you and your partner or for you alone?

How Lovemaking Heals Your General Emotional State

Our sexual drive differs from other basic biological drives such as hunger and thirst. Although we can't live without food or water, we can physically survive without making love or reproducing. That is, we can survive as individuals, even though our species can't. I say "physically survive" because I don't believe we are really living when this drive goes unfulfilled. Part of us, our sexual and emotional self, atrophies when it is not acknowledged.

Sexual expression may also contribute to a person's health in an indirect way. For example, sexual contact can provide a buffer against stress. Lovemaking is one form of what psychologists call "social support"—the human contact that people have available to them or that they believe is available to them. Having a person with whom you can self-disclose, a person with whom you can openly express and discuss feelings, is one of the most valuable forms of social support. A satisfying lovemaking relationship creates an excellent atmosphere in which to express feelings.

Another reason why sex will help you feel better has to do with the "placebo effect." The placebo effect is often brought up in a negative context, but in fact it is a testament to the healing powers of our minds. A placebo is a sugar pill, or "fake" pill, used in medical research. The term _placebo effect_ refers to how a medication often works if you believe it will, even if it is composed of an inert substance. This outcome is created by a person's positive expectation that his or her health will improve. The placebo effect can work for both physical and emotional problems.

Expectations are crucial in health care, and negative expectations are just as powerful as positive ones. For example, if you were ill and visited a doctor who said, "You know, you're probably not going to get better," or even, "You might as well try this—it *might* work," wouldn't you change doctors? Physicians provide treatment, often in the form of medication, for specific physical problems, but the major reasons why people visit physicians are psychological: stress, fatigue, anxiety, or depression. We really seek a physician's care to have another person convey a positive expectation that we will get better. Don't you always feel better right after you make a doctor's appointment? It's the placebo effect. Your immune system receives a huge temporary boost from your body when your mind knows you've done something to help yourself heal.

The placebo effect also works through touch. The "laying on of hands" has been a common medical treatment throughout history and in many cultures. In contemporary society, physicians and other health-care givers who touch their patients promote healing because they nonverbally convey the expectation that the patient will get well. The placebo effect occurs not only in health care, and not just in response to touch. The power of positive expectations in educational settings, in the workplace, and in personal relationships has been documented in many studies. Harnessing this power is the subject of books, seminars, and training.

Understanding mind-body phenomena is important because if you want to heal yourself or your partner of physical ailments, sexual problems, or emotional conflicts, you will need to learn to convey a sense of positive expectations. By imbuing your touch and sexual activities with positive, healthful expectations, you will make the most of the healing mindset you read about in the Introduction and Chapter 14.

If you want to use sexuality to heal yourself emotionally, I would suggest that you begin by doing the relaxation exercises in Chapter 16. Then do the sexual fitness exercises in Chapter 17. Also do the self-touch exercises in Chapter 18. From there, I recommend the peaking process. You could do it as described from the male standpoint (Chapter 23) or the female standpoint (Chapter 26).

I also recommend bodywork, which has its roots in somatopsychology. In particular, I highly recommend massage if you want to help yourself experience emotional healing. Because the mind-body relationship is a two-way street, bodywork, massage, and other types of somatopsychic treatment are very important for people who wish to heal themselves emotionally or deal with stress. There are many different types of massage, used for different purposes. By now you have experienced how sensate-focus, or sensual, massage can heal sexual problems. Well-known massage techniques, such as Swedish massage, are used for treating sore muscles and inducing relaxation. A number of lesser-known types of massage are used to increase both physical and mental well-being. They work by simultaneously easing tension out of the body and bringing up repressed emotions.

In addition to sensate focus, you may want to try other types of massage to heal you emotionally. Here is a list of some somatopsychic massage techniques:

* **Feldenkrais:** hands-on movements combined with a series of slow floor exercises to retrain the central nervous system and improve body functioning, awareness, and self-image

* **Rolfing:** a type of deep-tissue massage and manipulation that "untangles" the connective tissues and restructures the skeletal system to get rid of tension

* **Bioenergetics:** use of specific physical movements to work out chronically tense muscles and deepen contact with the body

* **Tragerwork:** gentle movement of muscles and joints to promote relaxation and playfulness

* **Shiatsu:** finger pressure placed on specific areas of the body to release tension and increase circulation of vital energy

* **Polarity therapy:** a system of massage, awareness skills, nutrition, and stretching exercises to balance the energies of the body

If you are searching for emotional healing, I also recommend meditation and yoga. None of the above practices are sexual, but you can use them in addition to the sexual healing techniques outlined in this book to accomplish healing of your emotions.

Too often people approach sex as an emotional one-way street. We may be insecure or have a restricted understanding of appropriate sexual expression. Some people use sex like a drug, to create certain emotions. Sex addicts, for example, use sex in an unhealthy way to relieve anxiety. Other people wait until they feel a certain emotion in order to have sex; they must feel in love or lovable to enter a sexual realm. But sex, when it is lovemaking, is a rich and multicolored emotional experience.

I think most of us could stand to be more aware of our emotions and be more honest about them when we make love. There is nothing wrong with using sex to explore your emotions—that is, to say, "I feel so angry tonight—I want to make love," or to desire to make love at apparently unusual times, such as after a funeral. Instead of putting your emotions on hold during sex, recognize that sex can be used to convey a multitude of emotions. If you use lovemaking to convey your existing emotions, you can often break down an emotional barrier and release energy. You may find that doing so causes uncontrollable weeping or laughing after sex, but it is nothing to worry about. Releasing these emotions while you are with your partner is potent and positive.

Other Emotional and Mental Benefits of Sexual Healing

Would you like to have a better body image or higher self-esteem? Perhaps you feel emotionally solid, but wish to improve your mental faculties. Maybe you suffer from boredom, and you want to recharge your inspiration. Perhaps you have a problem such as posttraumatic stress disorder, or wish to get past other toxic emotions such as hostility or negativity. Do you occasionally experience insomnia, fatigue, or stress? If so, you will benefit from introducing the healing power of lovemaking into your life.

Do you want to improve your mental capacity? Do you wish for a sharper memory, longer attention span, or deeper ability to concentrate? The basic sensate-focus exercises should help, since they provide a mental device that improves your focus. If after the basic self-touch exercises or partner exercises you want more help, try the more advanced sensate-focus exercise below.

∾ *Exercise 91.* SWITCHING FOCUS BY YOURSELF

There are a number of things you can focus on during sexual activity. A lot of people focus only on their genitals, but there is so much more. There are sights, smells, and sounds. An analogy is listening to an orchestra. Most of us probably hear the composition as a whole, but with more listening experience you become able to pick out the different orchestra sections and even the individual instruments. Here's another analogy: If you are an experienced cook (or, I suppose, an experienced diner), you are able to pick out subtle flavors in foods that most of us would not recognize.

To learn to switch focus, lie comfortably on your bed and begin to caress some part of your body—let's say your thigh. Be aware that you can be conscious of either your hand touching your thigh or your thigh being touched by your hand. As you focus on the sensations, see if you can switch your focus from how your hand feels to how your thigh feels and back again.

This skill takes a little practice. Don't expect to get it the first time. When you master this technique, try doing a genital caress, in which you focus on your hand touching your genitals, and then switch your focus to your genitals being touched by your hand. Practice consciously switching your focus back and forth as you continue a genital caress for fifteen or twenty minutes.

More Benefits

Making love can provide other mental benefits. It can inspire your imagination and increase your sensitivity. The sexual healing exercises teach you to channel your thoughts and energies in directions that you wish, thus multiplying their force. Lovemaking also helps you release the bonding hormone oxytocin. Oxytocin may help boost your creativity and heighten your senses, and it may also help increase your concentration, mental acuity, and focus.

Making love will make you less self-conscious and less concerned with what other people think about you. Many of the exercises in this book will raise your self-esteem by showing you that your partner finds your body—and you—desirable. Thus, you will become active and instrumental in gaining what you desire instead of waiting passively for good feelings to come your way.

Lovemaking can also build self-esteem through a more complex mechanism. Research shows that sexuality is tied closely to personality, and self-esteem is a huge part of one's personality. I do not mean that you can't feel good about yourself if you don't make love with another person—of course you can. But I do not believe that it is possible to feel good about yourself unless you accept your sexual feelings and accept your decisions about whether or not to act on those feelings. So sexuality can be a source of self-esteem, even if you choose not to make love with another person. The sexual healing program outlined in this book will build your self-esteem by helping you learn this self-acceptance.

I have tried to show you how sexual healing will work for you and your partner. But you may be surprised to know that it can also work for society in general. Lovemaking can help you get rid of performance orientation and competitive striving, behaviors that help us to be productive at work but are destructive in relationships. Lovemaking can increase your empathy—your ability to feel what another person is feeling—because it can hone your ability to read another person's nonverbal cues.

Lovemaking can also give you the energy to help others. Because it increases your sex drive or libido, it also increases your life drive, your *élan vital,* your *joie de vivre.* Because you will experience this healing energy and will also want to share it with others, making love could actually improve your character and make you a better person!

Other Attitude Issues

Do you have other attitudes that you believe are standing in the way of a fulfilling relationship with your partner? Common stumbling blocks are negativity, hostility, pessimism, and holding grudges or "carrying a chip on your shoulder." These are considered "toxic" emotions or attitudes—they contribute to physical illness. (In fact, depression, anxiety, and hostility are considered the "toxic triad" that tend to cause psychosomatic illnesses.)

I believe that the sexual healing program presented in this book can help banish these negative emotions. The only other cure I know for them is the "four G's"—giving, gratitude, graciousness, and the Golden Rule. If you need a quick attitude boost, do one of these things. Think about somebody who is a lot worse off than you are, realize how well off you are, and then figure out some way to help that person, even in a small way. Or show some class by being gracious to someone who isn't being very nice to you. And, finally, before you do or say something to somebody else out of anger or spite, stop and consider how that person will feel. These actions may sound sappy, but trust me, they work. If the person you end up being nicer to is your partner, then so much the better.

chapter 34

Healing Your Relationship: Bonding and Trust

The exercises in the next two chapters show you how you can use sexuality to heal your relationship. This chapter has to do with bonding and trust; the next chapter deals with play and verbal intimacy.

Bonding

When psychologists use the term *bonding,* they're referring to the emotional attachment that develops between an infant and its primary caregiver. Caregivers create this vital, intimate bond by spending lots of time holding, cuddling, hugging, and playing with their children. Sharing these activities gives children the love, security, and self-worth necessary to venture out into the world and mature fully.

As adults, we can bond with each other, too. The following exercises create and strengthen intimate feelings between partners. But I warn you: Don't try these exercises with your partner unless you are sure you want to feel closer to him or her. They will help you become relaxed with each other and attuned to your heart rhythms. They express your acceptance of your partner, and they help you feel accepted. It is easy to tell your partner, "I love and accept you," but that does not have the profound impact that holding, stroking, and physically calming your loved one does.

Many skeptics believe that an "exercise" for emotional intimacy is a gimmick, that intimacy just naturally happens with physical closeness over time, and that you can't do anything to force it or improve it. I disagree. These exercises are not gimmicks if they are done from the heart, with honest openness, and without manipulative intent. An emotional bond cannot be forced, but it can be given the opportunity to grow.

☙ *Exercise 92.* EYE GAZE

Lie together on your bed and face each other. Wrap your arms comfortably around each other and gaze into each other's eyes for several minutes without talking.

Sometimes it's hard to gaze into both of your partner's eyes at the same time when you're this physically close to each other. Try gazing into just one of your partner's eyes. It's best to gaze into the eye that corresponds to your partner's nondominant hand. In other words, if your partner is right-handed, gaze into his left eye, and vice versa.

I'll bet you two used to do this when you first met. Remember how good it felt? Enjoy the feelings that come up for you now. How have they grown richer with time?

☙ *Exercise 93.* NURTURING

Everyone needs a little nurturing from time to time. Too often we forget that it is okay to care for our loved one and that it is okay for him or her to care for us. If one of you has had a bad day, have your partner nurture you with this exercise.

You can nurture one another just about anywhere—in bed, on the couch, or on the floor leaning against the couch. One person sits with his or her back against the wall, headboard, or back of the couch. The other person lies down with his or her head or torso in the lap of the partner who is sitting, in whatever way is comfortable. The person who is sitting tenderly wraps his arms around the person who is lying down.

Share this embrace for ten minutes. Feel each other's warmth. Listen to each other's breathing. Feel your hearts beat.

☙ *Exercise 94.* LYING TOGETHER

Have you ever wanted to feel as much of your partner's body as you could at one time? So often we support each other emotionally, but what is it like to support each other in other ways?

Lie on your back on your bed, and have your partner slowly lower himself or herself on top of you. The person on top should gradually allow his or her full weight to be supported by the person on the bottom. You can move your heads around until you find a comfortable connection. Lie together like this for several minutes without talking. You can lie together nude or with clothes on.

Surprisingly, this position is possible and comfortable for most couples. It does not seem to make much of a difference if one partner is larger than the other, since your weight spreads out over a larger area (and the bed). If one of you is much larger than the other, move around until you find a position that works for you. Many couples like having their faces very close; others enjoy hearing and feeling their partner's heartbeat on their cheek.

ᐯ *Exercise 95.* PALM ENERGY

This is a wonderful way to become aware of the intangible energy in your relationship. Sit cross-legged facing each other. Gaze lovingly into each other's eyes. Don't let your gaze waver. Just as your arms can embrace each other's bodies, can your gaze caress each other's souls?

Raise your hands and place your palms against each other. Hold them there for ten seconds. Feel the heat running between the two of you. Now slowly move your hands apart so that they no longer touch but are just close enough so that you can feel a current of energy flow between you. Concentrate on that flow for five minutes.

ᐯ *Exercise 96.* PALM ENERGY AND BREATH SHARING

This exercise may sound innocuous, but it will really knock your socks off! The combination of palm energy and breath sharing sets up an energy exchange that gets your endorphins flowing and takes you to an altered state of consciousness.

Begin the palm energy exercise as described above. When you feel the energy flowing between you, lean together as if you were going to kiss. Keep your faces close enough together so that you feel your partner's breath. When one of you breathes in, the other should breathe out. Visualize your breath flowing in a circle—from your mouth to your lungs to your stomach to your pelvis, and then back into your partner and up through his or her pelvis, stomach, chest, throat and mouth. Now try to reverse this energy circle. Imagine that you are healing your partner by giving him or her the breath of life.

Trust

In Chapter 15 I talked about trust in the context of sensate-focus exercises. You build trust when you follow the directions and stay within the limits of the exercise. When your partner can predict your behavior, it builds trust.

Another aspect of trust is allowing yourself to stretch your limits or boundaries. That's what the next few exercises do. They have long descriptions because they are psychologically a bit more complicated than most of the other exercises in this book. Their payoff is not only an increase in trust between you and your partner, but also a reduction in performance pressure.

❧ Exercise 97. TOWEL OVER THE FACE

This exercise is especially good for women who have problems reaching orgasm and for men who have problems with erections. Often these problems are due in part to worrying about what your partner thinks of you. Searching our partner's facial expression for an indication of his or her response or feelings can distract us from our own enjoyment of a sexual encounter. Covering your partner's face removes a source of feedback and pressure about performance. This exercise can be done with either partner active or passive. Start with spoon breathing and focusing caresses, as described in Chapter 19.

To begin, let's have the man passive and lying on his back. Women, place a piece of clothing or a towel lightly over your partner's face, so that he's comfortable but you can't see his facial expressions. You are to pretend that you partner's body is a toy that you will be allowed to play with for twenty minutes to half an hour. He will remain completely passive. During this time, if you do something that bothers your partner, he will let you know, as in previous exercises. You can use any part of your partner's body to give yourself maximum enjoyment.

Here are some suggestions. Slowly rub yourself all over your partner. Lick his body. Masturbate with his penis. If he has an erection, climb on top of his penis and slowly thrust in and out. Experiment with different angles for thrusting. Masturbate by rubbing your clitoris on your partner's knees or hips. Use your partner's penis to find your G-spot.

Men, when you are passive, you are not to move or respond in any way. That means no talking, no moaning, no twitching, even if your partner is doing something that drives you crazy. Just focus on what she does and how you feel. If you become aroused, if you have an erection, or if you have an orgasm, just enjoy yourself. Your partner has been instructed to enjoy herself with whatever is available on your body. Don't push any arousal away, and don't try to make it better. Besides reducing performance pressure by eliminating facial feedback, this exercise allows you to give up all responsibility for the sexual interaction. When you are passive the only thing you can possibly do is relax and enjoy. Your partner is completely responsible for what happens. You do not have to respond at all.

Doing this exercise with the man passive and the woman active is helpful for men with erection problems and for women who have trouble becoming aroused and reaching orgasm. Reversing the roles can benefit men with inhibited ejaculation and women who try too hard to reach orgasm. If you want to do this exercise with the man active and the woman passive, have the woman lie on her back. The man then pretends his partner's body is a toy for him to play with. Have you ever had a fantasy about making love to a sleeping woman? Now is the time to indulge in this fantasy. The secret to doing this exercise is to use the sensate-focus techniques and to touch your partner gently and slowly. This isn't the exercise for you to work out your fantasies of porn movie sex. The man's mindset is very important in this exercise. Adjust your mindset so that you envision yourself healing your partner by awakening her sexuality while you are also touching her in ways that give you maximum pleasure.

To accomplish this, rub yourself all over your partner. Lick her body from head to toe, starting on the peripheral areas of the body and moving toward her genitals. Do oral sex with her if you enjoy it. If you want to have intercourse, gently spread or raise her legs. Your female partner will remain as quiet and passive as possible during this exercise. If you do something that bothers her, she will let you know.

Because this exercise really stretches the boundaries of trust, some people have a strong emotional reaction to it. If you are used to always having sex a certain way (for example, if the man always initiates intercourse), the woman's activity may cause the man discomfort. Some people are so uncomfortable initially that they stall out and do nothing the first time they are in the active role, or they drive themselves crazy trying to do something to force their partner to respond. In the passive role, they become upset because they want to respond. They think, "How can she really enjoy herself if I'm not doing anything?" For other people, being unable to see their partner's facial reactions is frustrating or feels unnatural. But with practice, this exercise can become extremely pleasurable. It is a relief to be able to enjoy yourself without having to do anything. I think all of us like the feeling of being "done to" once in a while.

This exercise can also reinforce the idea that you are responsible for your own arousal. It can encourage you to experiment with sexual activities you may not have done before because someone was watching. It can force you to pay attention to your own enjoyment because there is nothing else to pay attention to. It can wean you from being dependent on your partner's enjoyment in order to have a good time yourself.

It can also reduce some of your inhibitions about being "animalistic" during sexual activities. Sexual activity serves a number of purposes, one of which is to express love for your partner. There are other legitimate reasons for engaging in sexual activity, and one is to express the fact that sexual activity is also an animal activity. The active partner should always feel free to growl, grunt, or bare his or her teeth while touching and squeezing parts of their partner's body.

In another version of the exercise, the active partner also wears some type of blindfold. This forces the active partner to completely focus on sensations of touch.

Finish the exercise with spoon breathing and partner feedback.

◟ Exercise 98. ASKING FOR WHAT YOU WANT

This exercise begins the minute you enter the room; you do not do focusing caresses to prepare for it. The partner who is active asks for anything that he or she wants. Let's assume that the woman is active first. Nothing will happen in the exercise until she requests it. If she wants her partner to remove his clothes, she must say, "Take off your clothes."

When you are active, you need to tell your partner everything that you want him or her to do. You may ask for anything you can think of that you would like your partner to do, but you need to be specific. If what he does is not exactly what you wanted, say so and give him directions until he gets it right. Feel free to enjoy whatever you have asked your partner to do for as long as you want to. When active, you may also do whatever you like, as long as you tell your partner what you are going to do. For example, it you would like to be active for a while, you could say, "I want you to lie back so I can caress you for a while."

If you are the passive partner, do as your partner asks. You will have your turn later. Refuse only if your partner asks you to do something that you consider painful or unpleasant. Much as you might want to initiate something, don't. Try to do exactly what your partner asks, but do it for your own enjoyment and focus on it. The secret is to accommodate your partner's wishes while still doing the activities for your own pleasure.

This exercise can sometimes become awkward because many people are not used to asking for what they want. Sometimes a client and I have just sat and looked at each other for several minutes because he couldn't think of anything to ask for or was afraid to ask for anything. When you are the asker, be assertive and don't settle for something that is not really what you want. When you are the person being asked, accommodate your partner, but do everything for your own pleasure as much as possible by focusing on your own sensual enjoyment.

Make your requests clear. For example, instead of saying, "Would you like to give me a front caress?" say, "Please give me a front caress," or, "I want you to give me a front caress." If you do not want to do something your partner asks for, just say, "No." If your partner turns down some activity, it doesn't mean, "No, never, that's disgusting." It simply means, "No, I do not want to do that particular activity right now."

You can do this exercise with each person in the active role for half an hour. The exercise can be stressful, but it can also pinpoint problems you may have in asserting or enjoying yourself.

After the exercise, talk about how you felt. Use the guidelines outlined in Chapter 15 for partner feedback. Tell your partner if you had trouble knowing what you wanted, asking for it, or enjoying yourself. Tell your partner if you had thoughts such as, "I would have asked for such-and-such, but I was afraid you wouldn't do it." Your anxiety level during this exercise can give you real insight into whether you are still uncomfortable with accepting pleasure for yourself. If you are still uncomfortable, practice asking for one or two small things during other sessions until you become more comfortable.

Besides making you feel more comfortable with asserting yourself sexually, this exercise can help you feel a sense of equity in your relationship. If you do the exercise the way I have described, each partner has an equal chance to ask and to give.

∾ Exercise 99. THE ZOMBIE

The Zombie (also known as The Slave) is a more extreme version of the preceding exercise in that one person is in control throughout the session. One partner orders the other around for a half hour or an hour, and the "zombie" partner is required to do anything sexual the other partner asks (unless there is a severe objection to it). The zombie literally acts like a zombie—silent, obedient, and unresponsive.

This exercise is a way to experiment with loss of control. Some of your sexual problems may stem from your feeling that you have to be in control of your body or your sexual responses. A few minutes as the zombie may convince you that while you do not want to be out of control all the time, temporarily relinquishing some control of your body is not that bad. It can even be a relief not to have to be responsible for everything that happens.

The Zombie exercise is extreme and should only be done if you are comfortable with the idea. If done at the right time, it can build trust between partners. You may also find out some things about yourself that you didn't know. You may find that you are actually comfortable being totally in control or totally out of control. This exercise is a safe way to explore these feelings. Being a zombie with a person you trust is, in a sense, the ultimate in performance pressure. Can you deal with it? At the very least, you will find out if it is something you truly dislike.

Bear in mind that this exercise is not an excuse to be sadistic or to shock your partner. On the contrary: It is a way to build trust and to practice dealing with extreme performance pressure in a safe environment. When you are the zombie, do you try to perform or do you wonder if you are doing things right? Or are you so well trained in sensate focus that you are able to move into the sensate-focus mode right away and enjoy the interaction? If you become performance-oriented during this exercise, it will literally show you "how not to feel" during other sensate-focus exercises.

Finish the exercise with spoon breathing and partner feedback.

ᴄᴡ Exercise 100. STREAM OF CONSCIOUSNESS

What does a literary technique have to do with sex therapy? You can use stream of consciousness or free association to help yourself loosen up and deal with spectatoring.

Begin this session with spoon breathing and focusing caresses. I'll describe the exercise from the point of view of the man. Lie on your back. Have your partner caress the front of your body and your genitals in any way she enjoys. While your partner caresses you, talk out loud in a stream-of-consciousness style. This means that you say anything and everything that pops into your mind without censoring a word of it.

There is no way to plan or predict what you will talk about. Your stream may include random thoughts, grunts, moans, jokes, word lists, descriptions of how you feel, descriptions of how your partner is touching you, or descriptions of fantasies. Your partner will not comment on anything you say. In fact, she could wear earplugs or earphones so that she can't even hear what you say. That way you will be less self-conscious.

The first time you do this exercise you will be lucky if you let out a minute's worth of unedited and uncensored material during a twenty-minute exercise. This exercise is not easy! It is probably the most challenging exercise that I have seen clients do. But it is worth it, because the exercise can help you uncover unconscious material that may be interfering with erection or arousal processes. In addition, talking while you are receiving stimulation interferes with the worrying and spectatoring that can slow down your erection or arousal processes.

Finish with spoon breathing and partner feedback.

ᑐ *Exercise 101.* LISTENING TO MUSIC

The music-listening exercise is similar to the stream of consciousness exercise. It can help in cases of severe performance anxiety in people of either sex. Most people can learn to focus on sensations of arousal in their genitals. But for some people, it is impossible to "turn off their head" and stop worrying about erection, arousal, or orgasm. The solution is to provide some kind of stimulation that distracts your mind.

For this exercise, you will need a cassette player or CD player with headphones, and a cassette or CD of music that you don't particularly like. A good tape to use would be something that provides a constant low level of distraction, something that has little or no discernible musical quality, something that does not have lyrics, or even something that is mildly annoying. Don't use anything pleasant, such as a relaxation tape. A tape of white noise will work. (No offense to any fans out there, but when I used to do this exercise with clients, I used a tape of Black Flag. It was perfect.)

Begin with spoon breathing and focusing caresses. Next, the passive partner lies on his or her back while the active partner stimulates his or her genitals. As the active partner, you should still do the caress for your own pleasure. The music will distract the passive partner just enough so that he or she cannot worry about performance, but not enough to interfere with arousal and erection. As always, finish with spoon breathing and partner feedback.

❧

In addition to helping you along on your sexual healing journey, I hope that the exercises in this chapter have made you and your partner feel closer than ever.

chapter 35

Healing Your Relationship: Play and Verbal Intimacy

T his chapter continues the theme of using sexuality to heal various aspects of your relationship. An important part of sexual healing is the ability to be innocent, to appreciate simple pleasures the way a child does, and to comfortably express the closeness you feel to your partner.

Play

A lot of our unstructured lovemaking serves the same function for us that play does for kids. It lets us relax and take the pressure off ourselves. It is dynamic, creative, expressive, and not self-conscious. Unlike most activities in our adult lives, lovemaking isn't goal-oriented (or at least it shouldn't be). If you and your partner wish to enrich your relationship, one of the best things you can do is to play together. In fact, there are several forms of therapy (such as sand play) that use childhood activities to reconnect us with our ability to be playful.

You don't necessarily need any special equipment or expensive sex toys to play with each other sexually. You can often use things you already have around the house, such as food. Or the two of you could try a couple of the following romantically playful exercises:

↩ *Exercise 102.* SENSUOUS SHOWER

The sensuous shower is a whole-body caress that takes place in the shower. The purpose of the sensuous shower is not just to get clean (although you probably will) but also to enjoy your body and your partner's body in a different way.

There are a number of ways to savor a sensuous shower. You can share any of the caresses you have learned in this book, caressing each other's face, back, chest, or genitals. You can include oral sex. If you like, you can alternate taking active and passive roles. Or you can make this exercise a mutual caress, caressing each other at the same time. Don't forget that you can caress with all the different parts of your body, not just your hands.

Try using a liquid bath soap or fragrant bath gel, and caress any parts of your partner's body that feel good to you. When you caress, touch for your own pleasure. Focus on the silky sensations of your partner's wet skin and hair. When you receive a caress, concentrate on exactly where you are being touched, just as you would during any sensate-focus exercise. The only thing you have to watch out for is soap on the female genitals, because it can burn.

If you become aroused during the sensuous shower, simply allow yourself to experience the arousal. Don't try to make your arousal level go higher or push it away. Relax and enjoy the feeling of your partner caressing you and the water beating down on your skin. If you have an erection, ejaculation, or orgasm, welcome it. After your shower, pat each other dry with warm towels and a loving, healing touch.

If you prefer baths rather than showers, dim the lights in the bathroom, light a few candles, and take a bath together using scented bath oils or soaps. The sensuous shower or bath can be a relaxing prelude to healing exercises such as the genital and oral caresses.

ᴄ◡ *Exercise 103.* TOM JONES DINNER

Many of us gobble our food or eat while doing other things, like watching television or driving a car. We fail to take the time to enjoy the simple, sensuous aspects of eating. The ability to really take the time to enjoy food is highly related to a person's ability to enjoy sex. This is especially true for men who have difficulty with rapid ejaculation. Believe it or not, learning to eat more slowly trains you to focus more on all aspects of sensuality, including the ability to last longer during intercourse. The Tom Jones Dinner is named for the incredibly indulgent eating scene in the movie *Tom Jones*.

We did this exercise as part of surrogate training. Everyone in the class (ten to twelve people) brought some type of food that could be eaten with our hands. We spread a sheet out on the floor and arranged the foods beautifully. We were all nude (this was 1980) and there were three rules: no feeding yourself, no talking, and no utensils. Everybody fed each other.

Some of these dinners got pretty wild, with people eating food off of each others' bodies. This is much more fun than your normal potluck supper, believe me! The point of the dinner was not to have a wild food orgy, but rather to learn to enjoy the purely sensuous aspects of eating, free from the restraints of table manners.

You can create a delectable Tom Jones dinner at home for you and your partner. First, choose some sensuous foods. You might consider fruit (especially juicy ones, such as oranges and peaches), hors d'oeuvres such as cheese and crackers, any meat that can be pulled off a bone, and anything messy that can be licked off fingers and body parts. In general, anything that is creamy or juicy will feel especially good in your mouth. For beverages, serve wine or champagne, sparkling water, or fruit juice.

I've prepared this dinner many times, and one of my favorite foods for it is artichokes. They're fun to eat, and you can throw the leaves all over the place. If you are not into cooking or consider it a chore, go to a local bar or restaurant and buy a couple of orders of chicken wings, which work perfectly for this dinner. (This is starting to sound like a recipe book. Maybe my next book should be a recipe book for food to eat while you're making love. Not to mention, this section of the chapter is starting to make me hungry.)

To begin the Tom Jones Dinner, arrange the food on a sheet or piece of plastic to protect your carpeting and furniture. Or set the foods up outside if you have a private area. Take off your clothes. Relax and caress each other if you need a transition, then begin to feed each other. Go slowly, just as you would in a caressing exercise. Eat with the goal of feeling every sensation as the food passes your lips and through your mouth. Place food on your partner's body and slowly lick it off, or offer food to your partner on your body. If you want a drink, take one, and then, with a kiss, share it with your partner. Finish the Tom Jones Dinner by washing each other off with warm, wet towels or by taking a sensuous shower.

ᑫ Exercise 104. ACTING LIKE AN ANIMAL

A big part of being intimate is recognizing that lovemaking is playful and doesn't have to be serious, that you can really let your hair down with your partner. Sex is a basic animal activity, and sometimes you may want to use it just to express that animal urge. This exercise is based on an exercise called Wild Thing from one of my previous books, *Talk Sexy to the One You Love*. I used to call it Quest for Fire, and I have elaborated on it here.

One of you will be active while the other is passive. The passive partner lies on his or her back. The active person then uses the partner's body to indulge in and gratify his or her "animal urges."

When you are the active partner, lick, stroke, and suck your partner as if you were an animal. Make a lot of animal noises while you do this, such as grunting or moaning. Rub yourself against different parts of your partner's body. Groom your partner. If you are a woman and your partner has an erection, squat on top of him and thrust up and down. If you are a man, push your partner's legs back and penetrate her, or roll her over and enter her from behind. Be creative and have fun with this, but don't do anything that might hurt your partner.

ᐊ *Exercise 105.* SEX GAMES AND ROLE-PLAYING

You can be creative and make up your own sex games that may or may not involve role-playing. This is a sex game I made up called "Snake in the Sleeping Bag with Unsuspecting Camper." (And yes, I had been drinking when I made it up.) One person is the camper and one person is the snake. The "snake" crawls down to the bottom of the bed under the covers and lies there motionless. The "camper" then gets into bed and turns off the lights, pretending he does not know there is someone in the bed. As the camper relaxes, the snake awakens and slowly starts to slither and crawl up the camper's body, stopping to lick or squeeze at various points. The secret to enjoying this exercise is for the snake to go as slowly as possible and make a lot of creative movements involving oral sex and wrapping around the partner's body.

Verbal Intimacy

The following few exercises teach you to talk to each other in nonthreatening, productive, and intimate ways. The first three are incremental steps in a process to explore and improve your body image. The way you think about your body can have a profound impact on your sexuality. Sharing feelings about your body with your partner can also help you build trust.

ᐊ *Exercise 106.* BODY IMAGE, PART 1

The body-image exercises are not sensate-focus exercises. They are communication exercises or processes used to help each person learn to become more comfortable with his or her own body and with his or her partner's body. In these exercises, you will examine your nude body in detail in front of your partner, and you will tell your partner what you like and don't like about your body. You will also discuss whether certain parts of your body have positive or negative feelings associated with them.

For Part 1 of the exercise, the room should be well lit and should have a large mirror, preferably full-length. First, take off all of your clothes, and stand and gaze at each other for a minute. Stand about three feet apart and look into each other's eyes. Slowly take in your partner's facial features. Notice things that you have never noticed before or things that you haven't taken the time to notice in a while.

Now both partners should lower their gaze to take in the chest area. Think of this as a sensate-focus caress using your eyes instead of your hands. Let your eyes move slowly over your partner's body, as if you were caressing him or her. Take your time, and gaze at each body part for as long as it takes to visually enjoy it. Mutually shift your gaze downward over your partner's chest, abdomen, and legs. Take time to look at each other's genitals. Each partner should then take turns turning around so the other person can look at the backside of his or her body.

Your experience of this part of the body-image exercise will probably be different from my experience of the exercise with clients. When I did this exercise with clients, it was the first time we had seen each other nude. You may have seen your partner's body naked many times. If that is the case, use this part of this exercise (looking at each other) to appreciate, rather than to see things for the first time.

Even if you have seen each other nude many times, it may not have been acceptable in your relationship to stare at certain body parts, such as breasts or genitals. Or you may be in the habit of wearing sleepwear to bed, and sexual activity may take place only with the lights off. Partners may not be in the habit of walking around the house nude due to the presence of other family members. For whatever reason, you may not have much experience seeing your partner nude or being seen in the nude, so nudity itself may cause anxiety. If you feel anxious or self-conscious during this part of the exercise, take some deep breaths and tell your partner that you feel anxious. This is the only verbal communication in this part of the exercise.

If your partner expresses that he or she feels anxious, you should nod and say, "I understand." No other verbal feedback is necessary.

You may encounter other sources of anxiety during this part of the exercise. Men and women usually have different anxieties about their bodies and about being nude in front of a partner. For men, there are two common beliefs that may cause anxiety in this situation. The first is the feeling that one's penis is too small. Every male client I ever worked with expressed the belief during this exercise that his penis was not large enough.

A second source of anxiety for men during this exercise is whether or not they will have an erection. Men have different ideas about how long it should take them to get an erection when they are naked with a woman. Some men expect to have an erection immediately; others may allow themselves one minute or five minutes. Others think they should not have an erection at all and are embarrassed if they do get one. The body-image exercise is not a sexual exercise. Try to determine what your "time frame" is for having an erection, and take the pressure off yourself. If you do have an erection during the exercise, just enjoy it and keep doing the exercise. Don't try to make your erection harder, and don't try to make it go away. It is perfectly normal to either have or not have an erection during this exercise.

While men's anxieties tend to be about their genitals, women tend to worry about being overweight, and about whether their partner will find some of their body parts unacceptable. Most women tend to think that their breasts are too small or too saggy, and that their hips and thighs are too wide. Part of their reason for feeling overweight is that our culture and society place a totally unwarranted emphasis on thinness, idealizing a body that is quite honestly unattainable for the vast majority of women. Hopefully, doing this exercise and the ones that follow will help you to be more accepting of your body.

If you do feel anxious about whether your partner finds your body attractive, just accept the fact that you have these feelings for now. Doing the body-image exercise does not require a body that meets certain standards of attractiveness.

Your anxieties and feelings about your body and about your partner's reaction to it are real. These exercises will help you learn to accept negative feelings about your body and learn to not let those feelings get in the way of your sexual enjoyment. You will also learn how your partner feels about his or her body. I hope that the outcome of the body-image exercises is that you are able to develop an attitude that says, basically, "While there may be certain aspects of my body that I am not ecstatic about, my body is capable of feeling good. I can have sensual and sexual enjoyment of my body if I accept myself the way I am."

❧ *Exercise 107.* BODY IMAGE, PART 2

In the next part of the body-image exercise, one partner is passive and the other is active. Let's say the woman decides to be active first. She should take a long look at herself in the mirror and describe all the parts of her body and her feelings associated with each part. Her partner will sit comfortably and watch and listen.

While you are listening, you may find that you disagree with your partner's description or feelings about certain body parts. As the passive partner, you should not interrupt, make comments, or ask questions. You will have an opportunity for feedback when you are both through with the exercise. Try not to negate your partner's feelings; just accept that he or she feels that way.

When you are active, look at yourself carefully in the full-length mirror. Use a hand mirror to examine the back of your body. Starting with your hair, tell your partner whether you like or dislike it, what you like or dislike about it, any good or bad feelings or memories that are associated with it, whether you like to touch it or have it touched, and how it feels.

Do the same for all your other body parts. Here is a list so you don't leave anything out: hair, eyes, ears, nose, mouth, face, neck, shoulders, back, breasts/chest, arms, hands, stomach, waist, hips, thighs, buttocks, genitals, legs, and feet. Also include height, weight, body hair, and any characteristics such as moles, birthmarks, or scars.

After you have described your body parts and told your partner how you feel about them, examine your body as a whole. Tell your partner what your favorite and least favorite parts are. What do you consider your best and worst features? What parts of your body cause you anxiety to think about? Which parts do you like to have touched or looked at? Which parts don't you like to have touched or looked at, and why? If you could change anything about your body, what would you change? What would you like to look like, and why?

After you have switched roles and your partner has described his or her body, discuss the following. Did you feel that your partner was realistic about his or her body? Why or why not? Which part of your partner's body do you especially like? Finally, be sure to believe your partner's feelings about your body, even though they may not coincide with yours.

Please remember that this is not a time for bringing up any negative or critical feelings about your partner, or about your past or current relationship. It is a time to learn how you and your partner each feel about your bodies.

This is not an easy exercise to do because we don't usually discuss our feelings about our body with other people, even sexual partners we've been with for a long time. However, this exercise will accomplish several things. It will provide practice in communicating about your feelings, and it will provide information about how your partner feels about his or her body. This can be important, because a poor body image can cause people to shy away from sexual activities. In addition, your partner may have certain body parts that he or she is sensitive about. Getting your feelings and anxieties about your body out into the open can help eliminate further negative experiences. You may also learn that your partner's reaction to being touched may have much less to do with the way you touch him or her than with his or her own anxieties about body image.

A former client of mine, Alex, did not like to kiss, and it was causing a problem for him in relationships. During the body-image exercise, he revealed that as a teenager he had been in an accident and had broken his jaw. As a result he'd had to undergo major reconstructive surgery on his face, especially on his lips. The scars from the surgery were no longer visible, but the trauma stayed with him and made him self-conscious. He had never told a sexual partner that kissing created anxiety for him or why. The women he had been with had not known why he refused to kiss them. Consequently, they thought it was because of some problem he had with them, which made them anxious.

It is possible that either you or your partner endured a past traumatic experience that has caused you to feel uncomfortable about your naked body or embarrassed about a certain body part. For example, a woman may harbor discomfort on a deep level because of a molestation episode in her past that she had previously kept secret. She may decide to tell her partner about the trauma during the body-image process, and she may feel a great sense of risk in doing so. If this exercise brings up a powerful memory or issue for you, remember that sometimes just getting it out into the open can help to release it, although you might need the assistance of a qualified therapist to deal with it. If a painful memory comes up for your partner, try to completely accept his or her feelings and to be very supportive.

Another purpose of the body-image exercise is to find out if you and your partner have realistic views of your bodies. As a woman, you may find your body unattractive and think your partner is not telling the truth when he says that he likes your breasts or your thighs. If you are a man, you may feel that your penis is too small, when in fact your partner may like the way your penis looks and feels. These feelings about yourself and the way you look are probably not negative enough to stand in the way of doing sensate-focus exercises together. Problems arise when a person's body image is either totally unrealistic or so negative that he or she cannot relax enough to enjoy sensual arousal. An example of a person with an unrealistic body image would be someone who is actually fairly good-looking, but whose self-esteem is so low that she thinks she is ugly. I use the example of a woman because this sort of unrealistic body image is more characteristic of women. Another example would be a man who has completely let himself go, to the point of neglecting personal hygiene, yet thinks he is good-looking and appealing to women. Neither of these people is realistic about her or his looks, but this fact only presents a problem if it interferes with doing the sensate-focus exercises.

When I did the body-image exercise with clients, I found that most male clients had a positive attitude toward their bodies in general. Women are much more likely to pick themselves apart for not living up to a cultural ideal of attractiveness. I have worked with clients of all levels of attractiveness. I have never worked with a client who was so unattractive that it interfered with our ability to do the sensate-focus exercises. Both attractive and unattractive bodies feel good to touch. At the skin-to-skin level, it really only matters what your body feels like, not what it looks like. Looks have no bearing on sensuality, which has to do with touching and feeling rather than visual stimulation.

I know of no research on whether attractive people have more satisfying sex lives than unattractive people. However, it is possible that there is some aspect of your appearance that you would like to change. A number of excellent resources are available on skin care, health, exercise, and clothing choice. You are an adult, and you have a large degree of choice about how you look. While appearance may be given too much importance in our culture, making yourself more attractive can boost your self-esteem, and that is always worthwhile.

❧ *Exercise 108.* BODY IMAGE, PART 3

Here are some further suggestions for healing your body image. Many peo-ple have found that writing or journaling about a body-related trauma has been helpful. A good book to use as a guide to doing this is *Opening Up*, by James Pennebaker, Ph.D. (see Recommended Reading).

Sometimes a poor body image results from having no idea how you look to other people. If you have a body part you're particularly sensitive about, you generally feel that the whole world is looking at it. Chances are, however, nobody but you is paying attention to it. By focusing on a particu-lar body part, you've lost your sense of the big picture, which is the overall nonverbal impression you make on people who see you.

One way to help change your view of yourself is to enlist your partner's help and use a video camera. Have your partner tape you as you do various activities. When you watch the tapes, you'll be surprised how much better you look than you think you do.

As a further step to healing your body image, consider making a video-tape of you and your partner making love. If you're still self-conscious, use lighting and scenery to present yourself in the best possible light. (You obvi-ously should only do this if you are 100 percent sure you can trust your partner. You don't want this tape to end up on the Internet.)

❧

The next exercise will teach you and your partner how to communicate about sexual matters in positive ways.

❧ *Exercise 109.* GENITAL CARESS WITH VERBAL FEEDBACK

Remember the genital caress you did with your partner in Chapter 22? It was important that it be pressure-free, with no verbal communication. But now, in order to learn more about each other's sexual responses, you and your partner may also want to do a version of the genital caress in which you give each other verbal feedback about the types of genital touch you enjoy.

Start with spoon breathing and focusing caresses. Begin by doing a sensate-focus genital caress with either manual or oral stimulation, or both. When you are the passive partner, at the end of the caress tell your partner one or two things that he or she did that you found particularly pleasurable. Be specific. Then ask your partner to do these things again. (This is a bit similar to the Asking for What You Want exercise in Chapter 34, but easier to do.)

Allow yourself several minutes to enjoy what you asked for. If the touch is not exactly what you wanted, gently guide your partner's hand or face and give him or her more feedback until the caress is being done in exactly the way that pleases you. Then tell your partner something that he or she didn't do, but that you would like. You may take your partner's hand and gently guide it so that you can receive what you want. Enjoy this new caress for a few minutes.

When you are active and your partner asks you for more of something he or she especially liked, there is a constructive way to hear this feedback, as well as a way that's less constructive. Let's say your partner asks for a particular form of genital touch. You could think to yourself, "Of all the things I did, that was the one she liked the best?" Don't second-guess your partner. Instead, try to reframe the situation so that you think, "I'm really lucky, because my partner wants me to repeat something that I already did." Remember, as the active partner you always have the ability to say no to a request.

Similarly, if you are the passive partner and it's your turn to ask for a repeat of a caress, don't second-guess yourself. Trust yourself to think of something you want on the spur of the moment without having to plan your response. Try not to think, "Well, I'd really like a repeat of this, but he might not want to do that."

End the exercise with spoon breathing and partner feedback.

Now that you've had some beginning practice in verbally communicating your feelings in a positive and constructive way, you may want to go back and do some of the earlier sensate-focus exercises, adding in the dimension of verbal communication.

chapter 36

Be a Sexual Healer with Intercourse

Now is the time for you and your partner to come together in the ultimate healing connection. Intercourse means communication; depending on a couple's intentions, intercourse expresses a deep connection between two partners, among other things. This chapter will show you several ways to have intercourse with different healing mindsets and different healing goals.

As part of healing your other sexual problems, you and your partner have probably already had intercourse at some point in this program. The peaking and plateauing processes, which can benefit all of the sexual problems, can all be used during sexual intercourse. The exercises in this chapter are advanced exercises that use intercourse. Although I've provided short descriptions of different ways to have intercourse, these are not descriptions of different positions per se, as you would find in a typical sex manual. When you have intercourse, use whatever positions are comfortable for the two of you. The suggestions I make are simply that, suggestions. They are based on my experience with the positions that seem to best convey healing.

Before you try any of these exercises, it is very important that you have spent time spoon breathing and caressing each other with both nonsexual and sexual caresses. You may also wish to spend time with oral caresses and sensual oral sex. You need to spend time doing these things to get centered within yourself, to relax and focus on your arousal, and to get in sync with your partner. After intercourse, maintain physical contact and take time to spoon breathe together or nurture each other in an embrace. You will need a coming-down period to reground yourselves after the experience of healing intercourse. Finish with partner feedback.

If you decide to have intercourse after doing another, nonintercourse exercise, remember your basics. Relax and enter the healing mindset. Allow enough time so you do not feel rushed. And get centered together by beginning with spoon breathing, focusing caresses, and genital caresses.

ᶜ᷉ Exercise 110. GOAL-FREE INTERCOURSE

The theory behind goal-free intercourse is to escape the pressure to have, or to give, an orgasm. Intercourse without orgasm nurtures the mindset of continuity between skin sensuality, foreplay, and intercourse. As you enjoy goal-free intercourse, you learn to be more flexible and indulgent in your lovemaking, and to move away from thinking of intercourse as the result of foreplay, or of orgasm as the necessary end result of intercourse.

Decide who will be active and who will be passive. When the woman is active, she will begin by doing a sensate-focus caress with her partner—a front caress, genital caress, and oral sex. When he gets an erection, she will climb on top of him and begin intercourse using slow, sensuous strokes—as many as she desires. Her partner will remain passive and not move. His only responsibility is to focus on the pleasurable sensations he experiences.

There should be no performance pressure, no goals, no thinking ahead, and no orgasm. After this short exercise, the woman will maintain the sexual connection by lowering herself into an embrace with her partner and covering his body with hers.

When the man is active, the woman lies on her back. Her only responsibility is to focus on her own sensations. Her partner does a front caress and then genital and oral caresses. He can kneel between his partner's legs and use his penis to caress the outside of her vagina if this arouses him. When he is ready for intercourse, he can put a pillow underneath her, raise her legs, and enter her. This position, in which the woman raises her legs and the man kneels between them, brings both partners into a lovely face-to-face connection and offers greater stimulation for both. If you have trouble kneeling for any period of time, you can use the missionary position. The man does a few slow, sensuous strokes, as he desires, and when finished, lies lovingly on top of or beside his partner.

ᶜ᷉ Exercise 111. SENSATE-FOCUS INTERCOURSE

This is intercourse with a different focus: sensuality. In previous chapters you have practiced focusing on skin sensations in all parts of the body. Now you will learn to focus on the specific, erotic sensations of the penis inside the vagina.

Men, when you're in the active role, ask your partner to lie comfortably on her back. Do sensate-focus caresses, including a front caress, a genital caress, and oral sex. If you need direct stimulation of your penis to get an erection, use your penis to caress your partner's vagina, or caress yourself with your hand. When you are ready, start intercourse in the butterfly position. As the active partner, you will control the speed of the thrusting. Thrust as slowly as possible—try to caress your partner's vagina with your penis. Both of you should feel free to move, to thrust and roll with each other, while focusing on the exquisite sensations of your penis inside her vagina.

Next, try switching your focus to different parts of your penis. What can you feel? Both of you try to focus on the same sensations at the same time. Look at each other as you focus. There should be no pressure for either of you to have an orgasm, but if you do, that is okay. As the active partner, you decide when intercourse is over.

Women, when you're in the active role, ask your partner to lie on his back as you do a front caress, genital caress, and perhaps oral sex. When your partner has an erection, climb on top of him, insert his penis in your vagina, and begin slowly thrusting on his penis. Think of yourself as caressing his penis with your vagina. Both of you should focus on the sensations of his penis inside your vagina.

As the active partner, you lead with regard to the speed and extent of the thrusting, and your partner follows. It's like dancing—in fact, it is a dance, a love dance. As you make love, look into each other's eyes and try to match your breathing. The exercise is over whenever you decide to stop, regardless of whether either or both of you have orgasms.

ᥫᎯ *Exercise 112.* HEALING INTERCOURSE

This is another version of intercourse that is free from pressure or goals. In healing intercourse, you visualize and project healing sexual energy in a focused way.

If you are a woman in the active role, caress your partner while you both center your energies together. When your partner has a partial or full erection, climb on top of him and begin intercourse. While thrusting and focusing, visualize your vagina as a vessel that surrounds your partner's penis. Imagine that your vagina is hot, giving out a white, healing light that flows into your partner. This visualization will convey a positive healing energy from your vagina to your partner's penis. If your partner focuses on the same visualization, your vagina will actually begin to feel hot during the exercise. There is no goal, no pressure, and no time limit. You decide when the exercise is over. If you are able to reach a climax, give your partner the ultimate healing energy gift: you having a very intense orgasm.

If you are a man in the active role, begin with a front caress, a genital caress, and perhaps oral sex. When your partner is aroused and lubricated, begin intercourse in the butterfly position. Visualize your penis as a healing instrument, radiating white-hot healing energy to your partner. Or think of your sexual energy as a blue or white light flowing into your partner. Both of you should focus on this visualization. You can continue with intercourse as long as you want to, with or without an orgasm. You may actually feel your penis become hot.

Sometimes it is easier for a man to do this visualization than it is for a woman, because if he has an orgasm he actually is pouring something into his partner. So if you are a woman, when you have an orgasm, picture it as an energy gift—powerful, hot, and healing.

ᐁ *Exercise 113.* HEART-AWARENESS INTERCOURSE

This form of intercourse creates an incredible bond, especially if one or both of you have orgasms. During heart-awareness intercourse, you listen to your lover's heartbeat as the rhythms of your lovemaking build and climax. The exercise will sharpen your awareness of the rhythms of your bodies, your arousal, and, ultimately, each other. Alternatively, you can adjust your position so that your hearts are against each other and beat together as you make love.

Begin the exercise with focusing caresses. If you are the woman and you are active, when your partner has an erection, straddle him, begin intercourse, and thrust sensuously. While making love, lean over and rest your ear on your partner's chest. Feel his warmth. Listen to his heartbeat as you both become more and more aroused. See if you can cause your partner's heartbeat to speed up or slow down with the speed and force of your thrusting. As his heart beats faster, does his breathing quicken? Does your arousal climb? Does *your* heart beat faster?

If you are the man and you are active, when you have an erection, kneel between your partner's legs and enter her. As you slowly and sensuously thrust, lean over so your ear rests on your partner's chest. Feel her warmth and listen to her heartbeat. Does the speed and passion of your thrusting affect the beating of your partner's heart? Does her breathing quicken? Does your arousal climb in tandem with hers?

〜 *Exercise 114.* MUTUALITY INTERCOURSE

For this exercise, you can have intercourse in whatever position you choose. The idea is to try to see and feel the act of intercourse from your partner's viewpoint. In doing so you will find that you cannot tell where you end and your partner begins. You will feel ultimately unified, a greater whole than each of you individually.

There are two ways to experience mutuality intercourse. The first is to begin with peaking, so you are both at high arousal levels when you start intercourse. As you penetrate or are penetrated, ask yourself, "Is what I feel the penis or the vagina?" If you are a woman, see if you can put your consciousness in your partner's penis. If you are a man, see if you can put your consciousness in your partner's vagina.

The second way to experience mutuality intercourse is to pretend your physical positions are reversed. If you are on top, close your eyes and imagine that you are on the bottom. If you are on the bottom, close your eyes and imagine that you are on top. As you have intercourse and you mutually focus on this sensation, you may get the sense that the two of you are spinning or whirling through space.

A third option is to try to place your consciousness in the body of your partner and try to imagine what intercourse feels like for him or her.

Mutual and Multiple Orgasms

I am sure you have heard the phrase *simultaneous orgasm,* which refers to both members of a couple having orgasms at the same time during intercourse. In sex therapy, for a long time simultaneous orgasm was touted as the be-all and end-all of lovemaking. It eventually fell out of favor with sex therapists because many of them realized that this point of view placed too much pressure on couples, especially on men who had premature ejaculation problems and on women who had difficulty having an orgasm at all during intercourse.

Some of us, however, have not given up on the rare potential of simultaneous orgasm, which I prefer to call mutual orgasm because the term reflects so much more than simply two orgasms happening at the same time. The phrase *mutual orgasm* also reflects the idea that each lover enjoys his or her partner's orgasm as well as his or her own. With the techniques in *Sexual Healing*, especially peaking and plateauing, you and your partner can know so much about each other's response that you will be able to have mutual orgasms.

∾ *Exercise 115*. MUTUAL ORGASM

Begin with some unstructured foreplay or focusing caresses to awaken your senses. Then decide who will be on top. Bring your bodies together in an intercourse position in which you are face to face. Whoever is on top controls the speed of the thrusting and should start as slowly as possible.

As you roll through slow, sensuous thrusting, peak together up through levels 6, 7, and 8. Relax, breathe, and focus on the sensations in the penis and vagina. Men, think of yourself as caressing your partner's vagina with your penis. Women, think of yourself as caressing your partner's penis with the walls of your vagina. Keep your motion shared and mutual as you thrust together and slide apart. Gaze into each other's eyes as you move. If you've done many peaking and plateauing exercises together, you are probably very aware of your own and your partner's arousal levels. The best cues to your partner's arousal level are heart rate and breathing.

When the person on top climbs to the brink of orgasm, the other should follow. As you plunge into orgasm, take a deep breath, relax your body, open your eyes wide, and look into your partner's eyes. With practice you will find that you have the ability to either hold back slightly until your partner is ready or to accelerate your arousal slightly to match your partner's.

If you frequently experience mutual orgasm with your partner, you may think this is as good as lovemaking gets. But what if you could experience *multiple* orgasms together? Read on.

∾ *Exercise 116*. MULTIPLE ORGASMS FOR WOMEN

For women, the way to trigger multiple orgasms is similar to the plateauing exercise described in Chapter 26. Multiple orgasms may be strong, quiet, somewhere in between, or a combination of all of these. You can have multiple orgasms in any position. Most women find that being on top allows them to be more active and gives them more ability to control the strokes and the level of their own arousal. Other women find that having their partners kneel while they lie on their back provides more stimulation, particularly of the G-spot. I encourage you to try different positions and different types of orgasms with different trigger sites. You may want to try multiple orgasms alone first, with genital caresses or oral sex or a dildo, before trying them during intercourse with your partner.

Peak to levels 4, 5, and 6. Then, plateau at level 7 with breathing, pelvic movements, the PC squeeze, or switching focus. When you reach levels 8 and 9, instead of plateauing, let yourself go over into orgasm. Then continue the stimulation with peaking until you reach another orgasm. The more you are able to let yourself go and revel in your sensations, the more likely you will be to have multiple orgasms. The secret to multiple orgasms for women is when you reach an orgasmic peak, don't let your arousal go down very far before you start the stimulation again.

In _How to Make Love All Night,_ I wrote extensively about multiple orgasms for men, but I would like to explain the basics of it here, because for a couple, it is really the icing on the cake of mutual orgasm.

Contrary to popular expectation, it is possible for men to have multiple orgasms the way women do. To learn how, you have to realize that orgasm and ejaculation are two different bodily processes. An orgasm is a full-body response that includes spasms of the long muscles of the body, rapid heart rate, rapid breathing, and an intense feeling of release and pleasure. Ejaculation is a localized genital phenomenon that occurs when the PC muscle spasms and forces semen out of the penis.

Men can learn to become multiply orgasmic by learning to let their bodies go over into the sensations of orgasm while delaying or withholding ejaculation. You can do this by being intensely aware of the sensations that happen right at your point of ejaculatory inevitability (or "point of no return") and then keeping yourself from going over that point. Because you don't ejaculate, you can maintain your erection and continue making love, during which time you may go on to have one or several more orgasms. Many men especially enjoy having several nonejaculatory orgasms and then having an ejaculation with their final orgasm.

Becoming multiply orgasmic holds several benefits for men. By understanding the power of orgasmic potential, you gain insight into your partner's response and it becomes easier for the two of you to communicate about sexual matters. Also, women whose partners become multiply orgasmic delight in the sharing of this very special experience.

∾ *Exercise 117.* MULTIPLE ORGASMS FOR MEN

There are numerous detailed exercises in *How to Make Love All Night,* but try beginning with a preliminary exercise here. Some men have learned this technique in just a few sessions. Two things I have noted in working with clients is that men in their forties and fifties seem to be able to learn this process really well, and men who have a history of premature ejaculation also seem to do very well with this process.

First, bring yourself to orgasmic potential by trying this alone while doing a genital caress. Peak yourself up to levels 6, 7, and 8, and then do plateaus at levels 8 and 9. When you reach that split second before your PC muscle starts to spasm, squeeze your PC muscle as tightly as you can for five to ten seconds, open your eyes, take a few deep breaths, and consciously relax all of your other muscles. You may have an unusual sensation in which you have an orgasm but don't ejaculate. If you ejaculate a little bit, it just means you need to practice your timing.

Next, try the same exercise when making love with your partner. Most men prefer the butterfly position for making love in this way. I find that the men who learn the technique most quickly are those who are able to get rid of their performance attitude and make love because they enjoy it and enjoy their partners.

✿

How do you feel about the powers of sexual healing now that you've shared healing intercourse? Did you find that some of these approaches resonate with you and your partner more than others? You may wish to incorporate them into your general lovemaking. Be aware as you incorporate healing intercourse into your love life that you don't develop a performance attitude or lose touch with your partner's needs. Let the power of healing intercourse truly deepen and enrich your relationship.

chapter 37

Spiritual Healing Through Sexuality

Making love in a committed, intimate, mutual relationship can open up a vast spiritual dimension in which you and your partner connect with each other and with something larger than either—or both—of you. I am not religious and don't consider myself particularly spiritual, but I do know that you are missing something in life if you don't have a feeling for the transpersonal, even if the connection you feel is simply with nature. I have placed this chapter at the end of the book because it is an introduction to another dimension of sexuality—sacred sexuality—that some of you may relate to, while others may not. I encourage you to explore what this dimension can hold for you and your partner.

You may have already experienced the transpersonal or transcendental element of lovemaking. For example, have you ever felt an altered state of consciousness, in which everything looked clearer or brighter, after uniquely passionate sex? Physically we explain this state as resulting from the combination of hyperventilation and endorphin release, but that description shortchanges the profound effects that such a sexual connection can have on us. Many couples find that sexual union is a way to realize their connection with a higher power, whether that power is God, Goddess, nature, or goodness.

Sexuality in Religious Traditions

Most religious traditions have recognized the power of lovemaking and tie it into their cosmology, or theory of the universe. Judeo-Christian religions honor the Bible, which includes the Song of Songs, a lavish and beautiful poem that celebrates the eroticism of heterosexual lovemaking. Orthodox Jewish traditions refer to the Kabbalah, which also contains erotic passages. The Islamic religion includes erotic love poems. Buddhist, Taoist, and Hindu traditions all feature artwork depicting sexual scenes, and they include a focus on how sexual energy is a way to transcend this world. Have you ever seen pictures of some of the Hindu temple carvings in India and Thailand? They are very erotic, often illustrating copulation between the gods.

For some people, however, the idea that an organized religion could contain a tradition of sacred sex is very threatening. Many of us had a negative upbringing in a restrictive religious tradition in which sexuality was forbidden rather than celebrated. Many of us learned to avoid sex because our religious background taught us to associate the body and its sexual impulses with shame and guilt. I grew up in the Catholic tradition, where sex was strictly forbidden (and not even discussed) until you were married. Upon marriage, suddenly lovemaking became so special that it was a gift from God, a sacrament that reflected the relationship between Jesus Christ and the Catholic church. This was a challenging belief for my friends and me to try to understand and come to terms with, particularly as teenagers who were discovering our sexuality, often in the backseats of cars! It was very difficult to relate to sexuality in a sacramental sense when our entire sex lives up to that point had been governed by a "Don't ask, don't tell" policy.

Understanding the historical role of sexuality in our religious traditions can help heal any conflicts we may feel between spirituality and sexuality. Sexual healing can make it possible to deal with these conflicts and to allow your sexual relationship to enrich you spiritually as well as physically and emotionally. The following are exercises that can help you tap into the spiritual traditions you already have, and perhaps introduce you to some new ones.

ᐠᐰᐟ *Exercise 118.* SPIRITUAL AND EROTIC READING

If you are a member of an organized religion, find out what your religious tradition has to say about using lovemaking as an expression of your spirituality and your relationship with a deity or deities. Whether your religious background is Christian, Moslem, Goddess, nature worship, or something else, you will no doubt be able to locate some readings about sacred sexuality in your tradition. On a special night, read aloud to each other some of the erotic and/or spiritual writings from your tradition.

ᐠᐰᐟ *Exercise 119.* FOOT BATH AND CARESS

This exercise is not only sensual, it is also symbolic of humility and service. In the New Testament of the Judeo-Christian Bible, people wash each other's feet for this purpose. People often have negative feelings about

feet—that they are dirty or smell bad. This exercise can help change these attitudes. Practitioners of shiatsu massage know that putting pressure on various parts of the feet can result in healing of other areas of the body.

You may do this exercise clothed or in the nude, however you and your partner will feel most comfortable and close. You will need two towels, a basin large enough for a person's feet, liquid soap, lotion, and hot water. Unlike some of the other sensate-focus exercises, during the foot bath and caress you might want to create a special ambience. This can be done by dimming the lights, lighting candles, or playing soft music.

To begin, the passive partner sits in a chair with his or her feet on the floor. The bath itself includes only the feet and ankles. The active partner fills the basin with warm water and gently places the passive partner's feet in the water. Add the liquid soap and caress your partner's feet in the water. The foot bath and caress is like any other sensate-focus exercise. Use a light, caressing touch, not massage. Bathe one foot at a time, exploring how the different areas of the foot feel as you bathe them. Stroke the ankles, the arches, and the tender undersides of the toes. Although you touch for your own pleasure, believe me, your partner will like this exercise. As you touch your partner, draw the healing mindset around the two of you.

When you are done bathing both of your partner's feet, lift them from the basin one at a time, pat them dry, and wrap them in separate towels. Put aside the basin, then take one of your partner's feet from the towel, warm up some lotion in your palms, and caress your partner's foot with lotion. Again, caress for your own pleasure. I usually bathe each foot for about five minutes and then caress each foot for five to ten minutes.

As the passive partner during the foot bath and caress, the only thing you need to do is relax and enjoy. Allow yourself to be pampered. Relax your feet and let them hang from your legs. Your partner will lift them into the basin for you; you don't need to help.

ᥫ Exercise 120. THE FIVE SENSES

In this exercise, you use religious or spiritual symbols, such as earth, air, fire, and water, to gather just the right combination of elements that will engage all of your partner's senses in lovemaking. Each of you can take turns being the bearer of delights.

When it is your turn to be active, prepare your room for lovemaking with things that will stimulate all five of your partner's senses. For example, you could choose a jasmine-scented candle to appeal to your partner's sense of smell, wear something sexy that you know your partner would like to look at, and play some soulful music on the stereo. Then you could uncork your partner's favorite wine to stimulate his or her taste buds, and use your fingertips or palms to caress his or her skin. Make sure not to have *too* many things going on, as this can be distracting. One special stimulus for each sense is enough.

When your partner has prepared the room, as the passive partner you should try to empty your mind of thoughts and open yourself to your senses. Focus on each sense one at a time, then experience all of them together as a whole.

This exercise allows you to combine sensate focus with the sensual pleasures you know your partner likes, and also to make a symbolic and real connection between lovemaking with your partner and outward symbols of your spiritual tradition, such as candles or wine.

ᑐ *Exercise 121.* BODY DECORATION

Buy some paints that are suitable for use on the skin. You can find these at a bath shop, an adult store, or through a catalog. Try this in your bathtub or shower, or in a secluded, private area outdoors if you have one. Undress each other and offer each other your body. Your body may become a canvas for spiritual, sacred expression, or it may become a part of you that your partner is honoring. Each of you takes turns reverently painting your partner's body. You may wish to paint symbols that mean something to both of you. Or use designs that celebrate your body and body parts. You can turn this into a ritual if you wish. When you are both painted, do whatever you are inspired to do. If the paints are edible, lick them off.

ᑐ *Exercise 122.* SYMBOLIC DINNER

The breaking of bread and sharing of food can be a symbolic ceremony. For example, the Jewish tradition of Passover commemorates the Jews' flight out of Egypt; each food served at a Passover supper holds symbolic meaning. Have you and your partner gone through difficult times? Are there special times of rejoicing for both of you? Do you cherish special aspects of your relationship? Share a symbolic dinner that honors your history or sets the stage for your future together.

Consider this exchange a ritual or ceremony. Plan it in advance so it has a structure. Serve special foods that remind you of some aspect of your relationship or symbolize some aspect of your love. Make up a dialogue to go along with serving the food. For example, "As I'm pouring this wine, it reminds me of our wedding, when we shared this same wine with our close friends." As an alternative, you could prepare some readings to accompany each dish or course.

ᙡ *Exercise 123.* PERSONAL ALTARS

Practitioners of some Eastern religions often keep altars in their homes. They light candles or incense and meditate or pray before the altar. Some Christians also do this. In a similar way, try honoring your relationship. You could make your bedroom, or another private room in your house, a shrine to your relationship, using pictures and symbols. The following are some ideas:

Choose artwork with healing imagery, such as mandalas (Hindu symbols of the universe), spirals (symbols of an inner journey), or suns (symbols of life). Use statues and paintings that symbolize male and female fertility. Or use special photos that symbolize important milestones in your relationship. Play classical or New Age music, or music that mimics the heart's rhythms. For aromas, scent the room with essential oils of rosemary, lavender, eucalyptus, ginger, or clove. Make sure your room receives plenty of sunlight and fresh air. All of these will contribute to your spiritual well-being.

ᙡ *Exercise 124.* COUPLE RITUALS

Another thing you can do to heal your relationship spiritually is to start your own couple rituals. These are things that you make a commitment to do with each other every day, week, or month. By having rituals together you honor the importance of your relationship. Your purpose and your intention are key. With rituals, you can make the familiar unfamiliar and the mundane special. Here are a few of the rituals that have been shared by couples I know:

* ✳ If you are religious, attend a worship service together on a regular basis.

* ✳ Spend an evening savoring a meal in a favorite restaurant on a regular basis. Or make a special meal at home together on a regular basis.

* ✳ If you have a garden, plant a special area and tend it together.

* Spend an evening every so often reading favorite books or poems aloud. Alternate who reads and who listens.

* Make trips to a lover's point to watch the sunset together.

* Take dancing lessons, then go out dancing on a regular basis.

* Bathe each other and exchange massages.

The key to couple rituals is not what you agree to do together; it is that you commit to doing it regularly, that you both participate mutually, and that you both look forward to it. Your ritual could even be to talk about a particular subject at a particular time: the kids, your life goals, travel plans, your financial situation, things you think would improve your relationship. These are all rituals with which many couples have been successful. Lovemaking starts before you get to the bedroom and continues long after you leave it. If you think of everything you do together as adding dimensions to your emotional bond, you will discover new depths for both you and your relationship.

An important factor in any intimate relationship is what David Schnarch (the author of several books on relationships, including *Resurrecting Sex;* see Recommended Reading) calls *differentiation.* Differentiation means becoming fully yourself while continuing to relate intimately to another person. Couple rituals can help you and your partner learn to grow individually yet be close to each other at the same time.

Tantra

The religious or sacred tradition that has the most to say about making love is tantra, a form of yoga done in couples. The tantric cosmology features a theory of the universe created by the male and female forces. The universe springs from the union of the god Shiva (pure consciousness) and his consort Shakti (pure energy). The difference between most forms of yoga that you may be familiar with and tantra is that most yoga teaches asceticism (getting away from the worldly and the material) whereas tantra teaches how to reach the sublime by "debasing" oneself (becoming material, corporeal, or earthy). The most profound way to do this is through sexual intercourse.

In tantra, the man and the woman making love symbolize the male and female forces that created and power the universe. The male and female genitals are revered objects of worship. Tantra includes exercises, positions, rituals, and sexual postures that all have meaning in the tantric belief system. About ten years ago, I hosted a *Playboy* video entitled *A Guide to Tantric Lovemaking* that showed modern couples how to do some of these exercises and practices, some of which are quite weird by modern standards. For example, one of the tantric practices is to have sexual intercourse for twenty-four hours straight during a full moon with a woman who is having her period, and another is for a man to make love for many hours but withhold ejaculation. Some of the sexual practices that have their roots in tantra are very erotic and can help you appreciate the part of your relationship that is sacred.

Below are a few short tantric exercises. If you want more information, read one of the following excellent books: *The Art of Sexual Ecstasy* and *The Art of Sexual Magic,* by Margo Anand, or *Ecstatic Lovemaking,* by Victoria Lee. All are listed in Recommended Reading. In addition, if you would like specific training in tantra, with a bit of research you can find couples' tantric workshops.

ᥫ *Exercise 125.* CHAKRA MASSAGE

The chakras are centers in the body where various types of energy—physical, emotional, mental, and electromagnetic—are exchanged or connected to the world around us. Traditionally, there are seven chakras, which run along the spine and up to the head, reflecting the development of human consciousness. The seven chakras are located at the base of the spine, the pelvis, the navel or solar plexus, the heart, the throat, the forehead (or "third eye"), and the crown of the head.

To release energy from these centers for purposes of sexual healing, do sensate-focus caresses that start at the head chakras and move down to the pelvis chakras to concentrate energy there. Or do sensate-focus caresses that start at the base chakras and move up to the head chakras. This latter form of chakra massage helps kundalini (sexual energy, conceptualized as a serpent wrapped around the base of the spine) rise and be released, which can lead to some very intense orgasmic sensations.

ᥫ *Exercise 126.* TANTRIC INTERCOURSE

In tantric teaching there is a tremendous store of psychic and sexual energy that is locked or dormant in the "root center," at the base of the spine. Tantrics describe it as a coiled serpent named kundalini. When you become sexually aroused, kundalini energy starts to uncoil and slowly move up your spinal cord, energizing the other chakras as it goes. You may experience it as a white, hot light moving along your spine.

To awaken kundalini energy as you make love you should be in a position with a straight back, that is, sitting or standing or kneeling with your spine straight. Try a sexual position with one of you in a straight-backed position, then the next time you make love, switch positions so the other person is in a straight-backed position. Make sure you come together in a grounding embrace (see the next exercise) after any form of tantric intercourse.

ᕽ Exercise 127. GROUNDING EMBRACE

After any tantric exercise or tantric intercourse, it is very important to recenter yourselves or become grounded. After you have profound or spiritual or ecstatic sex, you will not feel like having a cigarette or taking a shower or rolling over and going to sleep. You may feel wide awake and vulnerable, and you probably will not feel like talking.

A good grounding exercise to do after tantric experiences is a version of the Eye Gaze bonding exercise described in Chapter 34. Lie quietly together face to face, hugging and holding each other, and simply gaze into each other's eyes. Let your breathing slow down naturally, let your sexual energy dissipate naturally, and feel your own heart beat as well as your partner's. This is a lovely finish to a tantric experience. You will find that as your breathing and heart rates slow, they will fall into sync with each other.

Ecstasy

As you and your partner may have already discovered while doing the sexual healing exercises, there is a level of sexual experience beyond arousal, and even beyond mutuality and intimacy. This is ecstasy. Sexual ecstasy is the feeling during a sexual encounter that you and your partner are so close that you temporarily transcend the material, physical plane of existence and enter into a highly spiritual realm as you have intercourse and reach orgasm together.

The way to find ecstasy together is to find balance between the male and female parts of yourselves. Ultimately, a woman is sexually healed by a man's worshipping her body, especially her vagina or "sacred space." Since a major aspect of a woman's sexual strength is to contain semen and give birth, the way she reaches sexual ecstasy is to expel energy by releasing it in a series of explosive orgasms. A man is healed by a woman's loving acceptance of his penis, his "wand of light," and by opening his heart. Since one aspect of a man's sexual strength is his ability to ejaculate, he reaches sexual ecstasy by learning to contain that energy in order to have multiple orgasms.

A couple will be healed together by learning to transmit love and respect to each other through their genitals. You will accomplish this through your presence with each other and through your healing intentions. During these tantric exercises, it is important that you also maintain an attitude of worship toward your own body and your partner's body. Worship your partner's body not only because he or she is your partner, but because his or her body symbolizes all that is male or female in the universe.

The exercises in this book lay the foundation for the healing mindset necessary to understand and open the doors to ecstasy. Spiritual experiences are always unique and highly personal, so I won't attempt to describe a typical ecstatic moment. Some people say they see intense colors or images, some have visions, others hear music, and some feel an overwhelming sense of connection with all creation. You now have all of the tools you need to use your loving partnership as a gateway to the spiritual part of yourself, and to help you connect with your partner's soul. The following two exercises can further open the doors to experiences of sexual ecstasy.

ᕙ *Exercise 128.* INTERCOURSE EXCHANGING BREATH

Let's have the man be active first. After he has done some sensual caresses with his partner, he kneels between his partner's legs and begins intercourse. As he continues to thrust slowly and sensuously, he leans over his partner and breathes into her mouth. They both visualize the breath flowing into her lungs, abdomen, and pelvis, back into him through her vagina, and up his spine. This creates a sensational energy circle that both partners can feel.

When the woman is active, she caresses her partner, and, when he has a partial or full erection, she climbs on top of him and begins intercourse. As she begins to thrust slowly and sensuously, she breathes into his mouth and they both visualize the healing breath flowing into his lungs, abdomen, and pelvis, and then through his penis back into her and up her spine. The breath is a golden light that fills them both until they feel it radiating out of them.

This can be a very intense exercise. End it by lying in a close grounding embrace until both of you are ready to release your touch.

❧ Exercise 129. EYE-GAZE INTERCOURSE

In this exercise you use your gaze to seduce your partner as you make love. This is seduction in a positive, beneficent sense. By gazing intently at your partner, you draw your partner in and seduce him or her with your focus.

Caress your partner as you both keep your eyes open and locked onto each other. Gaze deeply into his or her eyes as you climb on top and start to move, stroking up and down, in and out. Draw your sexual energies together as they build. Keep your movements flowing and sensuous, and force your partner to look back at you with the power of the sexual energy you create. To help both of you come down from orgasm, lie together in a grounding embrace.

chapter 38

Some Final Thoughts

I'd like to share a few more things that I think are important for you to know. First, be aware that the sexual healing program presented in this book is a very specific, cognitive-behavioral program for healing the most common sexual problems. However, it's not the only option available for dealing with these issues, and some people respond better to other strategies. Possibilities for other treatment options include hypnosis (a very advanced state of relaxation), visualization or imagery techniques, and intensive psychotherapy. There's also the very real possibility that in the near future virtual-reality techniques will be available to help people heal their sexual problems. I just hope I get invited to try out some of the prototypes!

If you do decide to give this program a try, know that an important part of any cognitive-behavioral program, whether it's to help someone stop smoking, lose weight, or change his or her sex life, is relapse prevention. Relapse prevention involves coming up with—and then actually implementing—a strategy to help you avoid falling back into your old habits after all the effort you've made to change them. In the sexual healing program, to prevent relapse you should continue to do the relaxation, sexual fitness, and self-touch exercises throughout your life in order to maintain your level of sexual health. In addition, know that many sexual problems seem to have dispositional components. By this I mean some people have tendencies to ejaculate quickly, some people have tendencies to be slower to reach orgasm, and some people have tendencies to be slower to get erections. If you have had any of these problems in the past, you'll still be vulnerable to them in the future, especially when you're under stress. Even if you have completed the program presented in this book and believe that your problems are a thing of the past, you will still have a vulnerability to your particular issues. For relapse-prevention purposes, it's a good idea to go back and do sensate-focus exercises with your partner once in a while to make sure you hold on to all the gains you have made.

We live in an era in which much of the information presented publicly about sexuality is negative. A focus on the potentially harmful aspects of sexuality (such as disease transmission, sexual coercion, and teen pregnancy) may cause us to overlook the overwhelmingly positive effects sexual expression can have on our lives. I hope the sensual activities you have learned here will help you to enjoy the many soothing and healthy aspects of sexuality, including increased sexual self-esteem, feelings of personal fulfillment, intimacy with your partner, and, possibly, sexual ecstasy. The pair bond between you and your partner is important; in fact, it's among the most important relationships you'll ever have. It is equally important to share with the rest of the world the energy, vitality, and goodwill you have created through the enriching effects of the sexual healing program. As you embark on your lifelong journey of sexual healing, let your health and happiness spread to others. And although I haven't said anything so far in this book about love, I recognize that love is the most important thing of all, isn't it? That's true for all of us. Choose this as the next direction in which to go. Learn what it means to be a great lover, in the broadest sense of the word. Learn to love not only in the bedroom, but also in your household, in your community, and in the world.

References

American Psychiatric Association. *Diagnostic and Statistical Manual of Mental Disorders,* 4th ed., Text Revision. Arlington, VA: American Psychiatric Association, 2000.

Annon, J. *The Behavioral Treatment of Sexual Problems,* vol. 1. Honolulu, HI: Enabling Systems, 1974.

Benson, H. *The Relaxation Response.* New York: Anchor Books, 1975.

Charlton, R., (ed). *Treating Sexual Disorders.* New York: John Wiley and Sons, 1997.

Gay, P., (ed). *The Freud Reader.* New York: W.W. Norton and Company, 1989.

Kaplan, H. *The New Sex Therapy.* New York: Brunner/Mazel, 1974.

———. *Sexual Aversion, Sexual Phobias, and Panic Disorder.* New York: Brunner/Mazel, 1987.

Levine, S. *Handbook of Clinical Sexuality for Mental Health Professionals.* New York: Brunner-Routledge, 2003.

Lowen, A. *Bioenergetics.* New York: Penguin Books, 1975.

Masters, W., and V. Johnson. *Human Sexual Response.* Boston, MA: Little, Brown and Company, 1966.

———. *Human Sexual Inadequacy.* Boston, MA: Little, Brown and Company, 1970.

Montagu, A. *Touching: The Human Significance of the Skin,* 3rd ed. New York: Harper and Row Publishers, 1986.

Reich, W. *Character Analysis.* New York: Farrar, Strauss and Giroux, 1945.

Recommended Reading

Anand, M. *The Art of Sexual Ecstasy: The Path of Sacred Sexuality for Western Lovers.* Los Angeles, CA: Jeremy P. Tarcher, 1989.

———. *The Art of Sexual Magic.* New York: G.P. Putnam's Sons, 1995.

Barbach, L. *For Yourself: The Fulfillment of Female Sexuality.* New York: Anchor Books, 1975.

Berman, J., and L. Berman. *For Women Only: A Revolutionary Guide to Overcoming Sexual Dysfunction and Reclaiming Your Sex Life.* New York: Henry Holt and Co., 2001.

Bodansky, S., and V. Bodansky. *The Illustrated Guide to Extended Massive Orgasm.* Alameda, CA: Hunter House, 2002.

Castleman, M. *Great Sex: A Man's Guide to the Secret Principles of Total-Body Sex.* Emmaus, PA: Rodale Press, 2004.

Ellison, C. *Women's Sexualities: Generations of Women Share Intimate Secrets of Sexual Self-Acceptance.* Oakland, CA: New Harbinger Publications, 2000.

Fisher, H. *Why We Love: The Nature and Chemistry of Romantic Love.* New York: Henry Holt, 2004.

Fulbright, Y. *The Hot Guide to Safer Sex.* Alameda, CA: Hunter House, 2003.

Hall, K. *Reclaiming Your Sexual Self: How You Can Bring Desire Back into Your Life.* Hoboken, NJ: John Wiley & Sons, 2004.

Katz, D., and R. Tabisel. *Private Pain: It's about Life, Not Just Sex: Understanding Vaginismus and Dyspareunia.* Plainview, NY: Katz-Tabi Publications, 2002.

Kaysen, S. *The Camera My Mother Gave Me.* New York: Alfred A. Knopf, 2001.

Keesling, B. *How to Make Love All Night*. New York: HarperCollins, 1994.

————. *Talk Sexy to the One You Love*. New York: HarperCollins, 1996.

————. *Sexual Pleasure: Reaching New Heights of Sexual Arousal and Intimacy,* 2nd ed. Alameda, CA: Hunter House Publishers, 2005.

Lee, V. *Ecstatic Lovemaking*. Boston, MA: Conari Press, 2002.

McCarthy, B., and E. McCarthy. *Rekindling Desire: A Step-by-Step Program to Help Low-Sex and No-Sex Marriages*. New York: Brunner-Routledge, 2003.

Milsten, R., and J. Slowinski. *The Sexual Male: Problems and Solutions*. New York: W.W. Norton and Company, 1999.

Pennebaker, J. *Opening Up*. New York: Morrow, 1990.

Schnarch, D. *Resurrecting Sex: Resolving Sexual Problems and Rejuvenating Your Relationship*. New York: HarperCollins, 2002.

Semans, A. *The Many Joys of Sex Toys*. New York: Broadway Books, 2004.

Sundahl, D. *Female Ejaculation and the G-Spot*. Alameda, CA: Hunter House, 2003.

Sources for Sex Toys

I don't endorse any specific company. I've listed the larger retailers that have websites in case you're too shy to purchase adult products in person. If you're not too shy, you can probably find an adult store in your area.

Good Vibrations
(800) 289-8423
www.goodvibes.com

Lady Calston
(416) 398-0999
www.calston.com

Xandria Collection
(800) 242-2823
www.xandria.com

Adam and Eve
(800) 293-4654
www.adameve.com

Index

More Hunter House Books on
SEXUALITY & RELATIONSHIPS

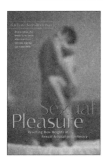

SEXUAL PLEASURE: Reaching New Heights of Sexual Arousal and Intimacy by Barbara Keesling, PhD ... Second Edition

To experience deep sexual pleasure, Dr. Keesling explains, you must explore your ability to enjoy basic touch. Focusing on touch and desire leads to greater passion, sensitivity, and fulfillment for both partners. Turning away from performance orientation, her book focuses instead on developing a wide range of sensation, a mastery of the erotic body, and a new sense of freedom in bed. This edition contains a chapter on oral sex and 20 new exercises including material about talking sexy and the unique pleasures of different sexual positions.

264 pages ... 11 illus. ... 16 photos ... Paperback $14.95

SEXUAL HEALING: The Completest Guide to Overcoming Common Sexual Problems by Barbara Keesling, PhD ... Third Edition

This third edition combines material from the first two editions with new research and is *the* definitive work on sexual self-help. It includes over 125 exercises to help treat sexual problems, from premature ejaculation and low sexual desire to sexual anxiety and sexual pain. It also describes how to use sexuality to heal your body, feelings, and relationship. The exercises can be used by people of any sexual orientation, and many are helpful for older people. Sex therapists will also find this book an invaluable resource for discussion and work with clients.

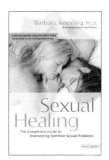

400 pages ... 4 illus. ... Paperback $18.95

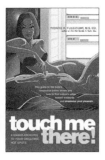

TOUCH ME THERE! A Hands-On Guide to Your Orgasmic Hot Spots by Yvonne K. Fulbright, PhD

Touch Me There! is the first book to focus exclusively on all of the body's erogenous zones, offering lovers a new realm of sexual exploration and experience. Sexologist Yvonne K. Fulbright gives readers a guided tour of the male and female body's wild attractions and explains how to maximize pleasure from head to toe. Contents cover a variety of sex acts and positions, sexual enhancers and toys, fantasy, and exercises for becoming more orgasmic and sexually satisfied.

240 pages ... 42 illus. ... 16 photos ... Paperback $13.95

FEMALE EJACULATION & THE G-SPOT by Deborah Sundahl

The G-spot is a woman's prostate gland. When stimulated, it swells with blood and emits ejaculate fluid, usually during orgasm. All women have a G-spot, and all women can ejaculate. Author Deborah Sundahl has led seminars on female ejaculation for 15 years, and this book is based on her research. Contents include:

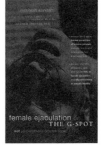

*   reasons why some women ejaculate and others don't
*   techniques, positions, and aids that help a woman ejaculate
*   how men can help their female partners to ejaculate
*   massage techniques developed to release emotional pain

240 pages ... 13 illus. ... Paperback $16.95

Visit www.hunterhouse.com to order — free media mail shipping on all web orders. For our FREE catalog call (800) 266-5592.

More Hunter House Books on
SEXUALITY & RELATIONSHIPS

EXTENDED MASSIVE ORGASM: How You Can Give and Receive Intense Sexual Pleasure by *Steve Bodansky, PhD, & Vera Bodansky, PhD*

In this hands-on guide to doing it, Steve and Vera describe how to take the experience of sex to a whole new level. They explain techniques and positions for extended orgasm, and how partners can help each other overcome resistance to pleasure.

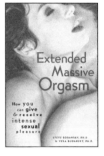

The authors disclose stimulation techniques and uniquely sensitive areas known only to specialized researchers, recommend the best positions for orgasm, and offer strategic advice for every technique from seduction to kissing. It's never too late — or too early — to make your partner ecstatic in the bedroom.

224 pages ... 5 illus. : 16 photos ... Paperback $14.95

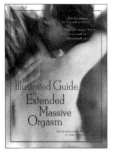

THE ILLUSTRATED GUIDE TO EXTENDED MASSIVE ORGASM
by *Steve Bodansky, PhD, & Vera Bodansky, PhD*

In this companion book, Steve and Vera Bodansky give much more detail about the best hand and body positions for performing and receiving EMO. More than 70 photographs and drawings illustrate genital anatomy and stimulation techniques, and the book covers new ground in the area of male arousal and orgasm.

Suddenly orgasm is no longer just a fleeting moment, but the beginning of lasting arousal that goes far beyond the bedroom.

256 pages ... 57 illus. ... 25 photos ... Paperback $17.95

INSTANT ORGASM: Excitement at First Touch!
by *Steve Bodansky, PhD, & Vera Bodansky, PhD*

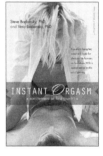

This book teaches readers to sensitize themselves to partners so they become instantly aroused when their partner touches them. This "first stroke" approach turns the idea of orgasm as a conclusion to lovemaking on its head. Readers learn how to get turned on at the first touch from their lover and stay at or close to peak arousal throughout their sexual encounter. Positions, techniques, and exercises are presented with illustrations, and the exercises follow an innovative sequence, developed for partners to train each other to reach instant arousal.

192 pages ... 24 illus. ... Paperback $16.95

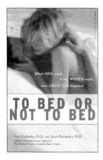

TO BED OR NOT TO BED: What Men Want, What Women Want, How Great Sex Happens by *Vera Bodansky, PhD, & Steve Bodansky, PhD*

This guide to seduction and better sex was written to help both men and women get it on. The authors have found that most men do not know what to do to get a woman to bed, or what to do when they get her there. Women also want to have sex but put up obstacles for men so as not to be considered "easy." This book describes, with examples and exercises, what people can do to make getting into bed and having great sex possible, easier, and a whole lot of fun.

240 pages ... 6 illus. ... Paperback $14.95

Visit www.hunterhouse.com to order — free media mail shipping on all web orders. For our FREE catalog call (800) 266-5592.